TRAUMATIC BRAIN INJURY REHABILITATION

The Lefaivre Rainbow Effect

TRAUMATIC BRAIN INJURY REHABILITATION

The Lefaivre Rainbow Effect

Christine Lefaivre

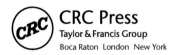

CRC Press
Taylor & Francis Group
Boca Raton London New York

CRC Press is an imprint of the
Taylor & Francis Group, an **informa** business

CRC Press
Taylor & Francis Group
6000 Broken Sound Parkway NW, Suite 300
Boca Raton, FL 33487-2742

© 2014 by Taylor & Francis Group, LLC
CRC Press is an imprint of Taylor & Francis Group, an Informa business

No claim to original U.S. Government works

Printed on acid-free paper
Version Date: 20151103

International Standard Book Number-13: 978-1-4822-2824-3 (Hardback)

Library of Congress Cataloging-in-Publication Data

Lefaivre, Christine, author.
    Traumatic brain injury rehabilitation : the Lefaivre rainbow effect / Christine Lefaivre.
    p. ; cm.
    Includes bibliographical references and index.
    ISBN 978-1-4822-2824-3 (alk. paper)
    I. Title.
    [DNLM: 1. Brain Injuries--rehabilitation. 2. Disabled Persons--psychology. 3. Disabled Persons--rehabilitation. 4. Patient-Centered Care. 5. Rehabilitation--economics. WL 354]

RC387.5
617.4'81044--dc23   2014000286

Visit the Taylor & Francis Web site at
http://www.taylorandfrancis.com

and the CRC Press Web site at
http://www.crcpress.com

TABLE OF CONTENTS

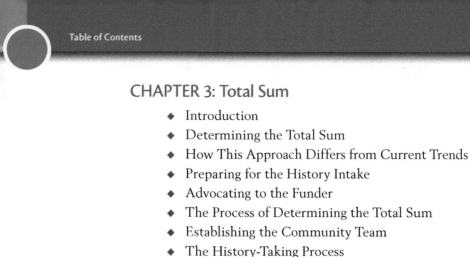

LIST OF ILLUSTRATIONS

LIST OF TABLES

DISCLAIMER

This book contains information obtained from authentic and highly regarded sources. While all reasonable efforts have been made to publish reliable data and information, neither the author nor the publisher can accept any legal responsibility or liability for any errors or omissions that may be made. The publisher wishes to make clear that any views or opinions expressed in this book by individual editors, authors, or contributors are personal to them and do not necessarily reflect the views/opinions of the publisher. The information or guidance contained in this book is intended for use by medical, scientific, or health care professionals and is provided strictly as a supplement to the medical or other professional's own judgment, knowledge of the patient's medical history, relevant manufacturer's instructions, and the appropriate best-practice guidelines. Because of the rapid advances in medical science, any information or advice on dosages, procedures, or diagnoses should be independently verified. The reader is strongly urged to consult drug companies' printed instructions and their websites before administering any of the drugs recommended in this book. This book does not indicate whether a particular treatment is appropriate or suitable for a particular individual. Ultimately, it is the sole responsibility of those in the medical profession to make their own professional judgments, so as to advise and treat patients appropriately. The author and publisher have also attempted to trace the copyright holders of all material reproduced in this publication and apologize to copyright holders if permission to publish in this form has not been obtained. If any copyright material has not been acknowledged, please write and let us know so that we may rectify in any future reprint.

FOREWORD

Amartya Sen, the 1998 Nobel Prize Laureate for economics, has an unyielding commitment to the fundamental tenets of social justice, social choice theory, and welfare economics that lead to the development of a theory and measures addressing the well-being of citizens of developing countries. His convictions were informed by experiences from his early years when he witnessed groups living in poverty. In his landmark theory of the *capabilities approach* developed in the early 1980's, he focuses on positive human development and freedoms arguing that these must be afforded to all citizens. At the heart of this work is the concept of *capability*, that is, a person's ability to participate freely in valued activities while recognizing the diverse nature of activity and the need for such opportunities to be accessible throughout society.

As with Sen, the like-minded occupational therapist Christine Lefaivre was influenced by her early experiences that led to the birth of the *Lefaivre Rainbow Effect*. Knitting together concepts to support her conviction that persons with brain injury could relearn and participate in valued activities is something that Sen would argue should be afforded to all human beings. Both authors are passionate about their work and focus on positive human development; for Sen, it was mitigating poverty and for Lefaivre, it is maximizing the potential of people with traumatic brain injury.

The *Lefaivre Rainbow Effect* provides an empowering, real-world, tangible, and systematic approach for specialized community-based traumatic brain injury rehabilitation that builds on the individual capabilities and social situations to extend their potential to re-engage in life and visualize future possibilities. This powerful approach embraces the essence of the issues without skirting the tough problems faced in the presence of brain injury. Deeply embedded in the *Lefaivre Rainbow Effect* is the philosophy of respecting the complexity of the human spirit and, as such, this approach does not heal but facilitates the healing process through collaboration and an implicit understanding of each person's unique circumstance. It was developed based on years of clinical practice and fluency with academic developments and has the potential for far-reaching application across borders, classes, and religions.

The nugget of the *Lefaivre Rainbow Effect* is conceptualized in a formula that is grounded, realistic, proactive, and honest. It is grounded as the formula fully appreciates and accounts for life pre-injury and is realistic by factoring in the diverse array of primary and secondary losses. The proactive aspect of the formula is realized in the nimble intervention that is tailored and responsive to the distinct client and family needs. It is through the expertise of the team that the full situation is collectively understood and translated into the functional everyday life of the client. Finally, the formula is honest because it acknowledges that all will not return to the way things were prior to the injury by accounting for the residual loss or the permanent deficits. Unique to this approach is that the formula includes both the client and the family unit in order to identify issues, educate all parties, and minimize the phenomena of the traumatically-induced dysfunctional family described by Lefaivre.

Discretely nested throughout the book are numerous clinical secrets and sage clinical experiences that Lefaivre shares to provide the reader with practical tips and numerous forms and templates on illusive subjects. There are guidelines on practical issues of how services are provided including medical legal work and establishing a professional practice as well as pragmatic, thoughtful lessons for using volunteers, accessing funding sources, and being alert to ethical issues. There is a superb use of broad-base cases to illustrate principles both of the *Lefaivre Rainbow Effect* and in the chapters that address medical legal and business practices. These case examples provide a rich tapestry of realistic scenarios that are useful to the practitioner and address the many difficult functional, medical, social, and legal issues confronted.

Through these pages, it is clear that the *Lefaivre Rainbow Effect* was developed from the heart with a true sense of urgency and immediacy to make a difference in the lives of persons living with brain injury. From the beginning to the end of this book, it is understood that the revolutionary development of the *Lefaivre Rainbow Effect* and the 25 years of implementation are just the beginning. It is for this reason that the *Lefaivre Rainbow Effect* is like a nova – we must explode its potential for the benefit of persons living with brain injury.

Susan Forwell, PhD, OT(C), FCAOT
*Associate Professor, Associate Department Head, and Graduate Advisor | Department of Occupational Science and Occupational Therapy
Research Associate, MS Clinic | Division of Neurology, Department of Medicine
Affiliate Investigator | Vancouver Coastal Hospital Research Institute
Principle Investigator | International Collaboration of Repair Discoveries
University of British Columbia*

REVIEWS

The *Lefaivre Rainbow Effect* is the vital piece that has been missing in the treatment of traumatic brain injury. I applaud Chris Lefaivre whose professional journey led her to these remarkable discoveries. Her work is universal to all countries and healthcare systems. The book is insightful regarding areas not commonly addressed, including the role of forgiveness in healing the spirits of patients who frequently blame others, not knowing that bitterness and resentment retard recovery. The *Lefaivre Rainbow Effect* brilliantly uncovers and develops strategies to manage the unique stress experience for each patient and makes insightful use of the brain's enhanced capacity to grow while pursuing pre-injury interests and motivations. Addressing the ups and downs while maneuvering inside the legal system—that often prevents healing—is helpful to survivors and caregivers alike.

The *Lefaivre Rainbow Effect* includes a unique concept of the traumatically induced dysfunctional family, working to maximize recovery and reduce the loss while preserving the family unit. The appropriate use of motivated participation of the TBI survivor makes this text stand out among those in the rehabilitation field. Like a cool breeze on a warm day, it gives refreshing new hope for brain healing.

> David I. Levy, MD, Clinical Professor of Surgery
> (Neurosurgeon), University of California, San Diego
> Author of *Gray Matter*

Dr. Levy is a recipient of the Patient's Choice Award in 2010–2012 and voted one of America's Top Surgeons in 2010–2013. He is the recipient of the Best Doctor Award 2007–2014.

This book transformed my understanding of traumatic brain injury (TBI) and the complexity of treatment programs. Chris Lefaivre's portrayal of working with her clients, their families, and the treatment team is inspirational. Her insight into the role of the human spirit and the importance of motivation and hope in determining outcomes a revelation.

This well written and accessible book is truly a must-read for all health and social workers, legal professionals, family members, employers, and indeed anyone involved in the support of traumatically brain injured individuals.

The author paints a fascinating picture of the practice of occupational therapy and treating traumatic brain injuries and shows how thoughtful approaches to therapy and support can result in extraordinary outcomes for patients. The book presents an integrated approach to treatment and care and to the business of occupational therapy. With its extensive resources and appendices it will become a standard reference for students, professionals, and families dealing with TBI.

This book could not be timelier—as we recognize the devastating effects of brain injuries in our society.

Deborah Buszard, PhD, Deputy Vice Chancellor
University of British Columbia, Canada

Deborah Buszard is Principal of UBC's Okanagan Campus, home of the Survive and Thrive Applied Research Facility (STAR), which brings engineers, neuroscientists, kinesiologists, and psychologists together to develop novel protective technologies to prevent head injuries and protect humans in hazardous environments and activities such as contact sports.

Brain injury is a most complex healthcare challenge, with its impact on all aspects of life and functioning. In this comprehensive volume developed through decades of first-hand experience with hundreds of individuals traveling the post-brain injury journey, Chris Lefaivre puts forth a framework that truly reflects the best elements of person-centered care. The *Lefaivre Rainbow Effect* is applicable across professional domains, cultural boundaries, and the continuum of care. The guidelines of the model are consistent with all rehabilitation fields, accreditation standards, and the World Health Organization's conceptualization of disability, functioning, participation, and health. The approach encompasses the biopsychosocial perspective of recovery and re-adaptation, emphasizing our common humanity and the value of the hopes, dreams, habits, roles, and connections that shape all of our lives. Lefaivre reminds us that the impact of brain injury exceeds a purely neurologic injury, and instead evolves across a survivor's contexts – as a member of a family, community, workplace, etc. This volume encourages the brain injury rehabilitation community to value tenets of lifelong living, purposeful activity, enriched environments, reduction of stress, forgiveness of self, listening deeply to clients and families, and other core fundamentals as key components of the healing process, a process that embraces joy, balance, and the unlimited potential of the human spirit.

Tina M. Trudel, PhD, Licensed Clinical Neuropsychologist;
President/Chief Operating Officer, Lakeview NeuroRehabilitation
Centers and Specialty Hospitals, USA; Assistant Professor of
Clinical Psychiatry and Neurobehavioral Sciences, University of
Virginia School of Medicine; Member of the Board of Directors –
Brain Injury Association of America (BIAA); Member of the Board
of Directors – North American Brain Injury Society (NABIS)

I am a personal injury lawyer who has restricted his practice primarily to brain injury litigation since the middle 1980s. I first retained Chris Lefaivre, in her role as a community occupational therapist, approximately in 1987, to assist me in identifying the future care needs of my client who had sustained a mild to moderate brain injury in a motor vehicle accident. My client had been working as a taxidermist at the time of the accident and wanted to continue in that role following his injury. I didn't know whether it was or wasn't possible, but my experience up to that point in time told me that there was likely little professional help available to assist him in achieving this goal. How wrong I was! It was at this time and through this client that I experienced firsthand the magic of the *Lefaivre Rainbow Effect* with its emphasis on first identifying, in-depth, the complete pre-accident profile of the brain-injured survivor and then building on that profile to deliver an effective and very personalized rehabilitation program, which Chris identified to me as the *Rainbow Effect* rehabilitation program. Chris advised me at the time of this retainer that she really didn't understand taxidermy and to my surprise, as I was to learn consistent with her program, she immediately researched this occupation so that she could better understand my client's pre-accident profile and abilities in order to deliver the most effective rehabilitation going forward. I'm proud to say that my client, with the appropriate supports identified and in place, did indeed return to the practice of taxidermy, something neither he nor I could ever have contemplated without his experiencing the *Lefaivre Rainbow Effect* delivered so effectively by Chris. Needless to say I subsequently endorsed the *Rainbow Effect*, for all cases, no matter the severity of the brain injury, because this program will identify any and all residual functioning remaining to assist the brain-injured survivor in achieving the maximum quality of life possible and how best to achieve this objective. From a litigation point of view, there is no better way to prepare your evidence for trial than to follow the *Rainbow Effect* rehabilitation approach. Whether you are a survivor, a family member, a medical/rehabilitation expert, or a lawyer, read this book – it was a game changer for me and it will be for you as well.

David Marr, QC, Personal Injury Lawyer, Kamloops
British Columbia, Canada

David J. Marr Q.C. graduated from the University of Manitoba in 1972 and was called to the Bar in British Columbia in 1973. He has practiced in the field of litigation for the past 30 years. He received his Q.C. in 1986. David has been a member of the Trial Lawyers Association since its inception and sits on the Board as a member at large for the County of Yale and, in recent years, has been very involved in its affairs. For the last 25 years his practice has been restricted to acting for plaintiffs involved in motor vehicle accidents and is now primarily related to acting for brain-injured claimants. Mr. Marr was the co-founder of the Kamloops Brain Injury Association in 1985 (approximately) and is currently its President.

The rainbow is a marvel of nature as is the brain. Not all the colors in the rainbow are real, our eyes are not quick enough to clear the margins, therefore the neuroplasticity of the brain translates the colors differently for each person. All of us will see a rainbow differently, depending on how each individual brain interprets the image.

Each rainbow is unique, every brain interprets stimuli differently; this is equally true for the therapeutic approaches described in this book for traumatic brain injury (TBI) survivors.

Despite the obvious progress in the capabilities of functional MRI imaging and the continuously rising knowledge of intracerebral communication paths, it is insufficient to merely visualize the primary post-traumatic organic damage.

This book fills the gap between what a radiologist can visually see on radiologic imaging and how clinicians observe the survivor's brain functioning in real life, with multiple stimuli.

Through her longstanding, extraordinary experience in the therapy of TBI survivors, Christine Lefaivre succeeds in transcending primary organic damage with a multi-modal therapeutic approach.

The various therapeutic levels amalgamate and ultimately form the foundation of a complex treatment approach for this patient group.

Due to the steadily rising number of patients who are frequently very young, in part due to the combat operations in Iraq and Afghanistan, this book has the potential to evolve into an interdisciplinary fundamental work for the therapy of TBI survivors.

With the interest of the patients in mind, I wish the book a wide circulation.

Dr. Michael Starke, Radiologist, Department of Diagnostic and Interventional Radiology, Federal Armed Forces Hospital Berlin, Germany

A complex, confused, and difficult world awaits the survivor of a serious traumatic brain injury (TBI). This complexity confronts the survivor's health-care providers, family members, and community. As a neuropsychologist, I know that understanding the injury effects can be challenge enough. But aiding recovery from TBI also requires consideration of the survivor's pre-injury environment and personality, of the shifting picture presented by recovery of function over time, and bringing together the panoply of professional services and persons that become involved. Complications are often the rule and come in many forms: medical setbacks, funding shortfalls, problematic family dynamics, and lack of availability of desired services, to name a few. Even geography can pose a formidable challenge to the recovery process when the survivor comes from an isolated rural area and the needed services are located in urban centers.

In her book, Chris proposes a systematic approach, the *Lefaivre Rainbow Effect*, to deal with these complexities. Recovery from a serious brain injury typically takes several years and Chris' book speaks to the challenges of coordinating a constantly evolving care plan that involves many individuals, interventions, and practical problems. The TBI survivor and his/her family are not constants either, as they adjust to the initial injury or as they move through the variable stages of recovery. The *Rainbow Effect* provides a multi-modal, multi-disciplinary model that stages interventions for the survivor, the family, and the community (eg., school, workplace), so that recovery is maximized. Chris highlights the role of the case manager in promoting collaboration and coordination among the various parties involved at any particular time in the recovery process. There are important sections in the book on the interplay between legal and funding agencies with execution of a treatment plan.

I think this book will be of particular interest to occupational therapists, but it will also be valuable to professionals and non-professionals alike who are involved in assisting the TBI survivor's difficult journey. While some impairments may persist following serious TBI, successful recovery of function is possible in many cases. I have worked with Chris using this model and have seen clients who initially had Glasgow Coma scores of 4-6 recover over a period of years, to the point where they could live independently, hold employment, and have normal relationships.

Bill de Bosch Kemper, PhD, Kelowna, British Columbia, Canada

The essential underpinning, and what makes the *Lefaivre Rainbow Effect* so therapeutically successful, is the belief that an in-depth understanding of the person's life prior to the traumatic brain injury offers the greatest value therapeutically. Further, it is the belief that this is the absolute foundation for optimal recovery. For too long we have focused on the specific, physical malfunction and not considered the person's historic, underlying mental health, and their pre-injury role in the extended family system and society in general.

The *Lefaivre Rainbow Effect* (LRE) teaches that it is essential that all care providers fully embrace the profound power of the human spirit. "Light the flame that sparks the spirit" is the rallying call for service providers, utilizing the LRE approach. Lefaivre's model, which is to base treatment on the pre-injury tapestry of the person's life by using an advanced knowledge of family system's theory, is brilliant. The approach captures the essence of the reality that having a critical understanding of how people derive self-worth can tremendously impact their ability to recover. As well, the incorporation of the unique theory of the traumatically-induced dysfunctional family sets the stage for a far more complete knowledge base of how to successfully treat the TBI patient. It is this understanding that is behind the thoroughness in a patient's data collection, which is then used to prepare and execute a top notch treatment program. The LRE's essential belief is that a human spirit is filled with hope. If that hope has been diminished, all caregivers need to gently nurture it along from the remaining historical embers to a new flame. The LRE consequently sees the family playing an absolute essential role in the traumatic brain injured person's recovery.

Lefaivre's original sensitivity, apparent when she paid mindful attention to the TBI client who was taking on the schizophrenic symptomology of the roommate when institutionalized, speaks volumes to her intuitive understanding of brain re-wiring and what is truly needed for the TBI patient's optimal recovery. That Lefaivre had the understanding 30 years ago, that the brain recalls best in a familiar environment utilizing old, familiar, cognitive stimuli, is a testament to her incredible awareness of the client's needs, long before the current understanding of neuroplasticity. As I read Lefaivre's work, I was astounded by her complete understanding that the best chance for functional recovery and optimal psychological benefit is when the TBI clients are in their pre-injury environment versus an institutional setting. Perhaps Dorothy from the Wizard of Oz was an inspiration to Lefaivre when she said "there's no place like home, there's no place like home…"

The LRE assumption that functional family members are integral to the recovery process for a TBI client, and the understanding that a family is at risk for becoming dysfunctional in the process of recovery, are the underpinnings of the success of this treatment approach. Just like a builder cannot erect an apartment building starting from the second floor without a complete understanding of the land and a well-dug, constructed, and pre-injury foundation and first floor, the TBI survivor is not optimally served without a well-documented understanding of his/her pre-injury life functioning. What a gift this text is to the world of traumatic brain injury treatment and patient care in general.

Gaye Gould, MSW, RSW, Mississaugua, Ontario, Canada

PREFACE

As a child of 13 I suddenly found myself in the Calgary Children's Hospital strapped into a Stryker frame—one of those sandwich contraptions that precluded any movement, flipping me over every 2 hours. It seemed impossible to me that only hours ago I had been at a gymnastics practice. After spinal surgery and then 6 weeks of immobility, I advanced to a body cast and then to a body brace.

An interesting note was not the offense of being in the Stryker frame but rather that I had gone from a budding competitive gymnast in my mind's eye to a disabled child in the eyes of my care providers. I suppose at face value I should have been able to understand that I didn't look like much of an athlete hanging in mid-air unable to move. I recall feeling misunderstood and devalued.

During my stay in hospital an outbreak of the measles legislated that all patients were quarantined; thus my social spheres were limited to those of us on the ward. I recognized that my experience of pre-injury identity was shared with the other patients—many much worse off than I was.

Fast forward to 1979 when, as a newly graduated occupational therapist, I chose to relocate to the sunny Okanagan. I committed to the only available job at the local mental health center, not because I had a burning desire to work with the psychiatric population but because I could pursue a certain lifestyle.

As my life journey continued to unfold, this was exactly where I should have been; with a love for neurology, I was excited to work with early brain-injured survivors who were placed in the mental health boarding home program. A young brain-injured client who shared many of the same passions as I, including gymnastics, was admitted to a group home with a severe brain injury and was living with schizophrenic roommates. In a wheelchair, aphasic, unable to speak, she began to mimic schizophrenic behavior. Watching this young lady struggle caused me to revisit those old 13-year-old feelings of being misunderstood and devalued. I was quite certain that she did not see herself as she presented, but rather as she was before this life-altering injury.

I reasoned that if a client with a traumatic brain injury could learn what she was being exposed to, then it appeared that learning was indeed taking place, I surmised "Shouldn't they be at home where things are familiar and they can relearn what they used to do?"

With the energy that only youth avails, I was a woman on a mission to advocate and secure funding for the brain-injured clients in my group homes to return home with support and supervision. The results were astounding. I began to document what scenarios were successful and which were more challenging. Sensory overload in many variations was frequently the culprit when there were suboptimal outcomes. If I could better understand how the brain was processing information up to the point of sensory overload, I could rewind the events so that, in the future, these hot spots could be avoided.

After years of careful observation I created a template that resulted in an in-house training program for my clinical staff that you will see unfold in the following pages.

The success of this approach was astounding; as a result, referrals came in from Western to Eastern Canada and from as far away as France.

Clients with Glasgow coma scores of 6 to 8 were getting married, having children, and becoming gainfully employed.

Clients with Glasgow coma scores of 5 or less were returning home, enjoying the community, and, on occasion, getting married.

I also witnessed that returning brain-injured persons home came at a cost to the family members, often resulting in health problems or relationship breakdown. I understood that if I could successfully advocate for service provision to the family as well as the client that the overall outcome and relationship breakdown could be averted.

It was an interesting process to advocate and find ways to educate funders to see the wisdom in approving funds to be spent on the family as well as the injured family member, thus protecting the family unit.

The purpose of this book is to share my 26 years of clinical experience with the traumatically brain injured; my hope is that more specialized training will be delivered at an educational level to any student who will eventually work with brain-injured survivors. I hope that this model will contribute to this need. Once understood, this method is simple and easy to carry out at little cost other than manpower. It is not bound by politics, religion, economics, or culture.

It has been rewarding to review worldwide research, which generally culminates in a conclusion that standards of care and protocols need to be established for more and improved universal standard service delivery for the traumatically brain injured. I would like this text to contribute to this discussion.

I hope this book will serve to provide structure to the varying levels of the recovery process and to inspire hope just as those very clients inspired me.

Chris Lefaivre

ACKNOWLEDGMENTS

I would like to express sincere gratitude to all those who assisted in the creation of this book—firstly to Susan Forwell, PhD, who has been encouraging me to get this work into publication since the early 1980s. Sue has donated countless hours of her own time and resources as well as the assistance of her work study students, Andrea Tomi, and Amanda Forwell. My sincere thanks to all of you for your help in the early days of the book's creation. Without your encouragement, insight, guidance, proofing, and editing of the first two chapters, this book would not have made it into the hands of the publisher. I remain grateful to you for your mentorship and support.

To David Marr, Q.C., who has proofed the legal and residual loss chapters for accuracy, my sincere appreciation for your time and support.

To Marjorie Lefaivre, who has provided invaluable insight by repeated proofreading of this book. Your practical, intelligent advice as well as candid and constructive feedback have been invaluable to the finished product—my heartfelt thanks.

To Ashley Schmidt, my research assistant, who at the time of the writing of this book, was a second year masters' occupational therapy student, I am extremely grateful for your diligence, commitment, organization skills, and strong work ethic. You will be an exceptional asset to any clinical setting you choose to work in.

To Karen Naumann—without her extensive understanding of the perplexing world of computers this book would not be possible. I am deeply grateful for your outstanding hard work and commitment to this project.

For the many others that have supported this work in various ways, my thanks to Wendy Bodsworth, Michael Bodsworth, Emely Pasqualotto, Sandra Halme, George Jacob, and Blair Forest.

My sincerest thanks to the incredible team at Taylor & Francis Group who believed in this work and brought it to fruition, including: Naomi Wilkinson, commissioning editor; Julia Molloy, editorial assistant; Laurie Schlags, production coordinator; Judith Simon, project editor; Maureen Kurowsky, copyeditor, Datapage Inc. Typesetting; Samar Haddad, proofreader; Nally Dookwah-Abrams, marketing manager; Matt Debono, Sr. marketing manager; and Dominique McMann, marketing executive.

And lastly and most importantly, to those amazing clients that I have had the privilege to walk the journey of life with, you have taught me much. I have witnessed courage and the resilience of the human spirit firsthand. I have marveled at your perseverance. I have felt joy at your accomplishments. I am humbled and grateful to have seen grace and dignity in action. You have modeled what is important in life and, in turn, you deserve the deepest respect.

NOTES TO PROFESSORS AND READERS

For the purpose of this book, the words "clinician," "health care provider," "service provider," or "professional" relate to any medical or clinical professional working with a traumatic brain injured (TBI) survivor.

The stories in this book quite typically represent scenarios that occurred in the author's clinical practice. To protect patient confidentiality, identifying details of specific cases have been changed to the point that the cases are fictional; the symptoms, however, are very real.

The following additional resources, family handouts, and an instructor's power point presentation are available for you to download and print at **http://www.crcpress.com/product/isbn/9781482228243**. Further information is available at www.christinelefaivre.com or LinkedIn Christine Lefaivre.

Family Handouts

1. Definition of Service Providers
2. Family History Questionnaire
3. Family Balanced Lifestyle Inventory
4. Family Stress Inventory
5. Brain Injury Associations and Useful Websites
6. The Brain: A Brief Overview
7. Sensory Overload: What Is It?
8. Energy Conservation
9. Diverse Funding Options
10. The Use of Volunteers

INTRODUCTION

BURDEN OF PROOF

Traumatic brain injury is the leading cause of death and disability in children and young adults around the world, and is involved in nearly half of all trauma deaths. Many years of productive life are lost and many people have to suffer years of disability after brain injury. In addition it engenders great economic costs for individuals, families and society [1, p. 164].

For the purposes of this book, a literature review was conducted; trends in TBI certainly are emerging, as is the noted burden on health care, family, and societal systems in general. There is a global consensus that TBI and the sequelae of TBI have become a serious problem worldwide. Due to the fact that criteria for gathering data varied study to study and country to country and that standards of care, protocols, and statistical measures are not consistent, the data cannot be uniformly compared, particularly in developing versus undeveloped nations.

Having said that, it has been projected that "traumatic brain injury (TBI), according to the World Health Organization, will surpass many diseases as the major cause of death and disability by the year 2020" [2, p. 341] with the male to female ratio estimated at anywhere from 2:1 to 3:1 [1].

"It has been estimated that after one brain injury, the risk of a second injury is three times greater, and that after a second injury, the risk of a third is eight times greater" [3].

TBI has an impact on greater society: A reported 53% of homeless individuals live with brain injury and the vast majority (70%) were injured prior to becoming homeless [4].

An estimated 82% of the prison population lives with the effects of traumatic brain injury [5].

TBI has been identified as the signature injury of the Iraq–Afghanistan conflict, with an estimated 10%–20% of returning US military personnel suffering from a traumatic brain injury, in addition to the several million North Americans each year surviving TBI. More people than ever are being affected by this life-altering injury [6, 7].

Considerations have been made toward traumatic brain injury as a "silent epidemic, as society is largely unaware of the magnitude of this problem" [8, p. 231]. Within industrialized countries "the number of productive years lost because of traumatic brain

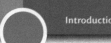

injury exceed those of cancer, cerebrovascular disorders, and HIV/AIDS combined" [9, p. 1698].

The primary causes of TBI worldwide vary with some commonality. Road traffic accidents, falls, workplace injury, violence, civil unrest, and sport are among the leading causes. Falls from roofs in Pakistan and falls out of unsafe bunk-beds in Hong Kong refugee camps for the Vietnamese are also common causes [1]. In low- and middle-income countries, pedestrians, cyclists, and bus passengers are at a higher risk for sustaining a TBI [1].

Costs of treating traumatic brain injury extend beyond the basic costs of hospital care and include costs of rehabilitation, care-giving, loss of productivity, and early retirement. These costs are exponential such that "if we prevent just one serious brain injury each year, over the lifetime of the first injury prevented, we realize a support care cost savings of over $90 million dollars" [10, p. 2].

The global estimated cost of TBI in 2000 was $406 billion [11].

The burden of proof chart in Table 0.1 cites the annual incidence of traumatic brain injury by nation, where available [2, 9, 11–16].

Without effective treatment, many of these people will lead lives of quiet desperation, isolation, and depression.

The *Lefaivre Rainbow Effect* is groundbreaking treatment for those suffering from a traumatic brain injury. This textbook is the culmination of more than 25 years of successfully implementing this transformative treatment by the author. What distinguishes this strategy from most others is that it is individually designed for each client and focuses on the cognitive retraining of the brain based on pre-injury lifestyle as well as the organic damage to the brain. This differs from most current techniques that focus on the disability alone. The intense preparatory work involved in developing a treatment strategy focuses on pre-injury function and motivations and the brain's capacity to relearn old, familiar information. The *Lefaivre Rainbow Effect* identifies and develops strategies to manage the confusing interrelated symptoms that arise as a result of the stress experience and those that originate as a result of the brain trauma, improving outcomes, and reducing secondary losses.

The *Lefaivre Rainbow Effect* includes the unique theory of the traumatically induced dysfunctional family with the aim to preserve the family unit and thus reduce the overall loss for the survivor of the brain injury. In the end, the *Lefaivre Rainbow Effect* maximizes the recovery process by tapping into the inner sanctuary of hope and positioning the TBI survivor to be a motivated participant in the arduous journey of recovery.

Table 0.1 Burden of Proof in Annual Incidence of Traumatic Brain Injury

	Statistic	Reference
North America		
Canada	500/100,000	10
United States	269.9/100,000	2, p. 346
South America		
Sao Paulo, Brazil	360/100,000	2, p. 347
Europe		
United Kingdom	453/100,000	2, p. 346
Germany	350/100,000	2, p. 343
France	281/100,000	13, p. 135
Sweden	546/100,000	16, p. 257
Finland	101/100,000	9, p. 1699
Turkey	300/100,000	12, p. 587
European Union average	235/100,000	2, p. 346
Africa		
Johannesburg, South Africa	316/100,000	2, p. 349
Australasia		
South Australia	322/100,000	2, p. 347
New South Wales, Australia	100/100,000	2, p. 347
New Zealand	790/100,000	11, p. 59; 14, p. 28
Asia		
India	145/100,000	15, p. 2146
Pakistan	50/100,000	2, p. 343
China	120/100,000	2, p. 344
Hong Kong	924/100,000	2, p. 348
Yemen	219/100,000	2, p. 348
Globally	200–558/100,000	11, p. 53

In these pages the health care provider is recognized as having the dual role of delivering care to maximize the client's recovery coupled with the necessity to submit medical legal reports to an adversarial system. These roles and an associated seamless ethical process are reviewed in detail, preparing the health care professional to be admitted as an expert witness and to have his or her testimony scrutinized under oath.

This textbook demonstrates how health care professionals, such as doctors, neuropsychologists, occupational therapists, speech pathologists, social workers, physical therapists, and educators, can use the *Lefaivre Rainbow Effect* in their practices to improve the therapeutic outcome for their clients and families as they integrate back into their homes and communities. The *rainbow effect* has been used in practice in the community with severe, moderate, and mild TBI survivors.

ABOUT THE AUTHOR

Christine Lefaivre has spent more than 25 years perfecting and implementing a unique treatment strategy for the traumatically brain injured as they return to their homes and communities. Lefaivre's clinical practice has provided consulting services throughout most regions in Canada and parts of the United States and France to third-party funders, such as litigators, insurance companies, and workers' compensation boards. She has employed many clinicians who were required to complete a comprehensive in-house training program lasting up to a year on the topic of the *rainbow effect*. Lefaivre holds a degree in occupational therapy from the University of Alberta and is a Clinical Assistant Professor in the Faculty of Medicine, Department of Occupational Science and Occupational Therapy at the University of British Columbia, Vancouver campus and an Adjunct Professor in the Faculty of Health and Social Development, School of Health and Exercise Sciences, at the University of British Columbia Okanagan Campus. At the time of this book's writing, Lefaivre was instructing a tutorial in neuroanatomy and neurorehabilitation to second year master's level students at UBC. Her alma mater has recognized her achievements with the University of Alberta Alumni Honor Award for her groundbreaking work with the traumatically brain injured and she has twice been named British Columbia Female Entrepreneur of the Year in the "quality plus" category. Lefaivre has been a consultant, lecturer, keynote speaker, member of advisory committee, and workshop leader on brain injury-related topics and courses, workshops, and conferences in Canada, the United States, and Europe.

LIST OF ACRONYMS

ADL:	Activities of daily living
AHRQ:	Agency for Health Research and Quality
AOC:	Alteration of consciousness/mental state
Ax:	Assessment
CAT scan:	Computerized axial tomography scan
COFC:	Cost of future care
CPR:	Cardiopulmonary resuscitation
FLS:	Frontal lobe syndrome
GCS:	Glasgow Coma Scale
GP:	General practitioner
Hx:	History
ICU:	Intensive care unit
IME:	Independent medical examination
IRS:	Internal Revenue Service
LMIC:	Lower middle income country
LTM:	Long-term memory
MRI:	Magnetic resonance imaging
MSP:	Medical services plan
NGO:	Nongovernment organization
NOCC:	Notice of civil claim
OT:	Occupational therapist
PET scan:	Positron emission tomography scan
PT:	Physical therapist
PTA:	Post-traumatic amnesia
PTSD:	Post-traumatic stress disorder
RDSP:	Registered disability savings plan
ROM:	Range of motion
Rx:	Treatment
SPECT scan:	Single photon emission computed tomography scan
SSDI:	Social Security disability insurance
SSI:	Supplemental Security income
STM:	Short term memory
TAU:	Treatment as usual
TBI:	Traumatic brain injury
WCB:	Workers' Compensation Board
WHO:	World Health Organization

CHAPTER 1

The Human Spirit

INTRODUCTION

Sustaining a traumatic brain injury (TBI) is one of the most devastating events that can happen to an individual. A TBI does not have a slow, insidious onset. Rather, it is abrupt, unanticipated, and alarming, intensifying the trauma experience for the individual and family. Sustaining a TBI can have severe repercussions cognitively, physically, mentally, emotionally, psychologically, spiritually, and financially.

This sounds encompassing but what does this really mean for the individual? For the person with the TBI, a myriad of symptoms may exist such as a physically awkward gait or decreased ability to ambulate, a hand or arm that is clumsy or has reduced function, feelings of depression or insecurity, being unsure about one's ability, cognitive confusion, and a possible lack of insight, judgment, and change in personality. There may be trouble in relationships with others. It may also mean not being able to get or keep one's job or continue in school.

We, the health care providers, need to walk hand in hand through the recovery process, developing creative treatment choices that focus on the individual's unique circumstances. We must be mindful that, like ourselves, persons with TBI and their families are as different as blades of grass. The tapestry of their lives is based on how they think, their cultural influences, what they learn, how they are loved, and their unique family dynamics and life experiences.

It is imperative to have a thorough understanding of the person's entire life pre-injury and how he or she derived self-worth, internally as well as externally. It is in understanding the nature of the person's life prior to the injury that we, as health care providers, can simulate cognitive tasks and functional activities that will reap the greatest value therapeutically and tap into the hope that will propel the person forward.

In doing so, it requires us, the health care providers, to step outside of our comfort zone. It requires the ability to connect intimately with our clients and commit to the lengthy therapeutic process.

Attending to the long-term therapy of a brain-injured person is not an easy task. The treatment can take 4 to 6 years before the residual loss is stabilized, bearing in mind that the learning process continues over the person's lifetime. Ethically working with a client who has sustained a TBI requires a commitment to the rehabilitation process. It is common that when there is a change of treating personnel that the person with the brain injury regresses, compounding the sense of loss.

As individuals we process our life experiences differently based on family dynamics, emotional health, where we live, how we were raised, and many other contributing factors that make us unique. We are also influenced by those we share our life journey.

To focus solely on the organic loss and physical consequences of the traumatic injury to the brain would leave the health care provider at a severe disadvantage, and the client with an unsatisfactory or at least suboptimal recovery. The remainder of this chapter describes the essential underpinning to the philosophy of the *Lefaivre Rainbow Effect* by discussing the critical concepts of the human spirit, forgiveness, primary and secondary losses, preservation of hope, and individualization of the therapy plan.

THE HUMAN SPIRIT

Underlying the *Lefaivre Rainbow Effect* is the belief that our motivation, our joy, and our zest for life are spawned from the human spirit. That is the life force that motivates us to be who we are—that part of us that can love and can experience sorrow and joy. This is the place where peace, acceptance, and motivation reside. To design a therapeutic regime without acknowledging the force of the human spirit would be missing a great opportunity and an essential component of the recovery process.

As we explore the concept of the human spirit, it will be abundantly clear that acceptance is the key to a person's ability to love himself or herself as he or she now is, and to forgive those who have caused pain. This acceptance and compassion will emerge despite the immense change these people find themselves facing. Elisabeth Kübler-Ross would say this is a stage of acceptance [17–19] (Appendix 1A) [20].

The very journey of life requires that we struggle at times in relationships with others. Relationships require ongoing negotiation, communication, compassion, respect, understanding, and at times reconciliation. If there were difficulties in a relationship prior to the injury, these problems will most likely fester and magnify after the trauma.

To embark on this difficult path of recovery it becomes imperative that we, as health care providers, assist our client to find peace in his or her new circumstance and, yes, even joy. If we are successful in understanding our client, we will bring realistic hope. It is important for health care providers to respect each person as an individual and not to treat our clients using a predetermined therapeutic regime.

It may cause us to step out of our comfort zone and step into our client's world. It is in doing this that we will find the essence of the person. If we have the courage to explore first the spirit, we will find what motivates clients in all aspects of life and help them to grow and accept the changes they are faced with. The risk of not doing so is imposing our values onto another and losing that critical therapeutic rapport in our relationship with the client.

Inevitably, the client's life will be emotionally and cognitively stripped down through this process. Some friends, family members, and employers will find the change in the person too difficult to handle and may withdraw or leave the relationship, compounding the loss and grief for the client. "As little as one year after the trauma, the parents, partners and children are the only members of the brain trauma patient's social network" [21, pp. 1006–1007].

There will likely be changes in function in many areas of the person's life that may include social/emotional skills, physical ability, cognitive function, and ability to work, depending on the part of the brain that has been impacted. To assist the client who survived a TBI to cope with this change or loss, health care providers must be in touch with the essence of what makes their clients who they are.

In the *Lefaivre Rainbow Effect* methodology we refer to this as their "spiritual self." The spiritual self is separate from physical beauty, financial success, material possessions, job status, and relationships with others. It is that part of us that can love and be loved. This is the part that forms a framework of how to live, how to believe, and how to hope, trust, and love.

When immense change occurs to an individual, these core beliefs may be challenged, particularly if a client's belief system is fundamentally connected to a job, financial success, material items, or another person for his or her identity. The adjustment can be more difficult as these key areas of identity are altered, possibly leading to hopelessness and suicidal thoughts.

The spiritual self holds the ability to say "I am OK just the way I am. My body may have changed but my heart and soul remain the same." This place within is what will foster hope, trust in the process, and, ultimately, lead to acceptance.

That sense of loving the "new me" and being grateful for "who I am" will emerge. It is an opportunity to live in the moment. The person may be stripped of the excesses, leaving those relationships with the most authentic value and allowing the client to reach the point of embracing, and being thankful for, the miracle that he or she has lived through a brain trauma, having emerged as a "new self."

It is astounding to hear that a brain injury can be a blessing. Some arrive at the place that, when stripped of all they know, the parts that are left are the best, particularly if remaining connected to the spiritual self, that place of self-acceptance, trust, and surrender. The superficial friendships and relationships that existed in the wake of a traumatic brain injury will fade.

Deriving self-worth from physical prowess or a high-powered job may not be viable post-injury. Escaping into busyness is very difficult, if not impossible. People in this situation are faced with the essence of who they are without extraneous sources of input, including material wealth.

Therein lies the mission of the health care provider to *light the flame that sparks the spirit.*

FORGIVENESS

The stressful legal process and examination for discovery that probes into one's life may contribute to perceived or real allegations of malingering, thereby deepening the wounds and hindering recovery. The very job of the defense attorney is to minimize the client's loss, oftentimes making the client feel that his/her new difficulties and troubles are invalid. Because the health care providers are commonly retained by insurance companies or litigators, this process can make it difficult for clients to trust their care providers. It is, in particular, during these times that a case manager will emerge and advocate for the client.

The area of unforgiveness becomes more complex when there is a third party who is responsible for causing the brain injury. In some cases, particularly in the cases of motor vehicle accidents, a family member or loved one may be responsible. In fact, the person with the TBI may find it necessary to sue a family member's insurance company, causing conflicting feelings and marked stress within relationships.

Another complicated scenario is when the person with the TBI caused the accident that may have injured himself or herself and others. In this case forgiveness of self and compassion for self and others become critical issues. The very nature of the adversarial litigation process, which in most cases accompanies the recovery process, can exacerbate unforgiveness, bitterness, and resentment for the client.

According to Dr. David Levy, "Emotions affect your immune system, for better or worse. Happiness heals like medicine. Bitterness kills like diseases. Releasing bitterness can dramatically help the underlying causes of many physical ailments often more than any pill or procedure" [22, p. 132]. The power of forgiving ourselves and others cannot be overestimated. In addition, Dr. Levy asserts that we have two choices; that is, "we can forgive and let it go or hold onto to it."

Similarly, Dr. Cloud and Dr. Townsend reiterate the idea that "forgiveness is very hard. It means letting go of something that someone 'owes' you. Forgiveness is freedom from the past; it is freedom from the person who hurt you" [23, p. 267].

Dr. Peck suggests that "the reason to forgive is for our own sake. For our own health, because beyond that point needed for healing, if we hold on to our anger, we stop growing and our souls begin to shrivel" [24, p. 48].

The *Lefaivre Rainbow Effect* methodology has long recognized that recovery is limited by pre-existing issues and issues arising from the trauma related to unforgiveness and emotional scars. This may be compounded by the legal adversarial process. It is, therefore, incumbent on the health care provider to assist the person to surrender, forgive, and let go of these emotional burdens. Introducing forgiveness into the therapeutic process allows the gateway of healing to open wide without emotional limitations.

There are boulders in the road to recovery that need to be moved or climbed over, or a new route needs to be taken. Forgiveness and letting go are critical for moving forward in the recovery process, to cope with changes, and to mitigate losses. Losses may be primary to the TBI or secondary in nature with both having a significant impact on the person with TBI and his or her ability to resume life.

LOSS

Primary Loss

Primary loss is the organic physical and cognitive loss that can be directly attributed to the brain injury. Typically, these are measured by radiologic brain scans and laboratory investigations, the impact of which can be quantified in the litigation process, such as wage loss, future wage loss, and cost of future care.

Secondary Loss

There are repertoires of secondary losses that are in response to the TBI and subsequent to the primary losses. These are typically difficult to measure objectively. These are the emotional and psychological changes for the person with the TBI as well as the family. Examples of secondary loss include but are not limited to stress, depression, anger, guilt, shame, isolation, sadness, fatigue, lethargy, emotional outbursts, loss of motivation, eating excessively, self-medicating with drugs and/or alcohol, sexual promiscuity that was not displayed before the TBI, an absence of joy, lack of peace, reduced self-esteem, decreased self-fulfillment, emotional and physical pain and suffering, loss of direction in life, broken relationships, loss of skill development, and a dysfunctional family unit.

In general, the primary and secondary losses become intertwined. There are a multitude of challenges for those faced with a myriad of life changes. The change of physical and cognitive status is daunting enough in itself. When that is compounded with the loss of ability to earn a living, absence of recreation, reduced social status, and loss of relationships, the consequences are overwhelming.

The stress attached to the primary loss may hinder the injured person's ability to move forward in recovery. The secondary losses can be as debilitating as the primary losses. If the secondary losses are not addressed at the same time as the primary losses, the situation can become very complex. Unforgiveness and hopelessness can develop deep roots that are difficult to break and will sabotage the therapeutic process. This new emotional, physical, and psychological state is an ideal breeding ground for depression. The secondary losses need to be avoided to capitalize on the recovery of clients, thus allowing them to mitigate their circumstances and move forward in life.

The method for avoiding secondary loss is to protect the uniqueness of each person by motivating the client through a balanced regime of familiar activity despite the injury and resulting symptoms. This approach is tailored to each client to facilitate self-acceptance and increase motivation on the difficult and arduous road to recovery.

PRINCIPLES THAT PRESERVE HOPE

Hope is found in the inner sanctuary of our being. It is an evasive quality that enters our lives when we believe we are where we need to be, in any given moment. Hope allows us to see the future with optimism while unforgiveness fosters pessimism. "Hope does not always mean cure, successful treatment or prolongation of life" [25, p. 82]. To heal from such a catastrophic event as a TBI requires a full-fledged action plan to dredge up that trickle of optimism in the most devastating of circumstances. Hope emerges when letting go and surrender happen. When we let go, we see the value in the life experience and the gift that each circumstance in life avails. We cease trying to deny or control the outcome and, rather, accept the situation, arriving at a place of gratitude for what is. Often persons with an active faith life do much better in letting go and surrendering to a higher power and to the process of healing. "Faith is a frequently used emotion-oriented coping mechanism that often provides the basis for effective coping" [21, p. 1009].

Hope is a feeling and therefore difficult to measure. A plan to produce hope may seem elusive. One must be mindful that a behavior precedes a feeling.

The principles for preserving hope embedded in the *Lefaivre Rainbow Effect* methodology are behavioral and measurable. To ensure success these principles are:

1. Facilitate acceptance both of self and of the circumstance by centering on gratitude for what is, rather than what is not. The mechanism will be the creation of a balanced lifestyle making adaptations where necessary.

2. Pay respect to how the change is impacting each member of the inner circle of the client's life.

3. Protect the family unit by advocating for services to preserve the pre-injury roles of all family members.

4. Focus on who the person was before the life-altering accident by making adaptations to recreate life while respecting the pre-injury routines, likes, and dislikes.

5. Tap into the wealth of the inner spiritual sanctuary of each client to assist him or her to cope with the loss and change. Assist the client to emerge from the painful emotions associated with both loss and unforgiveness.

Preserving hope is essential to recovery and the key to motivating the client to engage in the therapeutic process.

SUMMARY

The Lefaivre Rainbow Effect methodology embraces the notion that each of us is unique. Its foundation is built on lighting the flame that sparks the spirit. The flame is the hope that resides within, allowing us to experience change with dignity, grace, and, ultimately, acceptance.

The human spirit is the resilient part of the person, housed in the inner sanctuary of our being. If we value our uniqueness, as well as the diversity of our life experiences, we will value even negative experiences, thus learning to cope and ultimately find a new way of being following a catastrophic event such as sustaining a TBI.

Unforgiveness can inhibit us, robbing us of the lessons that each life event avails. As health care providers we need a skilled and sensitive approach not only to facilitate organic remediation but also to remediate a bruised spirit.

The concept of the uniqueness of our individuality accepts that each person, each neurological condition, and each life scenario requires a delicate balance of hope, forgiveness, and medicine.

It is only in honoring each person and family unit that we can understand the barriers to hope, with hope being the essential ingredient to healing and acceptance. For health care providers to attempt to treat the physical and cognitive loss without acknowledging the need to nurture and support the healing of a wounded spirit, would be akin to driving a car without filling it with gas.

It requires commitment, an astute sense of self, and the ability to envision walking the path with an individual and family who have experienced a TBI and the resulting devastating loss. It is also essential to realize that we do not heal, but rather that we facilitate the healing process.

To believe that we as health care providers can control our clients' clinical outcomes by imposing a template of our own values and interventions without tapping into their inner reservoir of hope would be missing the mark. Through the *Lefaivre Rainbow Effect* methodology, the client with a TBI is provided with an individually tailored, client-centered approach to recovery that is multi-focused.

While Kübler-Ross's stages of grief were originally written in relationship to the experience of the death of a loved one, the concept and stages also apply to traumatic brain injury and the sequelae to TBI. Grief becomes even more complex; for example, if, in a road traffic accident, death occurred to another person, coupled with the client's brain injury, the situation is fraught with emotion. As we assist our clients through the process of grief it is common to see that the client may succinctly move through the stages or dance back and forth until the desired stage of acceptance is reached.

APPENDIX 1A: KÜBLER-ROSS'S FIVE STAGES OF GRIEF

Five stages of grief	
Kübler-Ross stage	Interpretation
1. Denial	Denial is a conscious or unconscious refusal to accept facts, information, reality, etc. relating to the situation concerned. It is a defense mechanism and perfectly natural. Some people can become locked in this stage when dealing with a traumatic change that can be ignored. Death, of course, is not particularly easy to avoid or evade indefinitely.
2. Anger	Anger can manifest in different ways. People dealing with emotional upset can be angry with themselves and/or with others, especially those close to them. Knowing this helps to keep detached and nonjudgmental when experiencing the anger of someone who is very upset.
3. Bargaining	Traditionally, the bargaining stage for people facing death can involve attempting to bargain with whatever God the person believes in. People facing less serious trauma can bargain or seek to negotiate a compromise—for example, "Can we still be friends?" when facing a breakup. Bargaining rarely provides a sustainable solution, especially in a matter of life or death.
4. Depression	Also referred to as preparatory grieving. In a way it is the dress rehearsal or the practice run for the "aftermath," although this stage means different things depending on whom it involves. [It is] a sort of acceptance with emotional attachment. It is natural to feel sadness and regret, fear, uncertainty, etc. It shows that the person has at least begun to accept the reality.
5. Acceptance	Again, this stage definitely varies according to the person's situation, although broadly it is an indication that there is some emotional detachment and objectivity. Dying people can enter this stage a long time before the people they leave behind, who must necessarily pass through their own individual stages of dealing with the grief.

Source: David B. Wright Memorial Foundation. 2011. Five stages of grief by Elisabeth Kübler-Ross, http://www.davidbwrightmemorialfoundation.org/Pages/FiveStagesofGrief.aspx (accessed August 13, 2013).

CHAPTER 2

The Lefaivre Rainbow Effect

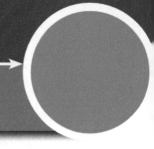

INTRODUCTION

The *rainbow effect* is an approach that offers a framework for clinicians to deliver quality, measurable health care. Embedded in this approach is that the human spirit is central to all aspects of life for the person with traumatic brain injury. The approach uses the spiritual dimension to capture hope, which leads to motivating the person throughout the recovery process. This approach is specifically individualized with an emphasis given to the client's pre-injury status, understanding all aspects of the emotional nature, values and belief systems, morals, priorities, character, intellect, interests, and relationships to others. The changes incurred because of the brain injury and the resulting rehabilitation will reflect the pre-injury profile of the client's life.

HOW THE *LEFAIVRE RAINBOW EFFECT* CAME TO BE

We need to go back in time to the late 1970s and early 1980s. This was the period prior to automobiles being fitted with driver and passenger air bags, legislated seat belt laws, bicycle helmets, and advanced emergency medicine procedures and technology. Brain injury, as a condition, was on the whole a new phenomenon, the consequences of which resulted in a lack of acknowledgment and understanding of the condition. There was no funding for long-term rehabilitation outside the acute care setting. The lack of funding also resulted in a severe shortage of professionals who specialized in traumatic brain injury community care. This was a new condition quickly reaching rampant proportions.

While the chance of survival was slim for persons who experienced severe TBI, those who did survive were initially treated in Intensive Care. As they emerged out of a coma, they were transferred to acute care and long-term hospital rehabilitation. When the goals of hospital rehabilitation were met, the person with the TBI would be discharged, despite the fact that many of the disabling symptoms persisted and life was in no way back to normal for the client and family in their home, community, work, and relationships.

The few solutions for discharge were complex and more often than not unsuitable. In the early 1980s, institutional care was standard practice for those with chronic, severely disabling conditions, many of which are now integrated into society. For persons with TBI, searching for a community-based care setting outside the hospital typically resulted in being placed in an extended care facility with seniors, a facility for the mentally challenged, or, most commonly, mental health group homes. At the time, the latter of these seemed to be the best match. This meant that persons with a brain injury would share their living space with individuals diagnosed with schizophrenia and other persons with chronic and persistent mental illness.

In the mid- to late 1980s in North America, a movement to mainstream back into the community and de-institutionalize persons with disabilities (physical, cognitive, or psychological) was adopted in legislation and social policy. To accommodate this social tsunami, numerous observable changes occurred in the community. For example, handicapped parking stalls have been designated, curb cuts on public sidewalks have become commonplace, public restrooms have wheelchair accessible facilities; public buildings have accessible entrances, auditory signaling has been installed at crosswalks, public signage is larger and better contrasting, etc. Schools began integrating individuals with physical, cognitive, and behavioral challenges into mainstream classrooms. Group homes, boarding homes, and private care homes emerged and received funding to provide housing and programs in a small, more family-oriented setting.

While these developments had an overall positive social impact, there were many that struggled with these changes, including families and the person previously living in the institutional setting. Some families wrestled with feelings of guilt recognizing that another family or family group would be caring for their loved one. This imposed a whole new thought process of "if they can manage then should we not have been able to all along?" Prior to this, families had some comfort in believing that their family member was well cared for in an institution.

For persons who had lived most of their lives in an institution and had developed institutional behaviors, the change to a community environment placed a new set of demands on them for which they were not prepared. Many were not successful in developing the independent life skills necessary for life outside a facility. The development of uniqueness and individuality had not been fostered in the institution; therefore, much direction and life skills work was warranted.

THE THEORY OF THE *RAINBOW EFFECT*

The author, an occupational therapist who supervised mental health boarding home programs in British Columbia, Canada, during the early 1980s, observed that persons with traumatic brain injury began to exhibit the same symptoms and behaviors as those with mental illness who also lived in the group homes. Lefaivre observed that those clients diagnosed with TBI were in fact beginning to model the behaviors of those clients with mental illness who shared their living space.

The group homes had a fixed set of protocols specific to the treatment of clients with mental health issues. In the early days these programs did not specialize in the treatment of traumatic brain injury. As such, in this environment a new "normal" was established for the TBI client. Everyone was expected to conform to the programs and follow the rules, despite diagnostic condition or abilities and whether it was appropriate to pre-injury skills, interests, and aptitudes.

It appeared that TBI clients living in the mental health group homes were not recovering well emotionally or cognitively; in fact, they seemed to lose motivation to participate in life in the group home and behaved as if defeated.

Lefaivre surmised that if a brain-injured client was capable of mimicking the behavior of a roommate with schizophrenia, then the brain was processing and integrating information and exhibiting new learning.

It appeared that brain-injured clients had the capacity to learn information based on what they were exposed to and what they observed. It seemed sensible at the time to theorize that because a person with a traumatic brain injury was able to learn behaviors observed in the institution, he or she would more easily be able to relearn skills and activities that were familiar to him or her prior to the accident and in a familiar environment. To test this theory and to advocate for the persons with TBI to be discharged home, the *Lefaivre Rainbow Effect* methodology for cognitive retraining was born. The reasoning was that persons with TBI would then be exposed to an environment that was familiar to them prior to their injury and to persons with whom they were familiar. The therapy plan would extend to their homes, community, and workplaces.

As a result, in the early 1980s, Lefaivre documented her observations by creating the framework for the *Lefaivre Rainbow Effect* theory. At that time specialized training facilities or private clinicians specializing in community-based therapy for persons with TBI were not the norm.

The programs that evolved using the *Lefaivre Rainbow Effect* theory were designed to utilize familiar information within the context of the person's pre-injury lifestyle and surroundings. The results were astounding. Practically speaking, it truly did appear that cognitive retraining was occurring using old familiar stimuli. The key to optimal recovery as operationalized by the *rainbow effect* was the incorporation of small, goal-directed measurable steps using pre-injury information while honoring the human spirit and the individuality of the patient. Every effort was made to allow the family to resume pre-injury roles and to protect the integrity of the family system. This was done by lobbying for funds to purchase care-giving services outside the family unit.

Based on early successes using the *rainbow effect* methodology with persons with TBI, it became essential to advocate in most cases for discharge into the client's home environment unless the client was in a persistent vegetative state or required 24-hour care. This was a foreign concept for the health care system and required considerable negotiation and education for the funder, client, and their loved ones.

THE APPROACH

The *Lefaivre Rainbow Effect* is a unique approach that looks beyond the obvious. This approach honors and builds treatment regimes based on the individuality of each client and his or her values. It analyzes how time is spent proportionally pre-injury. The therapeutic regime is designed based on the intake information of the client's pre-injury lifestyle as supplied by the client, family, and loved ones.

The *Lefaivre Rainbow Effect* is important to provide credible, reliable, creative, and effective intervention with measurable clinical results. The clarity of the rehabilitation reports will facilitate the settlement of the legal claim, thereby reducing costs and avoiding unnecessary stress for clients and their families. It will anticipate secondary losses and put supports in place to avoid the same. It will explore the use of rehabilitation workers as the most cost-effective personnel to provide day-to-day cognitive retraining with the professional team overseeing the treatment program.

Given the scope of the referral source requests, budgetary restraints, and the adversarial process, the plan may seem at face value to be unrealistic or daunting.

If, however, health care providers embrace their ability to case manage and work together as a team, it will become apparent that there are creative, cost-effective ways to lobby for funds and advocate for client care.

THE PHILOSOPHY

The philosophy underpinning the *Lefaivre Rainbow Effect* is the individuality and unique characteristics of each client. This approach aims to preserve the dignity of the client and maximize his or her performance. The belief is that "if we can *light the flame that sparks the spirit*," we can tap into the essence of the person—that part of us that makes us precisely who we are and different from all others. Despite horrific loss—perhaps physical, certainly cognitive—and often losing valued friendships, relationships, jobs, and finances, the resilience of the human spirit endures. It is a marvel.

Embedded in the philosophical position is the spiritual dimension of who we are, and this spills over into every other aspect of our life, how we view others, where we choose to spend our time, how we treat others, and how we expect to be treated. It guides our choices, goals, and selection of friends, jobs, and spouses. Our spirituality defines us and it makes us unique; the spiritual center is where hope lies. It is the source of our ability to love and be in relationships, to love others, and to love ourselves. It is the part of us that allows us to surrender to the process with peace in our hearts and hope for tomorrow.

It is this philosophical stance that supports the ultimate goal of moving through the many stages of recovery from traumatic brain injury. This recovery includes a grieving process of letting go of "what was" to acceptance of "what is, and what could be." The primary goal in therapy is to facilitate the client's path through to maximum recovery as well as fostering acceptance of the client's new self, despite the potential dire circumstances in which the client may find himself or herself. This is not something we can impose, but rather, through design, we can journey through the process of recovery with our clients setting goals that foster the process of self-acceptance so that if we:

◆ Are thorough and in tune with understanding the pre-injury self

◆ Gain the trust, support, and co-operation of clients and those around them

◆ Work hard to build a professional team that fosters the therapeutic regime

◆ Lobby for funds that will ensure a therapeutic regime that is meaningful

◆ Are creative and resourceful in that process

…then we have used ourselves therapeutically.

THE ASSUMPTIONS

Fundamental to the *rainbow effect* are these implicitly embedded underlying assumptions. They are not mutually exclusive but are described here at the individual, social, and organic levels:

- Individual
    - Respect of the human spirit will provide motivation and hope.
    - The individual has not maximized his or her potential in hospital.
    - The client remains in familiar home, work, and play environments.
    - Unforgiveness toward self or the person who is responsible for the injury or toward loved ones who abandoned the client post-trauma may cause a barrier to self-acceptance and lead to depression.
- Family
    - Family members are integral to the recovery process.
    - All efforts must be made to keep the family unit intact.
    - The approach is based on the belief that the family unit is at risk due to stress and role changes that trigger the phenomenon of the traumatically induced dysfunctional family.
    - If the family members become the primary care providers, there will be an increased risk of family breakdown, caregiver burnout, and health problems for the family members.
- Legal system
    - The adversarial system and the pending lawsuit may produce an adverse effect, focusing on the loss.
    - In the event that that there is third-party liability, the insurance policy and the ultimate settlement may offer the opportunity to finance rehabilitation both before and after the settlement.
    - When there is change there will be stress and when there is stress there will be secondary losses.
- Organic factors
    - Alcohol is not metabolized the same after a traumatic brain injury [26].

- ◆ Stress symptoms present similarly to or the same as organic symptoms and must be managed to treat the brain injury effectively.
- ◆ The brain has the capacity to relearn.
- ◆ The brain will process individualized goals based on the lifestyle before the accident most efficiently.
- ◆ The brain can process functional tasks in different ways using a variety of stimuli.
- ◆ Parts of the brain that have not experienced organic or lesional damage can be more effectively utilized to perform different tasks in a new way.

This respectful approach beginning with the initial contact and thorough assessment will focus on setting measurable goals and provide appropriate, timely, cost-effective treatment and follow-up.

THE *LEFAIVRE RAINBOW EFFECT* FORMULA

The formula that is the framework for the *rainbow effect* is conceptualized in four sequential, yet iterative, parts.

This formula is described succinctly as the "total sum" minus the "loss" plus the "intervention" equals the "residual loss" (Figure 2.1).

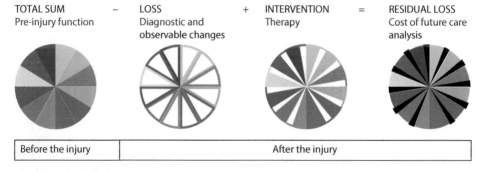

| TOTAL SUM | − | LOSS | + | INTERVENTION | = | RESIDUAL LOSS |
| Pre-injury function | | Diagnostic and observable changes | | Therapy | | Cost of future care analysis |

| Before the injury | After the injury |

Figure 2.1 The formula.

The total sum refers to the individual's pre-injury lifestyle, situation, and surroundings while the loss, intervention, and residual loss refer to the individual's status after the injury.

To best understand the formula, a description and purpose of each of the four parts is necessary.

The Total Sum

The "total sum" refers to the individual's abilities, lifestyle, and surroundings prior to the injury. The purpose of the total sum is to guide the team members in gathering information and administering comprehensive assessments to understand who the person was before this life-altering experience. It is this information that provides the framework to focus on the pre-injury status as the template to shape the intervention. There may be hot spots in a person's pre-injury life or relationships that will emerge during the history intake.

Insomuch as there is a process of assessing the client prior to introducing the intervention, one must weigh out the critical dynamics of care, particularly when it comes to relationship breakdown and client safety. For example, if the client's marriage is in obvious crisis it may be prudent to introduce a counselor, despite the fact that not all of the diagnostic reports and assessments are available and the formal community rehabilitation program has yet to commence. If the client is in a wheelchair, renovations allowing for accessibility to the home will need to be completed in advance of the client's discharge from hospital and possibly in advance of the history taking for the community team.

It is also important to note that cognitive remediation should not commence unless the neuropsychological assessment has been conducted and results reviewed. It is the "total sum" that differentiates this theory from others theories that typically focus on the organic loss rather than modeling the treatment from the fabric of the pre-injury lifestyle status.

Loss

The loss refers to the diagnostic definition of the organic/neurological damage resulting in the challenges, deficits, and changes the individual now faces as a result of the traumatic brain injury.

A review of the clinical team's standardized testing, diagnostic, radiological, and neurological reports as well as a functional assessment of the client's home and workplace will clearly outline the organic loss as well as the social consequences of the traumatic brain injury. This may include employment issues, role disruption, financial hardship, fatigue, difficulty sleeping, cognitive and motor impairment, irritability, depression, and mounting tension in relationships. It is important to note that when there is a catastrophic injury resulting in a TBI there may also be orthopedic, musculoskeletal, and other internal injuries. The "loss" section of the formula includes both primary and secondary losses.

Intervention

The intervention is the creation of a therapy plan by a multi-disciplinary team that is commensurate with the client's pre-injury function. This custom-made therapy plan will maximize recovery while reducing secondary losses as the client is discharged back home or to community care. It is at this point that a compatible one-to-one rehabilitation worker will be retained. It is important that this worker is age and interest appropriate. Special attention is focused on the emergence of changes in the family system and other secondary losses. The assigned goals, observations, and schedules are reviewed and amended weekly during this process. It is through careful interpretation of the one-to-one worker's observations of how the client is engaging in functional day-to-day tasks that patterns of sensory overload can be established.

The client's pre-injury level of activity and interest is carefully compared to the neuropsychological assessment findings. In areas where mild, moderate, or severe brain damage is noted in the neuropsychological evaluation, special attention must be paid to areas experiencing cognitive defect. The team must be careful when therapeutic tasks are introduced requiring the assimilation of cognitive stimuli where the client may be disadvantaged. When success is not experienced by the client, it is prudent to challenge other parts of the brain that are functioning within normal limits by modifying the task, with the expectation that a different part of the brain will assimilate this information in a new way for the same purpose. This stage requires the careful and thoughtful implementation of goal-directed steps while also utilizing aids and adaptations or making modifications to the environment.

Residual Loss

The outcome of intervention is the improvement gained by recognizing that there often remain residual deficits or losses. In Figure 2.1 the residual loss is represented by black areas or wedges. These are deficits remaining after the therapy is completed and they are accommodated through a number of compensatory measures. The residual loss represents the areas of function that have not been restored or remediated. These will inevitably be lifelong areas of challenge for the client.

The residual loss is also the basis of analysis for the cost of future care/life care plans for litigation purposes.

ELEMENTS OF THE *RAINBOW EFFECT* FORMULA

Having an understanding of the four-part methodology of the *rainbow effect* formula is the beginning of implementing the process. Provision of an overview is provided in Table 2.1.

Table 2.1 Elements of the *Rainbow Effect* Formula

Total sum	Loss	Intervention	Residual loss
Documentation of pre-injury status • Advocate to funder to engage in extensive history taking • History taking with the client and the family to establish a pre-injury baseline • Develop rapport with client and family • Conduct an assessment of the client's pre-injury living environment and lifestyle	Multi-disciplinary team gathers information to understand the client's deficits • Solicit and review medical reports • Interpret diagnostic loss as indicated by CAT, SPECT, PET scans topographical brain mapping, evoked potentials, and MRIs • Each discipline conducts baseline and standardized assessments • Review the findings of team members at a team meeting • Advocate to funder and introduce additional relevant health care professionals	Design, implement, and adjust a relevant therapeutic intervention program • Design therapy program based on clinical findings and pre-injury interests • Introduce a one-to-one worker that is age and interest appropriate to the client • Put family supports in place to assist the family to maintain their original pre-injury role in the family unit • Manage stress symptoms • Set goals • Observations • Color-coded weekly schedules • Each clinician follows up with client • Ongoing team meetings	Each discipline summarizes the client's gains and residual losses in a final report • A summary of all of the clinical team's concerns about the client's future needs is accumulated into a cost of future care/life care plan report, quantifying the lifetime losses • An actuary will index the lifetime costs to assist in quantifying the loss • Expert witness testimony may be requested by the clinical team or independent medical evaluators • In the absence of a lawsuit, a system of support is established for the family through volunteers and students

THE PROCESS OF THE *RAINBOW EFFECT*

The *Lefaivre Rainbow Effect* is user friendly to clinicians, the client, and family. The therapeutic outcome will serve to quantify the loss for legal purposes.

The most prudent process to structure the elements of the *rainbow effect* formula for favorable outcomes is the following:

1. Generally, a case manager is assigned by the funding source. This is frequently an occupational therapist or can be a case manager from another health care discipline.

2. This individual coordinates the efforts of the team and facilitates communication before and after the client is discharged from hospital.

3. The ideal is if the case manager can be retained at the time of the client's discharge from hospital to effect continuity of care. Team members from the hospital representing each discipline will review their hospital therapeutic goals at a discharge meeting and these goals will be transferred to the community team to be introduced to the real-life home, work, and play situations.

4. Any home renovations and vehicle modifications for accessibility should be completed prior to the client's discharge from hospital to reduce the client's frustration and ensure safety.

5. The family and significant others are provided with education, counseling, and support to reduce the stress on all family members and facilitate the family unit to stay intact.

6. The client is discharged home to the family and the community care team or, in the case of someone requiring nursing care, to a residential or long-term rehabilitation facility.

7. The family does not assume the role of care provider, but rather goes on with life as usual, maintaining their pre-injury roles and thus providing the framework of familiar activity and routine for the brain-injured family member.

8. To avoid family/relationship breakdown, funding is sourced out, or, in the case of lack of funding, volunteers are recruited and a myriad of support systems are put in place for the family to ensure they do not assume care-giving roles, to prevent burnout and negative health issues. To this end it is imperative that family members assume their pre-injury roles so that life is familiar to the TBI survivor.

9. Team meetings organized by the case manager are held regularly and should include the client, family, community health care providers, litigators, and funders. The purpose is for each discipline to review its testing results and incorporate its findings into the overall program objectives and goals. All care providers, as well as the client, and family should be in agreement

with the goals. Funding and volunteers need to be secured to avoid frustration for the client and disruption of care. These team meetings should be prepared for in advance and well attended to ensure cost effectiveness and enhance the efficacy of treatment.

10. In the event that third-party funding is not available, the same principles apply. Volunteers (see Figure 4.2 in Chapter 4) should be recruited and trained to provide care under the direction of the health care providers.

11. One-to-one rehabilitation workers may be introduced at various times in the recovery process to carry out the professionally designed, tailor-made program.

12. The rehabilitation worker should be contracted specifically for each client and should be age and interest appropriate.

13. The team commits to the duration of the treatment regime, which could last up to 6 years.

PROVIDERS OF SERVICES

The team for a brain-injured survivor generally includes a diverse cross section of multi-disciplinary health care providers through the multi-year recovery process. Some clinicians are consistently involved in the case while others join the team as their input is required.

In acute care the health care team is focused on critical care issues that include preserving life and medically stabilizing the client. When this is achieved, the individual is then ready to begin the initial stages of the rehabilitation process in an in-patient environment that may include a general neurology unit, a rehabilitation center, or other medical facilities. As the client improves, discharge to the community and home is orchestrated.

In the community the number and frequency of service providers will depend on the client needs and sources of funding. Ideally, the new community case manager and community occupational therapist should be in attendance at the hospital discharge meeting. If the professionals at the hospital discharge the client from their service and will not be following up long term, then a new team member from the same discipline may need to be added for continuity in long-term community follow up (see Table 2.2 and Appendix 1). Some clinicians are consistently involved in the case while others join the team as their input is required.

For instance, the hospital neuropsychologist may not engage in community work, so a community neuropsychologist will need to be retained. The neurologist, physiatrist, general practitioner, and possibly the neuropsychologist (if testing was completed in

Table 2.2 Service Providers in Health Care Settings

	Setting			
	Hospital		Community	
Health care provider professionals	Acute	Rehab	Typically	Adjunctive
Family physician	✓	✓	✓	
Neurologist	✓	✓	✓	
Neurosurgeon	✓			
Physiatrist	✓	✓	✓	
Neuropsychologist	✓	✓	✓	✓
Occupational therapist	✓	✓	✓	✓
Physical therapist	✓	✓		✓
Speech pathologist	✓	✓	✓	✓
Nurse	✓	✓		
Nutritionist	✓	✓		
Social worker	✓	✓		✓
Clinical psychologist			✓	✓
Pastoral care	✓	✓		✓
Pharmacist	✓	✓		✓
Case manager			✓	
Educator				✓
Vocational rehabilitation consultant				✓
Kinesiologist				✓
Sex health counselor		✓		✓
Lawyer (plaintiff/defense)	✓	✓	✓	✓
Insurance adjuster	✓	✓	✓	✓
Works under the direction of the professional team				
One-to-one rehabilitation worker			✓	✓
Volunteers			✓	✓

the hospital) would continue to follow up long term. All other hospital care providers will generally discharge the client to the care of a community team member of the same discipline.

In the early stages of recovery, depending on who was responsible for the accident/injury, additional players will become involved that may include plaintiff and defense lawyers, insurance adjusters, workers compensation, or victims' assistance.

Typically, much of the community care will be provided by private health care providers. There are many service providers merging in the marketplace, so it is important to choose reliable and reputable service providers with a proven track record, commitment to the client's long-term care, and credentials admissible in court.

Once the critical 4- to 6-year rehabilitation period has passed, the residual symptoms will be clearly defined. At this point, if funds have been awarded in a tort claim, assistance may be purchased privately by the client and family; specifically, rehabilitation workers, health care aids, and counselors may provide ongoing services. Periodic consultation may be required by the occupational therapist, physical therapist, and speech therapist as well as the neuropsychologist and physiatrist. The family doctor will be the primary case manager in the long term once the case has settled and the residual loss has been determined. In the event that funding is not available, the ongoing use of volunteers and community services will be necessary to provide assistance and respite for family members.

For the health care professional, the *Lefaivre Rainbow Effect* will provide a framework to engage in the roles of care provider and case manager as well as expert witness.

For the purposes of third-party funders and litigators, dollar figures can be attached to the outcome measures. This outcome can be quantified to produce a "cost of future care analysis." (This also may be called the "life care plan.") A cost of future care can then be indexed by an actuary to reflect the lifetime costs awarded to the client.

This measurable procedure will produce costs directly related to the injury and reduce secondary losses, which may cloud or discredit the client as a malingerer.

Most importantly, the plan will achieve the highest possible level of recovery for the client by designing a task-specific approach respectful of the values, beliefs, and skills of the client. The client will monitor progress through a simple color-coded technique (which will be reviewed in subsequent chapters.) This technique will provide a visual cue to the client and health care provider when stress symptoms interfere with the progress.

The client and family are integral members of the team as they work with the service providers to achieve a positive outcome. The purpose of the *rainbow effect* is for the client and family to emerge as the source of information, from which the therapy plan is constructed. The individualized program will reflect the client and family's pre-injury profile, including values and belief systems.

SUMMARY

The *Lefaivre Rainbow Effect* was designed originally to help those brain-injured persons who had been institutionalized. In advocating for a policy that supported return to home, Lefaivre found that persons with TBI experienced a marked functional recovery and psychological benefit when in their pre-injury environment. The brain appeared to find integrating old familiar information an easier task than integrating new foreign stimuli in foreign surroundings.

It was clear that a catastrophic event such as sustaining a traumatic brain injury resulted in marked stress for family members and the client. Immediate intervention to preserve the family unit was found to be most effective in reducing secondary losses.

A simple, user-friendly formula was developed that gave structure to the *Lefaivre Rainbow Effect* and assisted team members as well as the client and family. The formula is given in Figure 2.1.

A thorough intake procedure is used to capture the "total sum" that provides the health care provider with the relevant information necessary to tailor a therapy regime that is commensurate with the client's pre-injury lifestyle, thereby respecting who he or she was and assisting him or her in embracing "who I am now." Through standardized testing and diagnostic assessments, the "loss" identifies the primary and secondary challenges and deficits the individual experiences as a result of the traumatic brain injury. This includes the organic losses as well as the social consequences and stress symptoms resulting from the brain injury. The "intervention" then maximizes the recovery while reducing the impact of losses through the development of an individualized therapy plan that is in keeping with and relevant to the pre-injury function. The "residual losses" are deficits that remain after the therapy is completed and are accommodated through compensatory measures and adaptation to the environment, as well as continued relearning. The relearning can continue over the person's lifetime by teaching different parts of the brain to engage in a task in a new way.

The importance of hope as the integral ingredient to connect not just to our clients but also the clients to the process of healing has proven to be critical to positive outcomes.

A multidisciplinary team will provide intervention, guidance, and care during each phase of recovery from acute, rehabilitation, and community integration.

This method recognizes that continuity of care and consistency of care providers over the 4- to 6-year recovery process is critical to avoid unnecessary setbacks for the client.

A team approach facilitating clear and efficient sharing of information capitalizes on the expertise of all health care providers. A team of this nature needs a case manager to ensure that timelines and communication are streamlined. The formula will provide the framework for the community rehabilitation team; as we move to Chapter 3 we will explore the TOTAL SUM segment of the formula.

APPENDIX 2A: DEFINITIONS OF SERVICE PROVIDERS (See additional resource material: Family Handout Definitions of Service Providers (http:www.crcpress.com/product/ isbn/9781482228243.))

Case manager: Health care or social science professional who manages a clinical team and advocates for a disabled individual in the health care and social sciences fields.

Clinical psychologist: Assesses and diagnoses behavioral, emotional, and cognitive disorders; counsels clients; provides therapy; conducts research; and applies theory relating to behavior and mental processes. Psychologists help clients work toward maintenance and enhancement of psychological, physical, intellectual, emotional, social, and interpersonal functioning. Psychologists work in private practice or in clinics, correctional facilities, hospitals, mental health facilities, rehabilitation centers, community services organizations, businesses, schools and universities, and government and private research agencies [27, pp. 253–254].

Educator/teacher: Prepares and teaches academic, technical, vocational, or specialized subjects at public and private schools [27, pp. 247–248].

Family physician/general practitioner: Diagnoses and treats the diseases, physiological disorders and injuries of patients. They provide primary contact and continuous care toward the management of patients' health. They usually work in private practice, including group or team practices, hospitals, and clinics. Residents in training to be general practitioners and family physicians are included in this unit group [27, p. 211].

Insurance adjuster: Investigates insurance claims and determines the amount of loss or damages covered by insurance policies. They are employed in claims departments of insurance companies or as independent adjusters. Insurance claims examiners examine claims investigated by insurance adjusters and authorize payments [27, p. 115].

Kinesiologist: Uses techniques such as athletic, movement, art, or recreational therapy to aid in the treatment of mental and physical disabilities or injuries. They are employed by establishments such as hospitals, rehabilitation centers, extended health care facilities, clinics, recreational centers, nursing homes, industry, educational institutions, and sports organizations, or they may work in private practice [27, p. 223].

Lawyer (plaintiff/defense): Advises clients on legal matters, represents clients before administration boards, and draws up legal documents such as contracts and wills. Lawyers also plead cases, represent clients before tribunals, and conduct prosecutions in courts of law. Lawyers are employed in law firms and prosecutors' offices. They are employed by federal, provincial, and municipal governments and various business establishments or they may be self-employed [27, p. 252].

Neurologist: A specialist in the diagnosis and treatment of disorders of the neuromuscular system: the central, peripheral, and autonomic nervous systems; the neuromuscular junction; and muscles [28].

Neuropsychologist: A psychologist with specialized training in dealing with problems that result from some form of insult or injury to the brain. He or she is often called upon to do extensive assessment of the areas of emotional, behavioral and cognitive consequences of injuries to the brain. A typical neuropsychological evaluation will assess areas such as memory, problem-solving skills, attention, concentration, sequencing skills, abstract reasoning, motor speed, planning, organizing, task completion, and emotional/personality functions. This information is particularly important to rehabilitation following brain injury. The neuropsychologist can be available to consult regarding cognitive and behavioral rehabilitation that may help a loved one and can offer counseling and guidance with regard to issues of recovery [29, p. 7].

Neurosurgeon: Medical doctor specializing in neurosurgery.

Nurse: Provides direct nursing care to patients, delivers health education programs, and provides consultative services regarding issues relevant to the practice of nursing. Nurses are employed in a variety of settings including hospitals, nursing homes, extended-care facilities, rehabilitation centers, doctors' offices, clinics, community agencies, companies, and private homes, or they may be self-employed [27, p. 207].

Nutritionist: Dietitians and nutritionists plan, implement, and oversee nutrition and food service programs. They are employed in a variety of settings including hospitals, home health care agencies and extended-care facilities, community health centers, the food and beverage industry, the pharmaceutical industry, educational institutions, and government and sports organizations, or they may work as private consultants [27, p. 219].

Occupational therapist: Develops individual and group programs with people affected by illness, injury, developmental disorders, emotional or psychological problems, and ageing to maintain, restore, or increase their ability to care for themselves and to engage in work, school, or leisure. Also develops and implements health promotion programs with individuals, community groups, and employers. Occupational therapists are employed in health care facilities, in schools, and by private and social services agencies, or may be self-employed [27, p. 222].

Pastoral care worker: Conducts religious services, administers the rites of a religious faith or denomination, provides spiritual and moral guidance, and performs other functions associated with the practice of a religion. They work in churches, synagogues, temples, schools, hospitals, and prisons [27, p. 257].

Pharmacist: Community pharmacists and hospital pharmacists compound and dispense prescribed pharmaceuticals and provide consultative services to both clients and health care providers. They are employed in retail and hospital pharmacies, or they may be self-employed. Industrial pharmacists participate in the research, development, promotion, and manufacture of pharmaceutical products. They are employed in pharmaceutical companies and government departments and agencies [27, p. 218].

Physiatrist: A physician who specializes in physiatry (rehabilitation medicine) [28].

Physical therapist: Assesses patients and plans and carries out individually designed treatment programs to maintain, improve, or restore physical functioning; alleviate pain; and prevent physical dysfunction in patients. Physiotherapists are employed in hospitals, clinics, industry, sports organizations, rehabilitation centers, and extended-care facilities or they may work in private practice [27, p. 221].

Rehabilitation worker: Workers who provide one-on-one services to clients and assistance to health care professionals. They are employed in hospitals, offices of health care professionals, and nursing homes.

Sex health counselor: Provides counseling on issues related to one or more aspects of sexuality with the aim of understanding the underlying features of clients' sexual lives and how that affects their sexual and reproductive health. Such counseling requires the creation of a counseling environment where clients can express themselves and their concerns relating to sexual relationships and intimacy without fear of ridicule, discrimination, or other disrespectful treatment. Sexuality counseling tends to occur in organized one-on-one sessions between a counselor and a client, and is designed to solve a problem or give advice related to sexuality [30, p. 2].

Social worker: Helps individuals, couples, families, groups, communities, and organizations develop the skills and resources they need to enhance social functioning and provides counseling, therapy, and referral to other supportive social services. Social workers also respond to other social needs and issues such as unemployment, racism, and poverty. They are employed by hospitals, school boards, social services agencies, child welfare organizations, correctional facilities, community agencies, employee assistance programs, and Aboriginal band councils, or they may work in private practice [27, p. 254].

Speech pathologist: Speech–language pathologists diagnose, assess, and treat human communication disorders including speech, fluency, language, voice, and swallowing disorders. They are employed in hospitals, community and public health centers, extended-care facilities, day clinics, rehabilitation centers, and educational institutions, or may work in private practice [27, p. 220].

Vocational rehabilitation consultant: In the case of the traumatic brain injury survivor, the vocational rehabilitation consultant assesses the client's ability to return to work in concert with the occupational therapist and the neuropsychologist and facilitates the process of finding a job placement as well as supplying a job coach.

CHAPTER 3

Total Sum

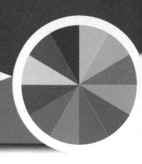

TOTAL SUM	−	DIAGNOSIS (LOSS)	+	INTERVENTION	=	RESIDUAL LOSS

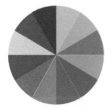

INTRODUCTION

In this chapter we will review the *total sum*, which is a system to analyze pre-injury information obtained from the client and significant others. The process will recruit pre-injury data by taking an extensive and comprehensive history.

To support the author's observation that brain-injured persons recover most effectively in a familiar environment utilizing old familiar cognitive stimuli, it is most important to understand *who the individual was* prior to the injury. Each topic area of the client's life is represented by a color. Figure 3.1 depicts an individual whose life was well balanced prior to the TBI. This may not always be the case. This pie represents on a weekly basis how much time the individual spent in each dimension of his or her life prior to the injury, such as:

- Who he or she was cognitively
- Who he or she was emotionally
- Who he or she was vocationally
- Who he or she was spiritually
- What he or she did for relaxation
- What he or she enjoyed socially
- What he or she embarked on physically
- Who he or she was in family relationships
- His or her involvement in the community
- His or her functional and day-to-day habits
- His or her leisure activities
- His or her sexuality

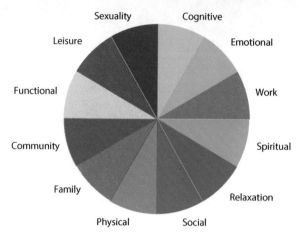

Figure 3.1 Life pie segments.

To gain this type of information, the client and health care provider must develop therapeutic rapport and trust. Information, with the permission of the client, may be gathered from the client as well as from family, friends, and employers with whom the client was involved prior to the injury. The initial gathering of information is ascertained through an intensive history-taking exercise (Appendix 3A). (See additional resource material, Family History Intake Form at **http://www.crcpress.com/product/isbn/ 9781482228243.**)

DETERMINING THE TOTAL SUM

We are the total sum of our values, beliefs, relationships, and activities. We live this out through how, where, and with whom we spend our time. Our priorities are reflected in the percentage of time we allocate to various areas of our lives.

Example 1: Mother's Percentage of Time

A mother may spend 50% of her time with her children/husband and related family activity, 25% of her time cleaning and cooking, 10% of her time keeping fit and 15% of her time with friends (Figure 3.2).

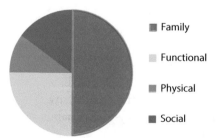

■ Family

■ Functional

■ Physical

■ Social

Figure 3.2 Mother's percentage of time.

Example 2: Father's Percentage of Time

A father allocates 40% of his time to work, 20% to family/wife, 20% to relaxation, 3% to his sexuality, 7% to functional activities, 5% to physical activities, and 5% to spiritual activities (Figure 3.3).

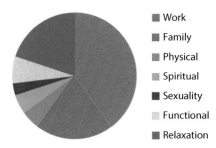

Work
Family
Physical
Spiritual
Sexuality
Functional
Relaxation

Figure 3.3 Father's percentage of time.

Example 3: A teenage girl may allocate 50% of her time to social activities, 20% to relaxation, 5% to chores/functional, 10% to physical activities, 10% to leisure activities, and 5% to work (Figure 3.4).

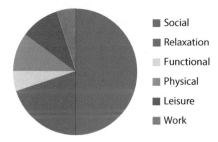

Social
Relaxation
Functional
Physical
Leisure
Work

Figure 3.4 Teenage girl's percentage of time.

In the world of therapy and stress management we know that a balanced lifestyle leads to a healthy mind, body, soul, and spirit. Ideally, an individual should strive to eat well, exercise regularly, and engage in healthy communication with spouse and family members. There should be time for work, fun, recreation, relaxation, community involvement, chores at home, family relationships, relaxation, emotional outlets, personal hygiene and grooming, sexuality, spiritual development, physical activity, and socialization. The association between stress and its impact on health and well-being indicates that "a balanced lifestyle would be one where stress is managed in a way that minimizes its long-term negative effects" [31, p. 12].

The concept of a balanced lifestyle seems to have widespread acceptance in the popular press. "The notion that certain lifestyle configurations might lend to better health, higher levels of life satisfaction and general well being is readily endorsed" [31, p. 9].

"Living a balanced life should yield positive states such as happiness, subjective well-being, resilience, and quality of life" [31, p. 10]. We spend a great deal of time at work, so we should engage in an occupation we enjoy, offsetting work with pleasurable leisure activities and rest. Taking time to nurture life-giving friendships is necessary as well as taking time to connect with our spiritual selves.

A balanced lifestyle promotes health, the ability to deal with stress, and an overall sense of well-being. Persons living a balanced life survive life's challenges much better and perceive their lives to be "more satisfying, less stressful, and more meaningful" [31, p. 11]. This balance is the key to staving off depression, anxiety, emotional shutdown, addictions, obesity…the list goes on.

However, most people do not have the ideal balance in their lives prior to the injury; if, upon initial consult with our clients, we impose a balanced therapy plan based on the ideal, without taking into account the measure of time spent by the client on pre-injury activities, we would be missing the picture of the person entirely. We then become part of the problem, imposing our own values rather than respecting the client's. This will jeopardize the therapeutic relationship that we need to establish.

The pre-injury profile pie is the template for the future therapeutic intervention.

HOW THIS APPROACH DIFFERS FROM CURRENT TRENDS

Current trends in how a client is discharged back to the home and community vary greatly worldwide with respect to the environment and amount of care accorded to the patient with traumatic brain injury. The literature indicates that the pathway of the patient after discharge relies heavily on the type of funding available and access to community resources and rehabilitation as well as severity of injury and amount of care needed [32–35]. Generally, patients will be discharged home from hospital to an inpatient, outpatient, or community rehabilitation program, which may or may not be covered under a public or private health care plan [32].

In today's health care market, funding—whether government, insurance, or other—begins at the point of the client sustaining the TBI. In emergency, ICU, acute care, and hospital rehabilitation, the medical status of the client is the key point of discussion—and rightly so, with previous history playing a minor role. It is the author's experience that the patient/client is quickly identified by his or her injury in hospital and the resulting sequelae as opposed to the unique individual he or she was prior to the traumatic brain injury.

Generally, a brief, possibly two-paragraph account of the client's pre-injury situation is referenced in the hospital medical reports with a strong focus being placed on etiology of the injury, diagnostics, and medical intervention.

In the case of community rehabilitation the *Lefaivre Rainbow Effect* initially places emphasis "on life before the injury," which is a much different framework from commencing the client/clinician relationship based on the deficits experienced by the client. In doing so, the functional impact of the traumatic brain injury on the client and family will be better understood for the purpose of re-engaging in life after discharge from the hospital.

PREPARING FOR THE HISTORY INTAKE

This is a unique and different approach for several reasons:

1. A strong focus is placed on taking an extensive pre-injury history to explore and understand the client's life before the brain injury. The future treatment will be shaped by this important information.

2. We, the health care professionals, may not be comfortable with this type of intimate history intake.

3. For this approach to be effective, it is important for the care providers to have their own emotional house in order. The difference in taking an in-depth history versus a cursory impersonal history is one of intimacy. Inevitably, when engaging in an extensive history-taking exercise with clients and families, we, the health care providers, will be triggered by our own life experiences. We must be evolved enough in our own lives not to personalize or project our own feelings onto the client's experience.

4. The health care team needs to be skilled and comfortable with exploring the client's pre-injury life, which will include sexuality, emotional triggers, possible addiction, sexual abuse, abandonment, etc. If these sensitive areas are not explored historically, the pre-injury template for cognitive remediation is not complete and therefore not compatible for rehabilitation purposes, rendering the treatment regime somewhat ineffective.

5. The funding source may not ordinarily allow for this type of time to be spent gaining baseline information.

We should be aware that we are placing ourselves in the middle of the client and family's grief process, often to be the target of misdirected frustration and anger. Understanding this unique therapeutic process will allow us to be comfortable enough to gain a working knowledge of all areas of the client's life—both strengths and areas of challenge.

ADVOCATING TO THE FUNDER

Funding may not be readily available for the required time to engage in an extensive historical intake. The health care provider must have a clear and thorough understanding of traumatic brain injury and understand why paving the way with historical information is essential to cost-effective and successful treatment, thereby allowing the clinician to lobby effectively for funds and advocate for permission to conduct an extensive history.

It is also important to respect and clearly understand the parameters and policies of the funding source. Generally, funding guidelines are clear, but may also leave room for flexibility. If a sound case can be made for a comprehensive intake, funds are generally granted—particularly if the clinician can support the case for short-term costs for long-term gain, resulting in cost effectiveness and better clinical outcomes.

To pursue an overall understanding of what motivated the client in the past will serve as invaluable information to platform toward the future, using this information to structure a personalized cognitive retraining regime. It is this cost-effective reasoning for taking an extensive pre-injury history that a funder will understand.

The *Lefaivre Rainbow Effect* will also unveil areas where a person has not been successful or happy in life before the injury, allowing for growth and avoidance of hot spots for the treating health care provider.

This heavily weighted intake will also provide the fertile soil for building trust and developing therapeutic rapport between the client and the health care professional.

This thorough intake procedure will also provide stable footing for the health care provider to be admitted as an expert witness in the litigation system. The history taking is not a 10-minute intake done in an office. It takes several hours of interviewing in a comfortable environment conducive to building trust. We need to have a clear understanding of family lineage, family values and dynamics, the client's role in the family, socialization likes and skill, recreation, physical activity, community involvement, evolution of spirituality, interests, sexual development, emotional health, aptitudes, intellect, career objectives, addictions, trauma, personality characteristics, vulnerabilities, schedules, responsibilities, and personal goals prior to the injury.

THE PROCESS OF DETERMINING THE TOTAL SUM

There is an ongoing, interactive, and simultaneous process occurring for the community and hospital teams during the hospital discharge planning period, which are the **total sum** and **loss** stages of the *Rainbow Effect Formula* for the community team (Figure 3.5). At this point the community team is determining the **total sum** while simultaneously preparing for determining the **loss** by soliciting hospital medical reports, preparing the client's home and vehicle prior to discharge, and having at least one community clinician attend the hospital discharge meeting.

It is important to note that the client's care is on a continuum (Figure 3.6).

The literature indicates that the path of a patient through the health care system is dependent on the severity of injury. Thompson et al. [33] found that length of stay for patients in acute wards with access to specialized neurorehabilitation services averaged 77.9 days compared to the group who did not receive specialized rehabilitation during their acute treatment, which averaged 112.7 days.

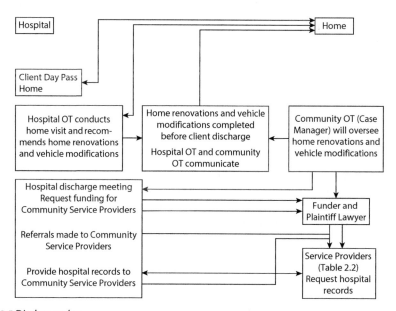

Figure 3.5 Discharge plan.

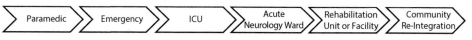

Figure 3.6 Client's continuum of care.

There is an interrelationship with the total sum segment (history), as well as an overlap in preparing for determining the loss (requesting the medical reports), which will then set the stage for the intervention. As a clinician it is important to anticipate what documents will be needed for each stage of treatment.

If there is a waiting period to receive a medical consultation or diagnostic reports, this will impact the continuum of care. Therefore, as we embark on taking the history, for the purposes of designing a community cognitive rehabilitation program for the future, we will be cognizant that as soon as the history is completed we will ideally begin to introduce a community rehabilitation program; therefore, we must also be in the process of requesting and receiving the previous emergency and hospital medical records pertaining to the client's TBI prior to commencing the community rehabilitation program.

Given the nature of the traumatic brain injury, it may be obvious that additional team members will be required for the community rehabilitation. Referrals for community practitioners should be made as soon as the need becomes apparent. For instance, if a client has a Glasgow coma score of 8 (Appendix 3E) he or she will most certainly need a neuropsychological assessment. However, the client may not have been able to tolerate this lengthy process while in hospital, so to avoid delays in community rehabilitation, a referral should be made for a community neuropsychologist to conduct this assessment upon discharge.

Practically speaking, there are wait lists for busy, reputable health care professionals; any lag in sending a referral or receiving a report puts the community team at a stalemate and puts the client at risk. Despite that, we are in the **total sum** stage, which is the pre-injury profile, we must also plan for the future intervention simultaneously. A team approach is critical to clinical success.

The neuropsychologist is a very important member of the team. It is important that this health care provider have the background and capacity to administer a full battery of assessments, which will profile the deficits that the client is experiencing as a result of the traumatic brain injury. With careful and thoughtful interpretation, this report serves as an invaluable tool for the community team members, providing a baseline of post-injury capabilities for the client.

The physiatrist and physical therapist are the team members with the expertise in physical performance, physical endurance, and stamina. It is through their expertise that the community team can reintroduce fitness, recreation, and activities requiring physical tolerance. Once completed in hospital and through the direction of the physiatrist and physical therapist, the physical program can commonly be transferred to a kinesiologist, fitness trainer, or rehabilitation worker. This information is also valuable to the occupational therapist, who can apply this knowledge to the client's function at home, work, and play.

The speech and language pathologist is important. Each clinician will begin commencing assessments, and it will be important to the team to have a working knowledge of the client's ability to receive auditory instructions and comprehend both written and verbal instructions. It will be important for the clinicians and family to understand and be prepared for any problems the client may have with expressive and receptive language.

The occupational therapist's home assessments will be important for the speech and language pathologist to understand how expressive and receptive language is impacting the client functionally at home and in relationship with significant others.

The occupational therapist and speech pathologist/audiologist will benefit greatly from reading the neuropsychological evaluation to understand how the brain is processing cognitive information and to be clear on the brain function that is impaired.

The pharmacist is important in that some of the client's medications may induce fatigue or altered sleep patterns. This knowledge is useful for the entire team as we challenge the client to expend more energy and become more active.

The family and client may benefit greatly from a clinical psychologist or social worker to assist in developing coping strategies as they navigate their way through these challenging life events. The entire team will be able to enhance the impact of the rehabilitation program as knowledge of the emotional sequelae of the traumatic brain injury is gained.

The neuropsychologist, speech pathologist, and social worker will benefit from the occupational therapist's report, which will profile the sensory and perceptual deficits as well as functionally indicate the impact of the brain injury (including safety risks) in a practical home or work setting. The inter-relationship of the interdisciplinary team is crucial. Not one clinician should embark in therapy as a sole practitioner if there is evidence that additional clinicians from a myriad of disciplines are warranted. Each discipline is a subspecialty of the entire community rehabilitation team. The team members can be involved consistently over the 4- to 6-year therapeutic process or intervene as necessary providing consultative expertise.

Remember that provision of a timely service is critical to avoid frustration, depression, and stress for the client and family. The process as shown in Figure 3.5 will outline the necessary approach to reduce or eliminate delays.

ESTABLISHING THE COMMUNITY TEAM

The human condition is multi-faceted and complex requiring an array of professional input from a myriad of disciplines as shown in Figure 3.7. This model capitalizes on the premise that there is a wealth of experience that ideally can be made available to the TBI survivor and his/her family, each discipline providing a unique perspective complementing the team and its effectiveness as a whole.

Each community clinician will have received a request to become involved with the client. It is important to note that the purpose of the request may vary from profession to profession. The timing of each discipline's involvement may vary.

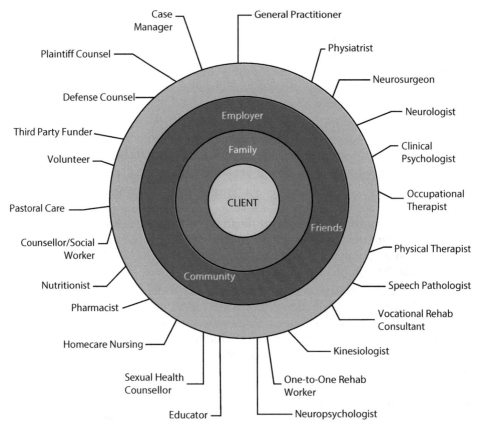

Figure 3.7 Clinical community team.

Secure Funding

Funding sources vary from country to country but generally fall within the following categories. The reasons for their involvement may include, but are not limited to:

1. Providing unbiased intervention funded by a no-fault or partial no-fault portion of an insurance policy
2. Providing intervention as part of a community health government-funded program
3. Providing intervention as part of a follow-up program from the hospital
4. Providing an independent medical evaluation for the defense lawyer
5. Providing an independent medical evaluation for plaintiff counsel
6. Providing intervention on behalf of a union
7. Providing intervention on behalf of veterans' affairs
8. Providing intervention on behalf of victims' assistance
9. Providing intervention as requested and privately funded by family
10. Providing intervention for disability insurance policies
11. Providing intervention on behalf of a nongovernment organization or nonprofit organization
12. Providing intervention on behalf of the military
13. Recruiting and educating volunteers where funding is not available

Requesting Emergency and Hospital Records

It is important that each clinician solicit copies of all available hospital records; tests; radiological reports such as CAT, PET, and SPECT scans; evoked potentials; topographical brain mapping; and MRIs, as well as the medical consultation reports in order to be well-versed on the etiology of the traumatic brain injury. It is very important to understand the nature of the brain injury from the hospital records before commencing a community assessment. This positions the clinician to avoid sensory overloading the client as we request the person to recount events of the past. There will inevitably be land mines.

Make a Request for a Neuropsychological Assessment

Be sure to request a neuropsychological assessment if one has not already been completed. This will be crucial to commence the next stage of intervention and may take time to complete.

Signing the Release of Information Form

It is the health care provider's responsibility to advise the client that insomuch as the code of confidentiality will be honored, whoever financed the report in essence owns the report and therefore becomes the gatekeeper of the confidential information. This information may be used in trial and become a public record and this should be explained to the client. It is important that the client knows who has requested the service as well as the limitations of confidentiality.

THE HISTORY-TAKING PROCESS

Preparing the Client

1. Ensure that transportation to the appointment is available.
2. Ensure that parking is easily and readily available, especially in the event that the client uses a wheelchair or has mobility limitations.
3. Be on time for the appointment to avoid frustrating the client.
4. Explain the process.
5. Ask if the client would like someone present.
6. Schedule the appointment at the time of day that the client is most alert.

Taking the Clinical History

1. The clinician will conduct the initial history intake in a comfortable environment—perhaps the client's home or an office where the client will feel at ease (Appendix 3A).
2. Upon review of the medical reports, the clinician may become aware of previous family difficulties. The clinician in concert with the client must discern who should be invited to participate in the intake procedure. This is a particularly sensitive area if previous neglect or abuse has been identified.
3. Generally, an effective approach is to see the client independently of other family members and then to interview the family alone to corroborate past and present information. Make a note if there has been a change in family roles since the injury. (See additional resource material, Family Role Changes Balanced Lifestyle Inventory http://www.crcpress.com/product/isbn/9781482228243.)
4. Typically, the client will be very fatigued. Disruptive sleep is a common symptom of traumatic brain injury; it is respectful to ask when is the best time during the day to engage in the assessment.

5. Pain and headaches may also be a factor. Take frequent breaks if necessary; multiple appointments may be required to complete the history.

6. Be aware of the other team members' expectations of the client to avoid double booking and overwhelming the client.

7. If there is a gap or loss of childhood memory this very well can be a sign that the client has experienced early childhood trauma. This needs to be explored gently, as the history taking will inevitably trigger emotions. However, when an individual experiences childhood trauma, there are already learned, pre-existing coping skills in place. The client will have a predisposition perhaps to deny or mask the brain injury symptoms, making it more difficult to get to the truth of the pre-injury life and thus losing the desired information on which to base the cognitive retraining program. "Dissociation is thought to be linked to a history of trauma in childhood" and is "associated with various forms of memory impairment" [36, p. 1277].

Confirm the length of the post-traumatic amnesia as well as the retrograde amnesia. The author has found that the post-traumatic amnesia is the best predictor of the therapeutic outcome and literature supports that the duration of post-traumatic amnesia can be useful in predicting the severity of the injury and the functional outcomes after injury [37,38] (Appendix 3D) [37].

Confirm the Glasgow coma scale (Appendix 3E) (39–42) or the Rancho Los Amigos scale (Appendix 3F) [43].

SUGGESTIONS FOR TAKING A CLIENT'S HISTORY

In the total sum phase, the clinician will conduct an in-depth interview. Generally, this will take at least 2 hours. It is through this process of history taking and assessment that the therapeutic relationship will be established (Figure 3.8).

When we commence taking a client history starting with early childhood memories, it is important to be discerning if there are gaps in memory recall as mentioned earlier. This could be a symptom of brain injury, but it can also be a symptom of childhood trauma, which will be important to understand. If there is a lack of childhood memory without a traumatic brain injury, this generally means there was some sort of high stress in the client's childhood environment or childhood trauma [36]. It is important to recognize this and gently probe to better understand.

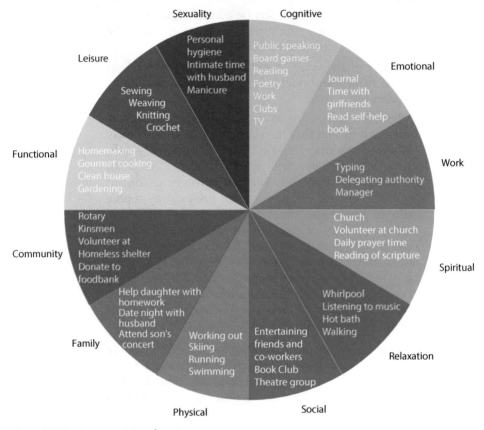

Figure 3.8 Total sum pre-injury function.

For example, if the brain-injured survivor has been sexually abused by the brother in the past, unbeknownst to the parents, and this brother is now placed in charge of the client for several hours a day post-injury, her behavior would change. If the pre-injury abuse is not revealed in the history-taking exercise, the symptoms exhibited while in the care of her brother could be misinterpreted as brain injury symptoms, resulting in the change of behavior. As a consequence, without this historical knowledge the clinical team may easily be misguided and thus redirect the therapeutic program in the wrong direction, possibly including an increase in unnecessary pharmacology intervention. This will also serve to break any trust or therapeutic bond if the client feels grossly misunderstood by the clinician.

When a history is taken, each of the questions asked leaves room for discussion, allowing the clinician to gather important insight and information. The clinician should expand the conversation by asking additional questions appropriately led by the segue availed from the answer to the first question. This will be additional information not found on the history-taking questionnaire (Appendix 3A).

This is therapeutic use of self. If you find that the client is not disclosing information, we will assume that a therapeutic bond has not been formed. This will result in insufficient information to commence a therapeutic program. It is important to conduct an ongoing therapeutic assessment of self (Appendices 3G and 3H).

It is a good sign if the client makes comments like, "I feel understood; no one has asked me any of this before."

BALANCED LIFESTYLE INVENTORY

The balanced lifestyle inventory (Appendix 3B) is a form that is filled out once the extensive history is taken. It provides the clinician as well as the client and family with a quick reference that is visual to the most blatant and obvious changes pre- and post-TBI in each area of the person's life.

At face value this may seem redundant in that the changes in the person's life will be obvious. However, at this stage the client and family have been traumatized by the injury and the fight for survival during the coma and ICU stage.

Patterns of minimizing or denying the aftermath of the TBI or rationalizing behavior may begin to set in; therefore, this form will provide a user-friendly summary to assist in providing realistic hope and insight.

The balanced lifestyle inventory will also start the color-coded process that will be carried out throughout the intervention.

CLINICIAN SELF-ASSESSMENT

It is important to take stock of our own comfort level as we embark on the lengthy recovery process with each client. At times our own biases, belief systems, confidence, and personal lives may impact our ability to be neutral and supportive.

These forms were created by the author for the purpose of accountability and quality control for use by clinicians. Each of us in the medical field has his or her own personal triggers and comfort levels. In conducting random file reviews for quality control in her company, the author found that each of her clinicians' levels of comfort and confidence was reflected in the quality of intake, as well as the quality of care for the client.

For instance, if a clinician is not comfortable discussing the client's finances, sexuality, emotional state, or relationships issues, a huge quantity of valuable information will be lost and the quality of clinical therapy will reflect this.

Another example would be if the clinician came from an alcoholic home and is now interviewing a client who has been an alcoholic: This may challenge the clinician's ability to be neutral or advocate for this client.

Periodic self-review is recommended. Appendices 3G and 3H are recommended to be placed on the front cover of the client's file for frequent reflection by the clinician.

SUMMARY

Chapter 3 is an important launching pad. The client is being transferred from hospital to home; the therapeutic relationship is ending with most of the hospital clinicians and has commenced with the community clinicians, and the family and client are beginning life as a "new normal." The process and importance of creating a thorough pre-injury profile has been laid out. The clinicians now have an understanding of life before the injury by using the history-taking template.

The inter-relationship of the community team members is being established at this stage. Timing is a critical issue in transferring the case from hospital to community and preparing for the community intervention. Excellent case management and communication will reduce timing lags, avoiding secondary losses for the client and family. The flow of information will allow each clinician to examine valuable information from every discipline's perspective.

The clinician's self-checklists are useful and effective to ensure that a therapeutic bond is established between the care provider and the client. These should be revisited throughout the therapeutic relationship.

The pre-injury profile will provide the clinicians with the necessary data needed to create a personal, meaningful, and therapeutic program using old information that is most familiar to the survivor. This old information will require less new learning, thus exacting more success and less frustration for the client.

The success in profiling the client's pre-injury life will directly impact the clinician's decisions as we move to Chapter 4 where "the loss" will show contrasts to life as the client knew it before the injury.

APPENDIX 3A: HISTORY-TAKING TEMPLATE

Please tell me a bit about yourself:

1. Where and when were you born?
2. How many siblings do you have?
3. What are their ages?
4. What are your brothers and sisters doing now?
    a. Where are they?
    b. Are they married?

c. Do they have children? If so, how many?

    d. What type of relationship do you have with your siblings?

    e. What was it like growing up in your family?

    f. Who were you closest to?

    g. What are the ages of your parents?

    h. What was their upbringing like?

    i. What was a typical week like in your house?

5. What type of work did your parents engage in throughout their careers? If this caused the family to move, where did you move to? How many times did you move? How did this impact you?

6. What did you enjoy doing during your younger years, as far as you can remember, from 1 to 6 years of age?

7. Socially: what types of things did you enjoy doing? Did you enjoy activities when you were alone or with others?

8. Do you have any memories of your early family life? What are they? (If there are issues, gently examine these further; this may reveal coping strategies adopted in early life.)

9. What types of memories do you have of your relationships with your brothers, sisters, and parents?

10. Was life at home happy? If there were conflicts, how were they resolved?

11. Did your family subcribe to a particular belief system?

From Grades 1 to 6

1. What was your favorite subject?

2. What was your least favorite subject?

3. What were the things that you enjoyed doing with your friends/siblings?

4. Were your parents working when you were in elementary school?

5. Was there any disruption within your home environment?

6. Did your parents use alcohol? If so, how often?

7. Did either of your parents have a problem with anger?

8. Were you able to communicate effectively with your parents?

9. What did you do after school with your friends?

10. What was your family's weekly routine?

11. Were there activities that your family routinely did together (i.e., church, prayer, golf, entertaining, swimming, etc.)?

From Grades 7 to 9

1. What did you do with your friends/family?
2. What did you do after school?
3. What did you do with your social time?
4. What was going on within the family environment during this time period?
5. When did you first become interested in sex?
6. When did you first become sexually active?
7. When, if at all, did you first begin using drugs and/or alcohol?
8. At what age did you become interested in dating?

From High School Grades

1. What did you do with your friends?
2. What did you do after school?
3. What career did you aspire to?
4. What did you do with your social time?
5. What was going on within the family environment during this time period?
6. How did you do in school? What were your marks? What were your least and most favorite subjects?
7. Did you have a significant relationship in high school or were you dating?

History of Work from First Part-Time Job to the Present Day

1. What was your first job?
2. How old were you when you secured your first job?
3. What hours and time of day did you work?
4. What were your responsibilities?
5. How long did you keep this job?
6. What was your reason for leaving?

History of Marriage Relationship

If the individual has been married more than once, include the history for each marriage.

1. Where did you meet your spouse?
2. What was your relationship like?
3. What did you enjoy doing together?

4. What did you enjoy doing at the beginning of the relationship?

5. What do you do with your spouse now?

6. What common values do you share?

7. How was your intimacy in the relationship?

8. How old were you both when you started a family?

9. What are the ages of your children?

10. What do you do with your children?

11. If the marriage or marriages ended, please describe the relationship at the beginning and at the end.

12. How did you cope during this difficult time?

13. What is the state of your finances?

Continue taking the history based on the theme of the individual's life socially, recreationally, emotionally, and cognitively—for example:

1. Have you taken medication for stress-related illnesses over any period of time?

2. Do you have any other medical problems?

3. Have you ever had any academic problems?

4. Have you ever had any altercations with the law?

5. Have you ever filed a claim at a Workers' Compensation Board?

6. Have you ever had any sports-related accidents?

7. What are your current goals?

8. What are your current complaints?

9. Have you ever had another car accident?

10. Have you ever had a previous brain injury or concussion?

11. Have you had previous surgeries if so what were they?

After the Accident

Please describe the changes that are most prevalent for you since the accident:

1. Have you had any difficulties with blurred vision?

2. Have you had any difficulties with double vision?

3. Have you had any difficulties with headaches? If so, how often?

4. Do you fatigue more easily?

5. Has your tolerance to alcohol decreased?

6. Do you have any ringing in your ears (tinnitus)?

7. Have you had any change in your sense of taste? (Be sure to ask about medications as they can also affect sense of taste.)

8. Have you had any change in your sense of smell?

9. Have you experienced decreased memory?

10. Have you experienced any changes in your concentration?

11. Have you experienced any changes in your attention span?

12. Have you experienced any changes in your ability to comprehend?

13. Have you experienced any changes in your personality?

14. Do you feel tearful more often than before?

15. Have you experienced any increase or decrease in your sexual desire? (Again, be sure to cross-reference with information regarding medications as some medications will also affect libido.)

16. Have you experienced any difficulty with balance?

17. Have you experienced dizziness?

18. Have you had any difficulties organizing tasks?

19. Have you had any difficulties sequencing tasks?

20. Have you had any difficulties following instructions?

21. Have you had any difficulties finding the appropriate word to use?

22. Do you ever feel overwhelmed?

23. Do you have difficulty following directions?

24. Have you ever had a seizure?

25. If so, how often?

26. Are you on medication for this?

27. Do you find that you often get agitated? If so, in what circumstance does this most frequently happen?

28. Do you ever feel confused or disoriented?

29. Do you get lost?

30. Do you have any difficulty finding the right words to use?

31. Are you having a hard time understanding what is being said or in expressing yourself?

32. Are you having any problems understanding written information or expressing yourself in written form?

33. Do you find that you are accident prone? Please give an example.

34. Are you hypersensitive to touch?
35. Do you have any problems sequencing tasks?
36. Do you have any changes in being able to mobilize?
37. Is it hard to initiate tasks?
38. Do you find that you ever perseverate when speaking?
39. Have you found yourself perseverating on a task?
40. Do you find yourself perseverating on a thought?
41. Is it hard to solve problems?
42. Do you have any problems swallowing?
43. Has anyone told you that your personality has changed?
44. Do you feel irritable or agitated?
45. Are you experiencing changes in your mood?
46. Do you have difficulty identifying objects and understanding what they are used for?
47. Is it hard to identify objects by touch?
48. Do you have any difficulty naming objects?
49. If you could change anything right now, what would it be?
50. Do you have difficulty understanding what someone is saying to you?
51. If I could help you with one thing, what would that be?
52. What are your top three priorities and how would you like to see me help you?
53. What are your concerns about the future? How would you like to approach these concerns?
54. How do you feel about being home? Is anything changing in the home environment or in your relationships?
55. What are the most important goals that you want to work on?

As you have gently uncovered the picture of the client's pre-injury life, you will have a sense of what is most critical in terms of rehabilitation goals; you will also know from the neuropsychological testing as corroborated by loved ones where the greatest challenges are. Begin to discuss with the client to assess insight.

It is important to work collaboratively with the brain-injured survivor; the initial goals set should be ones that challenge the parts of the brain that are functioning the best. Gently and creatively come up with examples of activities that you would recommend the client commence working on. It is through thoughtful and careful listening and internal problem solving that the initial goals will be broached with the client.

APPENDIX 3B: BALANCED LIFESTYLE SHEET

Physical		Family		Social interests		Sexuality		Cognitive intellectual		Emotional	
Before	After	Before	After	Before	After	Before	After	Before	After	Before	After

Leisure/recreational		Relaxation		Spiritual		Work		Community		Functional	
Before	After	Before	After	Before	After	Before	After	Before	After	Before	After

APPENDIX 3C: SEVERITY OF BRAIN INJURY STRATIFICATION

Mild	Moderate	Severe
Normal structural imaging	Normal or abnormal structural imaging	Normal or abnormal structural imaging
LOC = 0–30 minutes	LOC = >30 minutes and <24 hours	LOC = >24 hours
AOC = a moment up to 24 hours	AOC = >24 hours; severity based on other criteria	
PTA = 0–1 day	PTA = >1 and <7 days	PTA = >7 days
GCS = 13–15	GCS = 9–12	GCS = 3–8

Source: Dennis, K. C. 2009. *ASHA Access Audiology* 8 (4).

Notes: LOC = loss of consciousness; AOC = alteration of consciousness/mental state; PTA = post-traumatic amnesia; GCS = Glasgow coma scale.

APPENDIX 3D: POST-TRAUMATIC AMNESIA

Post-traumatic amnesia (PTA) has been well discussed in the literature and is described as the severity in disturbance of consciousness following a traumatic brain injury (TBI) [38,45]. In some instances the individual may experience a loss of consciousness, resulting in loss of orientation to time, place, or person. Durations of this amnesia have been shown to be an accurate indicator of severity of injury and can also be predictive of functional outcomes for the individual (Appendix 3C).

There are two types of amnesia: **retrograde amnesia** (loss of memories that were formed shortly before the injury) and **anterograde amnesia** (problems with creating new memories after the injury has taken place). Both retrograde and anterograde forms may be referred to as PTA or the term may be used to refer only to anterograde amnesia.

The duration of PTA is sometimes used, on its own or in conjunction with the Glasgow coma scale and other methods, to measure the severity of traumatic brain injury [37, p. 2].

- ◆ PTA = less than 5 minutes: **very mild**
- ◆ 5 to 60 minutes: **mild**
- ◆ 1 to 24 hours: **moderate**
- ◆ 1 to 7 days: **severe**
- ◆ 1 to 4 weeks: **very severe**
- ◆ More than 4 weeks: **extremely severe**

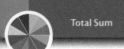

APPENDIX 3E: GLASGOW COMA SCALE

Activity	Score
Eye opening	
None	1 = Even to supra-orbital pressure
To pain	2 = Pain from sternum/limb/supra-orbital pressure
To speech	3 = Non-specific response, not necessarily to command
Spontaneous	4 = Eyes open, not necessarily aware
Motor response	
None	1 = To any pain, limbs remain flaccid
Extension	2 = Shoulder adducted and shoulder and forearm internally rotated
Flexor response	3 = Withdrawal response or assumption of hemiplegic posture
Withdrawal	4 = Arm withdraws to pain; shoulder abducts
Localized pain	5 = Arm attempts to remove supra-orbital/chest pressure
Obeys commands	6 = Follows simple commands
Verbal response	
None	1 = No verbalization of any type
Incomprehensible	2 = Moans/groans; no speech
Inappropriate	3 = Intelligible; no sustained sentences
Confused	4 = Converses but confused, disoriented
Oriented	5 = Converses and oriented
Total (3–15): _____	

Source: Jennett, B., and Bond, M. 1975. *Lancet* 1 (7905): 1.

GLASGOW COMA SCALE

The Glasgow coma scale (GCS) is an assessment used to determine severity of coma through various responses to stimuli including eye opening, motor response, and verbal response. The patient is rated on a scale with a minimum possible score of 3, indicating least responsive, and a maximum score of 15, indicating most responsive [39–41]. Severity of damage according to the Glasgow coma scale is scored as follows [42]:

- ◆ Severe brain injury (3–8 points)
- ◆ Moderate brain injury (9–12 points)
- ◆ Mild brain injury (13–15 points)

The GCS is a measure to determine severity of coma and is a predictor of mortality and morbidity in the acute phase of traumatic brain injury [42]. It is commonly used to guide decision making in emergency triage. A second assessment, the Rancho Los Amigos scale (RLA), is used to measure cognitive functioning in relation to level of awareness, environmental interactions, cognition, and behavior. This scale is used to determine different levels of recovery in the patient and can be used to guide treatment planning [46].

APPENDIX 3F: RANCHO LOS AMIGOS SCALE: LEVELS OF COGNITIVE FUNCTIONING [43]

Cognitive level I: no response. Person will be unresponsive to environmental stimuli.

Cognitive level II: generalized response. Person will demonstrate some response to environmental stimuli and may respond inconsistently to the stimuli or show a delay in reaction. Individuals generally respond in the same way to stimuli and may include chewing, sweating, faster breathing, moaning, moving, and increased blood pressure.

Cognitive level III: localized response. Level of alertness may vary throughout the day, drifting in and out of wakefulness. The person may begin to make more movements in response to stimuli but reaction will still be slow and inconsistent. Individual may begin to recognize family and friends and can begin to follow simple directions and respond to simple questions with head nods.

Cognitive level IV: confused, agitated. Individuals will appear confused and frightened, and may not understand what is happening around them. They may lash out in response to stimuli, including hitting, screaming, or using abusive language. They will be highly focused on their basic needs but may not understand that people around them are trying to help them. They may demonstrate difficulty with concentration and may demonstrate difficulty following directions. They will recognize family and friends some of the time. They can begin to do self-care tasks with some assistance.

Cognitive level V: confused, inappropriate, non-agitated. Individuals will have difficulty making sense of what is happening around them and may not be oriented to the date, their location, or why they are in the hospital.

The person will be able to pay attention for a few minutes and may begin to do more self-care tasks with step-by-step instructions. The person becomes overwhelmed and restless when fatigued or when there are many people around. He or she will have poor memory and may attempt to fill gaps in memory through confabulation. The individual may demonstrate perseveration with tasks or ideas.

Cognitive level VI: confused, appropriate. Individuals will still demonstrate confusion due to memory and problems with thinking. They can remember main points from a conversation but may forget or confuse the details. They can follow a schedule but will become confused by changes in routine. They are oriented to the date and year and begin to demonstrate longer spans of attention, but they can become distracted with noises or complex activities. Individuals complete self-care activities with assistance and may demonstrate more awareness of physical problems rather than thinking problems.

Cognitive level VII: automatic, appropriate. Individuals can follow a set schedule and can complete self-care tasks independently. They demonstrate problems with planning, starting, and following through with activities. As well, they may have problems in new situations and become frustrated as a result. Stressful or distracting situations can result in difficulty paying attention. They may not demonstrate awareness into how their thinking and memory problems will impact future plans and goals. Supervision may be beneficial since individuals may demonstrate lack of safety awareness and judgment. They think more slowly in stressful situations and may be rigid or stubborn. They may overestimate their own abilities to complete a task.

Cognitive level VIII: purposeful, appropriate. The person has insight into problems with thinking and memory skills and will demonstrate compensation techniques for these problems by being more flexible in his or her thinking. The person is able to learn new things at a slower rate and may be ready for driving or job training evaluation. He or she is still overwhelmed in difficult, stressful, and rapidly changing situations and is likely to have poor judgment in these new situations and may require some guidance for decision making. The person may still experience thinking problems that may not be noticeable to others who did not know the person prior to the injury.

APPENDIX 3G: FORM 1: CLINICIAN SELF-CHECKLIST FOR ESTABLISHING THERAPEUTIC RAPPORT

Have I understood the unique characteristics of the client?

Rate the following on a scale of 1–10:

1	2	3	4	5	6	7	8	9	10

If, from my perspective:

1. I feel that I have been able to preserve the dignity of the client by understanding the pre-injury lifestyle. ☐
2. I feel that I can advocate for the client. ☐
3. I feel that I can be objective about the client. ☐
4. I have information in each piece of the pie. ☐

_____/40

If, from the perspective of the client/family:

1. The client is disclosing to me. ☐
2. The client is responding to me with openness of speech and warmth. ☐
3. The client respects and understands my feedback. ☐
4. The family members have opened up to me. ☐
5. The client is willing to cooperate with the assessment process. ☐

_____/50

If, from the perspective of team members:

1. Other team members respond to the request for team meetings and return my telephone calls. ☐
2. Respectful, prompt, and informative communication is engaged in. ☐
3. Co-operative planning takes place in the establishment of the therapeutic goals. ☐

_____/30

If, from the perspective of the referral sources:

1. The referral source understands the need for therapy and values it as well. ☐
2. The referral source approves funding for the teams proposed therapeutic regime. ☐

3. The referral source is giving positive feedback. ☐
4. The referral source is sending new referrals. ☐

____/40

Total   ____/160

APPENDIX 3H: FORM 2: CLINICIAN SELF-CHECKLIST FOR DETERMINING THE TOTAL SUM

Questions to ask yourself to measure if you have understood the "total sum" and have established rapport.

Rate yourself from 1 to 10, where 1 is the lowest and 10 the highest.

1. As the clinician, it is my responsibility to understand that clients who are in difficulty may be difficult. Did I develop rapport in spite of this?

1	2	3	4	5	6	7	8	9	10

2. Do I have a genuine positive attitude toward the client?

1	2	3	4	5	6	7	8	9	10

3. At the end of the client assessment, do I have a clear picture of the client's pre-injury profile?

1	2	3	4	5	6	7	8	9	10

4. Do I understand the needs of the family? Have they opened up to me?

1	2	3	4	5	6	7	8	9	10

In order to build therapeutic rapport,

    5. Did I make the client feel comfortable?

1	2	3	4	5	6	7	8	9	10

    6. Did I build trust with the client?

1	2	3	4	5	6	7	8	9	10

    7. Was I able to get enough information to advocate for the client?

1	2	3	4	5	6	7	8	9	10

    8. Was I able to inspire and motivate the client to proceed with therapy?

1	2	3	4	5	6	7	8	9	10

    9. Do I clearly understand the client's goals and priorities?

1	2	3	4	5	6	7	8	9	10

    10. Do I clearly understand the family's goals and priorities?

1	2	3	4	5	6	7	8	9	10

        Total   ____/100

CHAPTER 4

The Loss

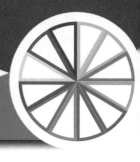

TOTAL SUM   –   DIAGNOSIS (LOSS)   +   INTERVENTION   =   RESIDUAL LOSS

 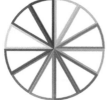

THE LOSS

The *loss* or the *change* is the second stage of the *rainbow effect* formula. The loss will define the primary and secondary changes resulting from the TBI. The organic or primary loss will be determined by radiological tests such as MRI, PET, SPECT, and CAT scans topographical brain mapping and evoked potentials as well as standardized and nonstandardized assessments administered by the hospital and community clinicians. The secondary psychological losses will be determined by the history taking and functional information gleaned from loved ones as well as the clients themselves.

As mentioned in Chapter 3 there is continuum of care that has overlapping portions during the *total sum* and *loss* stages.

THE PROCESS OF TRANSFERRING THE CLIENT FROM HOSPITAL TO HOME AND COMMUNITY

By now the client is in the process of being discharged from hospital. The **hospital** clinicians are, from their own disciplines' perspectives, preparing discharge summary reports. These reports will be kept as a permanent record at the hospital and will also be requested by whoever will be funding the community-based portion of the clients care as well as potentially subpoenaed by the litigators.

Some hospital clinicians, such as the physical therapist, social worker, or the neuropsychologist, may continue to see the client on an outpatient or private basis; however, the client is typically discharged to a new team of professionals that are community based with the family doctor providing the continuity (see Table 2.2 in Chapter 2).

A great deal of organization is required as the client goes home and the team responsibilities are transferred from the **hospital** to the **community clinical team.** The goal is to provide continuity from the **hospital** to the **community** and client's home.

The funding source for the community care should be established prior to the client's discharge from the hospital (see Figures 4.1 and 4.2).

The first order of business is safety. Any home renovations— such as making the home and vehicle wheelchair accessible,

> ◆ Motor vehicle insurance
> ◆ Tort claims
> ◆ Insurance settlement
> ◆ Government including
>> ◆ Long-term care
>> ◆ Community care
> ◆ Labor unions
> ◆ Veterans affairs
> ◆ Victims assistance
> ◆ Aboriginal affairs
> ◆ Private disability insurance
> ◆ Workers' compensation
> ◆ Homeowner insurance
> ◆ Private funding
> ◆ Nonprofit organizations

Figure 4.1 Third-party funders.

> ◆ University students/independent study
> ◆ College students/independent study
> ◆ Service groups
>> ◆ Rotary
>> ◆ Kinsmen
>> ◆ Lions
>> ◆ Gyro
> ◆ Cultural societies
> ◆ Church groups
> ◆ Nonprofit organizations

Figure 4.2 Sources of volunteer support.

installing grab bars in the bathroom, etc.—should be completed before the client is discharged from hospital.

The hospital occupational therapist (OT) will have assessed the client in a simulated environment in hospital or, in some cases, in the client's actual home environment. Ideally, while still residing in hospital, the client will have returned home for an outpatient visit to reveal any safety or accessibility concerns; the hospital occupational therapist may have been present, determining and anticipating any safety issues that might arise when the client ultimately returns home.

It is common practice for the **hospital** occupational therapist to forward on findings to the **community** occupational therapist, who will generally be the person to ensure that the home renovations are completed. Because of this, it is common practice for the community occupational therapist to be invited to the hospital discharge meeting, to ensure that the hospital team's safety concerns in relation to the client's return home can be addressed before the client is discharged from hospital. It is also common, because of the early involvement, for the occupational therapist to become the community team case manager.

All members of the hospital team, the funder, client, and family as well as the community OT, will be in attendance at the hospital discharge meeting.

As the hospital program is transferred from acute care to community care, it will be agreed that requisitions for service will begin to be sent out to a variety of community clinicians as recommended by the hospital discharge team.

In most cases a neuropsychologist is a very important clinician at this stage. The neuropsychology assessments are lengthy and take time to be administered and interpreted; therefore, the request should be made as soon as the client is able to tolerate this lengthy assessment. This assessment may be done in hospital or by a community neuropsychologist depending on the client's readiness and tolerance.

The neuropsychological assessment (Figure 4.3), for example, is of the utmost importance. This detailed and technical report, when translated into function, can serve as an invaluable launching pad for the entire team. The author has found that the most helpful neuropsychological reports were ones where the complicated technical information was synthesized into a useable practical guide for the rest of the team—if the psychometrics showed evidence of deficit in, for instance:

◆ Auditory comprehension
◆ Sequencing
◆ Impulse control

This function would then be graded on a sliding scale.

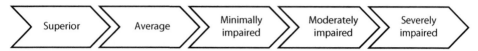

Figure 4.3 Neuropsychological sliding scale.

This document provides the other team members with invaluable information. Armed with this knowledge, the severely impaired components could be avoided or gingerly approached therapeutically. In addition, those areas of function that were categorized in the superior range could take on a greater responsibility of relearning.

The community rehabilitation program should not commence intervention until this assessment is completed and the report has been dispersed to the entire community team, as it sets the baseline in terms of the client's brain function and areas of deficits. The team is fortunate, indeed, if the neuropsychologist goes one step further and also sees the client in the home environment, corroborating test findings with real life.

This information is knowledge that will allow the growing community team to avoid therapeutic regimes, which will sensory overload the client and avoid unnecessary costs for the funder and setbacks for the client.

The family will most likely be exhibiting symptoms of stress, so counseling support provided by a clinical psychologist or social worker may be warranted to execute the transition home successfully. This is generally organized by the hospital social worker and funded by third parties or government.

The hospital physical therapist may recommend a home program to be followed up on an outpatient basis or as overseen by the rehabilitation worker or kinesiologist.

CASE MANAGER

The case manager will function from his or her own discipline's perspective as well as assume the role of case manager. The role of the case manager is to ensure continuity of care and advocate for the client, as well as to act as an organizer for the complicated community team. This person will ensure that time lines are met, and will co-ordinate the clinical team's completion of assessments, and ensure that the reports are dispersed to all community clinicians, as well as facilitate communication through well organized team meetings.

The greatest challenge for the new team is one of communication. Unlike the hospital, each of the community clinicians is operating out of a different work site, disallowing for convenient exchange of information. Each community clinician will conduct his or her own battery of tests and assessments, revealing information pertaining to function and deficits in each area of the client's life as it relates to his or her own area of expertise and as reflected in the color-coded pie.

The community rehabilitation program does not start immediately.

The community team is actively engaging in setting up appointments to conduct their own assessments from a community reintegration perspective.

The initial community team is now established, generally including a neuropsychologist, occupational therapist, social worker or clinical psychologist, physiatrist, speech pathologist (if appropriate), and general practitioner. They will each solicit and review the hospital medical records and consultation reports.

The tapestry of the client's losses and the etiology of the traumatic brain injury symptoms will begin to become clear as the hospital reports are reviewed and augmented by new information revealed by the community team's tests and assessments.

There are a myriad of diagnostic assessments that will provide each community clinician with relevant data about how the client's brain is functioning. The point is not which assessments to use, but rather to ensure that information is gathered from each part of the person's life from each discipline's perspective, as presented in the color-coded life pie. The only criterion is that the assessments used by each discipline are current and credible, pursuant to common industry standards. Just as the color in the *total sum* represented pre-injury life, the absence of color represents *the loss,* or the changes resulting from the traumatic brain injury.

Regarding the *Lefaivre Rainbow Effect,* the loss of color in each piece of the pie in Figure 4.4 indicates the change from the pre-injury status to post-injury status without therapeutic intervention.

Perhaps the most difficult part of understanding the client through assessment is in the interpretation of the results. If the clinician only takes the test score but neglects to see the inter-relationship to other tests conducted, the review of the medical reports, and information gained from the other team members and client history, then the picture is lost. It is in synthesizing all of the formal and informal tests, radiological findings, and assessments as well as the history that a template for the therapeutic regime can be determined.

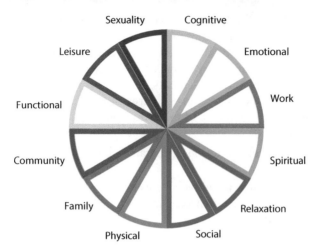

Figure 4.4 Pie segment (loss).

For instance, if a manual dexterity assessment is conducted and the findings reveal that the client is having bilateral coordination problems (more significantly, when using his right-dominant hand), this will be noted in the report—most likely including a standard deviation score in comparison to the norm. If, however, this text score is not cross-referenced with the client's real job description, leisure interests, and aptitude tests as well as the functional home assessment, then it is simply a score withholding functional implications for the client.

The very word "clinical" would indicate that we, the clinicians, will make a clinical profile based on numbers, measurements, and test scores. However, this alone does not suffice in imparting knowledge that will build a cognitive remediation program that will be practical and effective. It is in weaving the outcomes of the formal assessments with the in-depth pre-injury history that a true reflection of the client's situation will emerge.

The accrued information is only useful therapeutically when it is woven together as a tapestry through interpretation of the results and then corroborated with observation and practical application in real-life situations in the client's home.

If we take the previously mentioned example of the dexterity test score, a more realistic interpretation would be the following example:

> This 28-year-old chef is experiencing reduced dexterity in both of his upper extremities, more notably in his right-dominant arm and hand. In comparison to the norm, his right-dominant hand demonstrates a unilateral dexterity score that places him in the 26th percentile while his bilateral dexterity score places him in the 46th percentile.

This reduced ability to coordinate fine motor tasks indicates that if this young gentleman were to return to his work as a chef at this point, his performance would surely not be met with a positive outcome in terms of his performance as well as the safety risk of using sharp knives and working with hot elements and heavy pots.

Further complicating the functional impact of the client's reduction in dexterity is the fact that when cross-referencing these findings with the results from the leisure activity survey, the interest profile, and the functional home assessment, it is found that the client requires the use of fine and gross motor movement in virtually all of his recreational and home activities.

It is recommended that the client not return to work at this time and commences a rehabilitation regime involving the use of a one-to-one rehabilitation worker. The program will involve repetitious use of both his right and left arms and hands through meaningful activity as revealed in his pre-injury history, until such a time as the client's dexterity improves to a 75% ratio bilaterally.

In the meantime to avoid failure and accidents and to capitalize on his motivation, it is further recommended that services be put in place for meal preparation at home as well as handyman services for the functional chores that the client would normally be required to complete. A remediated leisure program will also be introduced.

This case indicates a more functional approach to synthesizing the findings of a variety of test scores into function rather than simply reporting the standardized deficit of the dexterity problem.

When the other team members read this report, the dexterity deficit takes on a greater meaning as it applies to real-life function.

INITIAL CLINICAL REPORTS PRODUCED BY COMMUNITY CLINICIANS

The initial reports provided by each respective clinician should be clear, documenting all results from standardized and non-standardized tests and assessments.

For those practitioners conducting assessments within the home, these findings will be incorporated as well. Unlike brief hospital reports, community-based clinicians will write sometimes lengthy reports to profile their findings.

When a specific test result is summarized, it should be integrated into a meaningful conclusion as it relates to the interrelationship of each segment of the life pie. The goal for each clinician is to better understand the etiology of the brain injury and the functional outcome for the client pursuant to his/her area of expertise.

For this protocol to work, clinicians will conduct their assessments and then integrate their results so that the information can ultimately be broken down into sections of the rainbow pie as it relates to real-life function, including the anticipated challenges for the brain-injured client. Then each clinician will write a report that will be circulated to all team members and reviewed in a team meeting. The information will be assimilated as the team moves toward implementing the therapeutic intervention.

It is through the expertise of the team that we will collectively understand how the organic brain damage is translating into function and everyday life for the client. We will then be able collectively to design a therapeutic regime targeting each area of the client's life for full therapeutic impact. Each professional will have therapeutic strategies that will be integrated into the program to be carried out by a one-to-one rehabilitation worker. These suggestions will be amalgamated and discussed during the first team meeting as the initial community goals are established for the client's return home.

Once the multidisciplinary assessments have been completed and the findings dispersed to the entire team, the case manager should advocate for authorization to conduct a team meeting. It is during the team meeting that the team will problem solve and develop a strategy of setting goals aimed at community reintegration, starting with those that will reap the highest level of reward and safety for the client.

PREPARING FOR THE TEAM MEETING

This is a time of settling in for the client and family: They are back home, busy with the testing appointments and forging new relationships with the community medical team. The occupational therapist or case manager should at the same interval be conducting an education session for the family, significant loved ones, and client as reviewed in Chapter 5.

Meanwhile, the community team is preparing to share its findings at the first team meeting after discharge.

The case manager will prepare the client and family; they will be informed of who will be at the meeting and what the roles are. They will be educated on the purpose of the meeting. The case manager will assist the client and family to prepare their own list of questions that will be sent out in advance to the team so that they can be prepared to address the client's and family's concerns.

It is important that each clinician be prepared for the team meeting; these meetings are costly. In preparing for the initial team meeting, the case manager should ensure that all clinicians working on the case have completed their assessments and that the reports have been distributed to each team member in advance.

An agenda should be sent out in advance with relevant questions from all team members. This enables thoughtful discussion and will produce cost-effective decisions.

SUMMARY OF HOW THE CASE MANAGER WILL RUN A TEAM MEETING

- Ensure that funding has been approved for each community clinician.
- Ensure that referrals have been made by the funder to each required clinician from various disciplines.
- Ensure that each discipline can conduct its assessment in a timely fashion.
- Set a date for a team meeting in a convenient location.
- Ensure that each team member has completed his or her assessment and written his or her report.
- Ensure that all reports have been circulated to the team members in advance of the meeting.
- Ensure that the family's and client's questions have also been circulated to the team in advance of the meeting.
- Confirm each team member's ability to attend several days in advance of the meeting.
- Prepare an agenda and send out at least one week in advance.
- Ask each clinician to give a brief review of his or her findings at the team meeting.
- Establish therapeutic goals with potential barriers being addressed from each discipline's perspective.
- Establish whether a one-to-one rehabilitation worker will be used to carry out the program with the client.
- If so, confirm the required number of hours per week for the worker and ensure that the client and family are in agreement to having a worker.
- Solicit funding for the one-to-one worker. (Ideally, the funder is present at the meeting.)

- The case manager will co-ordinate the team to set the therapeutic goals that the worker will carry out initially.

- The case manager will agree to meet with the one-to-one worker each week to review the goals, observations, and weekly schedule.

- Each discipline will introduce components from its area of expertise to the therapeutic plan and advise the worker on what to observe regarding the client's ability to integrate cognitive stimuli while attempting to accomplish each goal.

- A system of communication and a schedule of future meetings will be established.

- Each clinician will continue to see the client in private appointments to follow up with issues pertaining to his or her expertise.

It is interesting at the team meeting to observe how each clinician extrapolates meaning from a brain injury symptom from his or her own discipline's perspective. The findings of each different discipline will overlap but may be interpreted differently. For instance, the neuropsychologist may identify agitation as an issue for the client; this may be interpreted as a result of damage to the frontal lobe. For the occupational therapist, agitation will be credited to the frontal lobe damage as well, but may be observed at home with more intensity when coupled with a great deal of auditory stimuli such as listening to the television or having verbal discussions at the dinner table. Therefore, the combination of the frontal lobe damage and receptive language produces an unanticipated functional and emotional result.

This additional functional information is useful to the neuropsychologist as it corroborates the diagnostic findings, but also lends functional credibility as the client's damaged brain is attempting to assimilate multiple stimuli in a real-life situation rather than in a quiet testing environment.

The team will then report this finding to the speech and language pathologist for suggested intervention strategies related to receptive language. It is important that this information be shared among all members of the team and that intervention strategies be established that will be practiced by all team members, including the family.

As mentioned, this information is only useful therapeutically when it is woven together as a tapestry through interpretation of the results and then corroborated with observation and practical application in real-life situations.

SUMMARY

The *loss* is the second stage in the *rainbow effect* formula. The multidisciplinary team will administer assessments both standardized and non-standardized to establish a clear reflection of the diagnostic losses and the functional implications for the client.

The organic (primary losses) and any emerging secondary psychosocial implications will be identified. The process at this stage is one of transition moving the client from hospital care to the home and community, relearning life as it used to be. The flow of medical information travels with the client from the hospital team to the new community clinicians.

The priority now shifts from acute care to one of integration back to the home, family, and community—it is a stage of transitions. The flow of medical information is disseminated to the new community team. The reality is that timing can be an issue, so heightened communication between the family, client, funder/volunteers, and clinical/hospital team is necessary to ensure the transference of information. To this end a case manager will be determined.

The case manager will ensure the seamless flow of information as well as co-ordinate the growing team of community care providers.

The decision to hire a suitable one-to-one rehabilitation worker will be determined at this stage. From his or her own discipline's perspective, each clinician will be establishing baseline knowledge of the client's sequelae to the traumatic brain injury. Therapeutic relationships are forged to build trust and gain information for each area of the client's life as reflected in the life pie.

An effort is made to educate the community clinical team in the complicated task of assimilating test scores and transcribing the statistical data into a report that reveals the functional day-to-day implications of the findings for the client. The chart in (Appendix 4A) has been used in practice by clinicians to ensure that the report is not only clinically oriented but practical as well. This example is for use by occupational therapists but the template can be modified for each service provider (see Table 2.2 in Chapter 2).

The clinical findings of the team at this stage are organized to create a therapeutic regime suited to the client's home and community reintegration plan.

The cooperation of the family and client is integral to achieving clinical success. As we move to Chapter 5 we will explore the importance of educating the family and significant others.

APPENDIX 4A: CROSS-REFERENCE OF ASSESSMENT TOOLS AND SECTORS OF BALANCED LIFESTYLE EXAMPLE FOR AN OCCUPATIONAL THERAPIST

Assessment	Functional	Leisure	Sexuality	Cognitive	Emotional	Work	Spiritual	Relaxation	Social	Physical	Family	Community
Constructive leisure activity		×		×	×	×	×	×	×	×	×	×
Lifestyle inventory	×	×	×	×	×	×	×	×	×	×	×	×
Personal assessment			×	×	×	×	×	×	×		×	
Assertiveness inventory			×	×	×	×			×		×	×
Activities of daily living	×	×	×	×	×	×	×	×	×	×	×	×
Interest inventory		×		×		×						×
Career assessment		×		×		×						
Physical capability inventory	×	×	×			×				×		
Occupational career profile				×	×	×			×			
Gross dexterity assessment	×	×		×		×				×		
Fine motor dexterity test	×	×		×		×				×		
Perceptual and sensory	×	×	×	×	×	×	×	×	×	×	×	×
Leisure lifestyle		×			×			×	×	×	×	×
Bilateral coordination	×	×		×		×				×		
History	×	×	×	×	×	×	×	×	×	×	×	×
Balanced lifestyle inventory	×	×	×	×	×	×	×	×	×	×	×	×

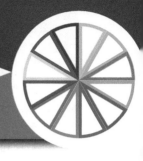

CHAPTER 5

Educating the Family

TOTAL SUM	−	DIAGNOSIS (LOSS)	+	INTERVENTION	=	RESIDUAL LOSS

 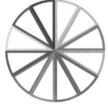

INTRODUCTION

The families at this stage have maneuvered themselves through uncharted waters in hospital and are ready for a semblance of order. The client's return home is a milestone for all who have been impacted by the client's traumatic brain injury. Prior to commencing the community rehabilitation program, it is helpful to have a family meeting. This is an excellent time to educate the family and client, listen to their concerns about the return home process, and inform them of the team's proposed plan.

It is important to respect the fact that the family has been sitting bedside through the trauma in emergency and there has been a stressful vigil in the intensive care unit with the client in a coma. Hopefully, the client has spent time in the rehabilitation unit at the hospital or in a specialized neurorehabilitation facility but this is not always the case. The family will be exhausted and traumatized. They are thrilled that their loved one is alive but at the same time very concerned about the future for their loved one and also concerned about how this will impact their lives in the future. We must be mindful that clients from rural areas have most likely been treated away from home in a major center. Therefore, the family has the extra stress and financial burden of being away from home.

When sitting bedside, the prayer is for survival; this is now real life. The injured person is ready to come home. The person may well be someone the family does not recognize in terms of behavior or cognition—particularly if there is frontal lobe or limbic system involvement. The physical changes are easy to identify because they can be visually seen. However the finer neurological symptoms will be a mystery to the family. The physical changes may require home renovations if the motor center in the brain or spinal cord has been affected. The family may notice personality changes, inappropriate sexual advances, outbursts, or difficulty with impulse control. In this case this will exact a response from the family, possibly embarrassment, rejection, hurt, or anger. There may be problems with sequencing tasks, memory, amnesia, executive function, seizure activity, poor initiation, poor judgment, impaired impulse control, difficulty with organization, language problems, and the list goes on. All in all, the return home can be exciting and filled with joy while coupled with fear and apprehension.

In the case of mild to moderate brain injury the stay in hospital may be brief or, perhaps, the client has not been admitted at all. It is not uncommon that a traumatic brain injury is not identified in the initial hospital visit. This appears to be more common in mild TBI cases or when other injuries such as orthopedic injuries occur as well. These physical issues may override the subtle TBI symptoms, which frequently go unattended.

In this case, when the client returns home without a diagnosis of traumatic brain injury, the family becomes confused and less understanding of the cognitive and behavioral changes, placing them at greater risk for family breakdown.

The brain injury survivor can easily become frustrated and understands that something needs to shift to avoid the conflict. Masking of symptoms and the emergence of maladaptive coping mechanisms can commonly occur in this scenario.

The health care team must have a thorough working knowledge of family systems to be able to identify the risk factors.

The community team needs to understand the dynamics of the family members prior to the client's TBI. Typically, when a youth has been in a coma for any length of time, the focus is shifted to the injured child and attention is not equally demonstrated to the other children in the family.

This may result in changes in feelings and behavior of the other siblings; feelings of resentment, anger, and bitterness possibly start to flavor the family interactions.

These role changes are discussed at length in Chapter 6 but are noted here as well. The care provider must be keenly in tune with the family's reaction to the effect that the TBI has had on family relations. Each family member will adjust in his or her own unique way:

◆ "Parents and partners of patients experience other difficulties. A TBI has a greater impact on partners than on parents. The relationship becomes less stable and the stress experienced is greater.

- Partners voice more health and psychological complaints, score higher on depression scales and face crisis situations more often than parents.
- Siblings have lower self concept, behavior problems, symptoms of depression and their relationship with the child with TBI becomes more negative than before the injury.
- Young families with several young children are the most vulnerable. If, in addition there are financial problems and there is little social support, the stress is so great that it becomes impossible to function normally." [21, pp. 1006–1007]

Adopting the hypothesis that the brain relearns old, familiar information more easily, then changes in family interactions will prove foreign and confusing to the TBI survivor.

As the symptoms of change arise the clinicians will need to introduce education—first to build trust and diminish family anxiety and then to introduce the therapeutic intervention.

Once the client is discharged to the community team we need to diffuse any anxiety, providing the family with education—preferably in the format of a family meeting where questions and concerns can be discussed. The meeting should be run by the case manager. The less mystery and surprise the family encounters, the better the outcome will be.

The first family meeting to plan for the introduction of the brain-injured loved one back home will most likely be energy charged. There will be immense relief that the client has indeed survived the TBI and is coming home. There may be an indication of denial that, once the loved one is home, all will be right with the world and life will resume as it was before the injury. There will likely be fear as the family is unsure of what to expect.

There is a great deal of change happening at this stage. The client is transitioning from the hospital back home. In many instances the safety of the hospital and the familiarity of the hospital staff have brought comfort to the family. Saying goodbye to care providers in the hospital can be difficult for the client and family.

The new community team members may seem casual in comparison as the sterility of the hospital environment has been traded for more casual home and office visits. Gone are the white lab coats. The practical goals of the community team are much different from the life-saving measures the family experienced in the hospital. At initial glance it is not uncommon for the family and client to question the wisdom and sophistication of the community team. It may also appear that the client is more at risk in the uncontrolled home environment—particularly if the client exhibits orientation and memory problems.

In light of the fact that a preponderance of survivors are young males, in the first team meeting the client will frequently express a desire to return to driving, sporting activity, and independence. This often exacts a price of panic on behalf of significant others.

The case manager does not have a long relationship history with the client and family at this point. The initial family meeting forges into this important arena.

At this juncture there is a risk of the client being identified by the family and himself or herself as "brain injured," which is quite different from being the loved one he or she was before. At this point any evident fear on the part of the family members may translate into overprotection and co-dependency; this can be a delicate situation for the case manager to maneuver through.

FAMILY MEETING

How to Prepare for the Family Meeting

1. At this point the extensive history has been conducted; therefore, "hot spots" in family relationships and pre-existing historical trauma have been identified. There could be evidence of overprotection on the part of a family member. There could also be the emergence of anger and resentment. This is often seen when a child or adolescent is injured and other children in the family have felt neglected because the focus for months has been on the injured sibling.

2. Be cognizant of the fact that if there were family members in the vehicle at the time of the accident there may be survivor's guilt—particularly if there has been a death as a result of the accident. Be aware of ongoing tort claims—particularly if they involve a family member's insurance policy.

3. During the long convalescence in hospital some family members may be taking the brunt of the family's stress by way of becoming the "scapegoat" and, yet, another family member may emerge as the "hero."

4. We, the community health care team, will want to set the family up for success. It is important to be prepared to explain the proposed rehabilitation plan, which is based on the hospital and community teams' assessments and how this might translate into concerns for the family and client.

5. The education process begins by having all significant loved ones present (the client may also choose to have employers and friends present). This is a time to answer their many questions. Typically, the initial concerns will be voiced by asking, "When will he be back to normal?" "How long will the rehabilitation take?"

6. It is important that the client not be addressed as a third party during the meeting. When this happens, they can feel like their life is not their own—like they have ceased to exist. They can become anxious and confused about what will happen in the future. It can impinge on their ability to be able to trust.

7. It is important that only one person speaks at any given time and is cognizant that these are early days for the client; speaking slowly and avoiding extraneous noise will help.

8. Members in attendance should avoid finger or pencil tapping, keeping movements to a minimum. Ensure that the environment where the education meeting is occurring is quiet with little if any moving visual stimulation (e.g., kids playing in a swimming pool outside the window).

9. Conducting a general discussion in a comfortable home or office setting encouraging questions and interaction is helpful. It is important that the element of shame be averted through open and honest sharing of information. Hope will emerge as the central aspect to move forward to the next step.

10. Oftentimes the fear, frustration, and anxiety need to be diffused by open discussion. A brief and basic description of the TBI should be reviewed. Handouts should be available to family members, describing in layman's terms how the brain functions (Chapter 8). (See additional resource material, Family Handout the Brain A Brief Overview at http://www.crcpress.com/product/isbn/9781482228243.)

11. Practical concerns, such as safety and financing of the rehabilitation, should be addressed early in the meeting.

12. Once the emotional concerns have been put in abeyance, the real understanding can commence.

13. The use of static flip charts (which adhere to any wall or window) is effective in providing visual education in any environment.

14. The analogy of presenting the recovery of a physical problem such as a burn helps the family put the recovery process into perspective. This is because a burn can be seen.

15. The proposed plan should be introduced to the family and client to ensure their cooperation.

16. An emphasis is placed on the family returning to pre-injury roles as much as possible.

17. Supports such as family counseling and homemakers will be put in place.

18. A plan should be set out and agreed upon to hire a one-to-one rehabilitation worker.

19. Literature that is user friendly should be left with the family. (See additional resource material, Family Handouts Sensory Overload, Energy Conservation at http://www.crcpress.com/product/isbn/9781482228243.)

20. The case manager who ran the team meeting should be on call to answer any questions or concerns the family or client may have after the meeting.

21. The case manager will follow up with the client to answer any questions and to see how the client feels about the proposed plan.

22. A therapeutic plan integrating the multidisciplinary team's therapeutic goals will be set and agreed upon.

23. A follow-up meeting should be set.

24. The family should be made aware of supports in the community, such as brain injury associations (Appendix 2). (See additional resource material, Family Handouts Brain Injury Associations at http://www.crcpress.com/product/isbn/9781482228243.)

BURN BLISTER ANALOGY

Stage One: The Blister Stage—Natural Healing

If we use the example of a burn, it can assist the family in understanding visually the invisible process that is happening inside the brain. For instance, when we burn ourselves, our body immediately reacts by developing a blister, pain, and redness. This happens whether there is any medical intervention or not. It is the body's natural healing response. The outcome is best when the area is kept sterile and dry, preventing infection. If we surmise that the brain does the same, then the first stage of natural recovery for the brain lasts approximately 6 to 9 months; it is during this period that we see spikes in recovery, emergence from the coma, recognition of family members, the beginning of speech, and eye tracking. The swelling in the brain is reduced, the bleeding will cease, and the brain will begin its recovery. The body's reaction to the trauma happens with or without medical intervention, but can certainly be facilitated and expedited toward a better outcome with medical intervention, such as medication or performing a shunt to reduce intracranial pressure.

Stage Two: The Scab

The second stage for a burn is where a scab is formed. Again, there is natural healing—however, less pronounced—and this healing can be accelerated with the introduction of antibiotics and dressings and keeping the wound clean. In the case of the brain, stage two involves spontaneous natural recovery where the brain is restoring its function; along with this spontaneous natural recovery, the brain can relearn through cognitive retraining and adaptations to the environment. In the author's experience, this phase generally lasts about 6 months to 2 years, depending on the injury.

Stage Three: The Scar

At this stage in the burn analogy the wound has healed; the cleanliness of the wound has facilitated the healing process and prevented infection, but there is still a scar. If there has been an infection, then the scar will be greater. When comparing this to the recovery process of the brain, in stage three the natural spontaneous process has been completed and the only course of action is relearning through cognitive remediation or teaching a different part of the brain to do the same task in a different way, as well as modifying the environment. The scar represents the residual loss. This residual loss is the end result. The symptoms that exist will most likely be permanent; therefore, any changes in function will occur because of alterations to the environment or use of remediation tools or relearning through alternate approaches to cognitive function. It takes 2 to 6 years for the residual loss stage to be reached. The process of cognitive relearning can go on for a lifetime. The scar or the residual loss represents what the litigators commence a legal action against (see Table 5.1).

INTRODUCING STRESS

The question we need to ask ourselves is how we, as health care providers, make the scar (as described in the burn example) or residual loss as minimal as possible.

Again, if we look at the analogy of the burn, if the burn gets infected the scar is larger. In this context what would serve as infection in the case of a brain injury? The answer is stress. Stress is the agent that will cause the scar or residual loss to be greater. The author has observed, not surprisingly, that the greater the change, the greater is the stress.

We therefore need to define what stress is. In the mid-1960s Holmes and Rahe produced a social adjustment rating scale measuring the impact of change on a person's health [47]. In the case of brain injury this is complex; the very core of the injury exacts a price of change that, in itself, will produce health risks. Change

Table 5.1 Analogy of the Burn

	Blister	Scab	Scar
Burn	Swelling, fluid-filled sac Keep clean, antibiotics, bandage, keep dry	Crusty, sore, itchy Bandage, antibiotics, keep clean and dry	Smooth, shiny skin; heightened color without infection If an infection has occurred, the scar is larger and angrier in appearance
Brain injury	Natural healing Coming out of the coma, eye tracking, face recognition, initial movement of extremities	Natural healing plus cognitive retraining; mobility improves, sequencing organizing, executive function; improved attendance to activities of daily living	Adaptation to residual loss Community reintegration; independence with assistance
	If stress is dynamic, the healing is compromised	If stress controls the situation and the family members become primary caregivers, the family unit is at risk, as is the health of family members The interplay between the stress symptoms and the TBI symptoms will compromise the rehabilitation process	If the stress is not managed, the relationships break down, more loss is incurred, independence and skill development have been greatly compromised. Funds may have been squandered as a result of the stress; there is an absence of joy and hope The traumatically induced dysfunctional family symptoms become evident
	0–9 months post-trauma	9 months–2 years post-trauma	2 years ongoing

in physical, cognitive, emotional, recreational, sexual, social, community and work relationships, etc. can be seen post-TBI. The brain injury causes massive change. How can we avoid the toll that stress caused by change will take on the recovery process?

1. Identify the change (balanced lifestyle sheet) (see Appendix 3B in Chapter 3).

2. Put supports in place to reduce the change when the client returns home.

3. The family resumes their pre-injury roles, ideally playing a minor role in care giving.

4. Remediate and modify the client's pre-injury leisure, recreational, and social interests.

5. Restore life balance for the client and family members.

6. Educate the client and family to understand the similarity of stress symptoms and traumatic brain injury symptoms.

7. Avoid sensory overload and practice energy conservation techniques as outlined in Chapter 8.

THE INTERPLAY BETWEEN STRESS AND ORGANIC SYMPTOMS

The risk of allowing the stress to go unattended is that the physiological symptoms produced by stress could easily be confused with the symptoms arising out of the TBI.

One can see in looking at this list of stress symptoms in Table 5.2 that it would be easy to confuse the origin of symptoms that appear the same as brain injury symptoms but with different causation.

Table 5.2 Some Examples of Stress Symptoms [33, 47–49]

• Appetite change	• Flatness of affect
• Headaches	• Anger
• Fatigue	• Resentment
• Insomnia	• Emptiness or loss of meaning
• Muscle aches	• Doubt
• Digestive upsets	• Looking for magic
• Pounding hearing	• Needing to prove self
• Accident prone	• Cynicism
• Teeth grinding	• Loss of hope
• Rash	• Self-loathing
• Hives	• Lethargy
• Restlessness	• No purpose
• Anxiety	• Feeling unlovable
• Frustration	• Feeling useless
• Mood swings	• Untrusting
• Nightmares	• No vision for the future
• Crying spells	• Forgetfulness
• Irritability	• Dull sense
• Depression	• Poor concentration
• Worrying	• Lethargy
• Easily discouraged	• Whirling mind
• Impatience	• Boredom
• Guilt	• Spacing out
• Tearfulness	• Negative self-talk

Continued

Table 5.2 (*Continued*) Some Examples of Stress Symptoms [33, 47–49]

• Nervous, tense	• Nail biting
• Pre-occupied with specific fears	• Picking
• Irritable	• Hair twisting
• Cranky	• Increased substance use
• Over-enthused	• Procrastinating
• Poor memory	• Lack of ambition
• Poor attention	• Impulsive actions
• Disorganization	• Diminished work output
• Large margin of error	• Sleeping
• Difficulty organizing tasks	• Avoidance
• Poor task completion	• Accident proneness
• Intolerance	• Easily embarrassed
• Loneliness	• General social withdrawal
• Lashing out/hiding	• Verbal abuse, swearing
• Clamming up	• Sensitive, thin skinned
• Lower/higher sex drive	• Defensive
• Short tempered	• Apathetic
• Excitable	• Whirling mind
• Critical	• Impaired judgment
• Inappropriate behavior	• Self-medicating
• Isolation	• Acting out
• Nervousness in social situations	• Poor work performance
• Laughing inappropriately	• Poor articulation of verbal thought
• Being late	• Loss of insight
• Mixing up plans	• Poor initiation
• Fewer contacts with friends	• Limited attention span
• Lack of intimacy	• Low stress tolerance

To this end the clinical team must make every effort to reduce or totally eliminate the stress for the client early on in the recovery process. Literature supports the idea that "conflicts with professional careers should be avoided" and that "support from professionals reduces the stress being experienced and encourages people to cope effectively" [21, p. 1004].

It is very important for us as care providers to establish therapeutic rapport with our clients; to do this we need to be available to the client and to be able to see the client in a timely fashion. We, as health care providers, will write our reports very soon after having seen the client to ensure the flow of information is shared with each team member. We must also see the therapeutic regime through to completion. The clinical team will be cognizant of the fact that any delays, poor time management, wait lists, or procrastination of report writing can add to the already stressful situation and compromise our therapeutic relationship with the client and his or her family.

If we identify stress as change, then we need to reduce the amount of change for the client. (See additional resource material, Family Stress Symptom Inventory at http://www.crcpress.com/ product/isbn/9781482228243.) We do this by understanding what life was pre-injury for all family members and keeping life as much the same as possible. The family's roles should not change if at all possible; above all else, they should not become primary caregivers. The literature is clear that caregiver burnout is a risk as well as the increased risk for occurring health problems of family members that become primary caregivers. A major health issue for a family member would further complicate this already complicated situation. The literature reveals that family caregivers of persons with TBI report increased stress and unmet needs over time [50]. Stress scores for family caregivers can remain high for as many as 10–15 years after the initial injury [21].

This is where the role of advocacy comes in for the community team. We, as health care professionals, need to plead the case to the funding sources, educating them to better understand that, if we can reduce or minimize the stress for the client and family in the early stages of recovery, then we can improve the outcome by reducing the residual loss over the lifetime of the client and family. We also capitalize on the natural healing that is taking place for the TBI survivor, therefore reducing the overall long-term costs. When translated to the insurer this means more cost-effective treatment, allowing the client to mitigate his or her circumstances and reducing the claim by providing a better quality of life for the injured party and facilitating the family system to stay intact.

In the case where there is no third-party liability, the care provider needs to utilize community and volunteer resources. Utilizing university/college students as volunteers (gaining them credit in course curricula) is a great option, as well as utilizing reliable volunteers from churches and service groups (Figure 4.2 in Chapter 4).

SUMMARY

The client has now returned home, and the family will be making every effort to establish homeostasis by creating a new normal. At the same time as the new clinical team is conducting their assessments, the family will be craving information on how this is going to work at home. The natural gravitation at this stage is for family members to protect the TBI survivor and to become care providers themselves; this may seem to come without a price in the initial stages of reintegration home, but over the long term this strategy puts the family unit at risk for burnout and health problems. The community team will work toward providing intervention to assist the family to return to their pre-injury roles, advocating for assistance by the funders to provide help in the home maintaining the original family roles.

The case manager or another community health clinician will have an educational meeting with the client and loved ones, preferably within the client's home. This clinician will be well versed on the client's TBI and will be armed with knowledge gained from taking an extensive history and understanding of the medical reports.

The analogy of the burn provides a concrete example of the body's ability to heal as well as the risks of infection, which in the case of TBI is stress. For the purposes of this discussion, stress has been identified as change. The body's natural physiological reaction to change produces symptoms that appear similar to or the same as brain injury symptoms. Left unattended, these stress symptoms will confuse the rehabilitation process and put the family unit at risk. The impact of stress and, particularly, how it impacts the family unit will be explored at greater length as we proceed to Chapter 6.

CHAPTER 6

The Loss...Stress

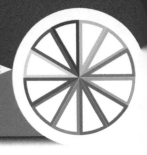

TOTAL SUM   –   DIAGNOSIS (LOSS)   +   INTERVENTION   =   RESIDUAL LOSS

    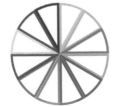

STRESS

Most of us have experienced stress in our lives. I am sure you can recall a close call, perhaps when a child ran out in front of your car and you swerved to avoid hitting her. Your autonomic nervous system kicks into high gear. Your adrenal glands produce an increase of adrenaline. Your heart races, your pulse quickens, there is a rise in your blood pressure, you begin to perspire, you have an increase of saliva production, and you may feel your face flush and feel a bit light headed. Our body prepares for fight or flight and automatically responds at a physiological level.

Our body reacts similarly when we are faced with illness. Our immune system mobilizes into action to fend off the foreign organism, our body temperature rises, we may feel fatigue or nausea, and we will have an increase in white blood cell count.

Our body physiologically reacts to stress. We know that stress can be positive or negative but stress will always involve change.

In the case of positive stress, the stress may have been planned for and may be welcome; for example, it is common to hear that the first year of marriage or a new job can be joyful and stressful until an element of familiarity and routine can be established. Despite the fact that it is positive stress, the body will still inadvertently react and produce some stress symptoms as identified in Chapter 5.

For example; a teenage girl may be very excited about her first date with a star football player, but her body may react to this positive stress producing such symptoms as a breakout in acne or menstrual cramps.

A father may be thrilled with his new job as a superintendent of schools but may experience a sleepless night before his first day at the new job coupled with symptoms of acid reflux.

A mother may be absolutely in awe at her son's graduation from medical school and his job offer 1,000 miles away from home at a prestigious hospital, but just before attending the ceremony she has an outbreak of colitis.

Our body internally and physiologically reacts to the changes that inevitably occur in life. The literature is clear that if we can control these life changes through balance and planning, then the ability to manage these life changes and reduce the negative physiological symptoms can be thoughtfully controlled.

It is not uncommon to hear that we should only make one major change a year. The more magnitude the change has on an individual and family, the more carefully it needs to be handled. For instance, if a family moves to another country, they will no longer be speaking in their native tongue and everything in their environment will be new, including food, currency, customs, and geographical terrain. There will inevitably be challenges within the family system as each member struggles to regain balance and a sense of homeostasis.

There is nothing familiar about a traumatic brain injury; many aspects of life over and above the TBI will change. The survivor most certainly changes, and finances, recreation, daily routine, community involvement, friends, emotional capacity, personality, activities of daily living, and ability to work may add to the new mix of life changes.

The changes and the uncertainty of the future are stressful. The family and client are in a full-on war to bring life back to a place of sameness.

The client's coming home is causing loved ones and the client to feel hope, as well as fear and anxiety. It is very common for the roles of family members to have a tendency to shift in an effort to try to keep things the same. Children can find themselves parenting an injured parent; spouses can begin to feel like caregivers rather than partners and lovers. We, the health care providers, from our vantage point can identify these changes and intercept before a new family system overtakes the old familiar one.

For the client the "new normal" can be hope filled and realistic, embracing the "new me" and being thankful for "what is." Or the change can produce maladaptive coping mechanisms such as anger, depression, suicidal ideation, resentment, denial, codependency, alcohol and drug use, and abandonment—to name a few.

It is of great importance for the community clinical team to put supports in place, either funded or through the use of volunteers, to maintain the familiar pre-injury family roles, responsibilities, and routines as it was before the loved one's TBI.

The traumatic brain injury has happened to an individual but it impacts the entire family. It is not uncommon to witness a family member:

a. Protecting
b. Caring for
c. Doing for
d. Possibly abandoning the situation

To assist the family in avoiding any maladaptive coping mechanisms, the clinical team practicing the *rainbow effect* has expended great effort in understanding the family unit and the client's life as it was before the TBI to ensure a working knowledge of sameness.

The goal now of the community team is to reduce the stress, protect the family system, and provide therapy for the survivor—a delicate balance for the new community clinicians as they make every effort to gain the trust of the family and client.

The first step (as reviewed in Chapter 5) of having an educational meeting has set the foundation.

The care providers will have a full understanding of the negative repercussions of the stress the family and client have experienced. Research has shown that "the level of stress experienced by the family members of patients who have traumatic brain injury is such that professional intervention is appropriate even after 10–15 years" [21, p. 1004].

"If there is a disruption in the rules of the existing pattern within the family system, it does not disrupt just the identified person; it affects and disrupts all participants in the system. Finally every system is unique; the system of one family is different from another family system" [21, p. 1006]. This research supports the need for an individualized approach specific to each client and family situation.

"Traumatic brain injury brings along more stress, greater dysfunction and more problems, which, in turn give rise to more stress, greater conflict, etc." [21, p. 1007].

The author has found, as the research supports, that appropriate client and family support reaps the greatest reward when the client returns home.

"Family members cope better with out-patient rehabilitation than with residential treatment even if the severity of the injury is the same" [21, p. 1008].

The research further supports that "family members shut themselves off from the outside world and thus avoid unpleasant reactions from their entourage to, for example, the victim's socially inappropriate behavior" [21, p. 1009].

"Various surveys have established that some 30% to 50% of couples divorce within 8–10 years following the trauma" [21, p. 1009].

It is frequently thought in various regions of the world that the family is indeed the best care provider for the TBI survivor. However, with research indicating that family breakdown is a risk factor, as well as caregiver burnout and resulting health issues for family caregivers, it makes sense to provide supports to the family and make every attempt to preserve their pre-injury roles. Despite the fact that the author believes that the family should not assume the major role in care giving or be the primary provider of therapy or case management, it would be naive to think that the family has no role at all.

In reality and in light of the major changes resulting from the family member's injury, the household workload will inevitably shift. If a father is injured, the functional tasks of the father, such as mowing the lawn or shoveling snow, as well as earning a living will now fall to other family members.

If a mother is injured, laundry, cleaning, baking, cooking, bringing in a second income, and nurturing younger siblings will fall to other family members.

The husband of the injured wife may become solely a parent or care-giving figure and lost will be the romance/sexuality and mutual partnership they once shared.

If a child or youth is injured, other siblings may assume their chores while the parents focus most of their attention on the injured child. "The better the family members can cope with the situation, the better the patient's recovery" [21, p. 1004].

There are quite typically limitations when third-party funding is involved that limit the intervention or support solely to the TBI survivor. However, with effective advocacy from the community team, the funder quickly becomes aware of the benefits in providing supports to the entire family, possibly in the form of counseling, lawn maintenance, homemaker service, handyman service, transportation, childcare, etc., depending on the pre-injury role of the TBI survivor. The family can then assume their pre-injury primary role as family members—whatever that was before the loved one's brain injury. The team educates the funder, supporting their position with the realistic knowledge that if the family unit breaks down or the family burns out and becomes ill then, indeed, the costs of funding for the TBI survivor will rise.

It is to this end that it is in everyone's interest to reduce the stress caused by the changes for the family as a unit as well as for the client.

Returning to how the *rainbow effect* is taking shape in the **total sum** stage, the team has gained the working knowledge of the client's pre-injury life. In the **loss stage** an understanding of the etiology and ramifications and sequalae of the client's TBI is understood. It is a reality that the family has experienced immense change and stress thus far; as we look at the impact of stress, please note that we are still in the **loss stage** of the formula.

The stress and change need to be managed. Things are not the same as before; however, through education and family/client support, we move toward bringing the family back to a new kind of homeostasis with hope being a central motivator.

At this point we are still positioning the client and family to engage in the community rehabilitation process. Timing is critical: The client has just returned home, the obvious safety supports are in place in the home, but the program of intervention—including cognitive retraining—is still at the preliminary stage. The family and client should be on board at this stage, understanding that the urge to "do for" the client may be counterproductive unless there is a safety hazard.

This process may seem arduous and the tendency may be to dive directly into the rehabilitation plan but that is foolhardy without addressing the interplay of the stress and organic symptoms. In reality this educational process will take place within the first or second day of the client's returning home.

The plan at this stage is to:

1. Ensure that all home renovations and vehicle modifications have been completed.
2. Continue educating family members on the effects of stress.
3. Identify what stress symptoms look like (Chapter 5).
4. Identify what areas of the brain engage in certain functions (Chapter 8).

As we look at the *rainbow effect* formula, we will see the absence of color in the second **loss** pie. The absence of color represents the absence of activity, production, or the change in activity level from the client's pre-injury status.

With our knowledge that change = stress, then, the absence of color in the loss stage of the formula represents the magnitude of the stress experience and the associated risks.

THE PROCESS FOR MANAGING STRESS

A pre-injury profile has been conducted arming the clinicians with the knowledge of life as it was before (Appendix 3A):

1. A review of pre-injury family roles and responsibilities has become clear.

2. Through the process of educating the family the fear and anxiety will have been disclosed to the clinicians. This emergence of therapeutic trust will allow the case manager to observe shifts in family roles positioning the team to put counseling in place.

3. The clinicians take on the role of advocate and present to the funder the risks to the family system.

4. Services are put in place to allow the family to resume life as it was before. Any family members who are having a hard time disengaging with a care-giving role will receive additional support and education.

5. In the case of lack of funding, volunteers and community support will be solicited.

6. The client will be ready to embark on the community therapeutic journey. Goals will have been established that have meaning to the client and produce the cognitive remediation required to achieve independence, preparing the client for the next step in the formula— the **intervention.**

7. As the family settles into life at home and resumes their pre-injury roles, the client begins the job of cognitive remediation at home and in the community; the roles and familiarity of routines and dynamics will position the client for success.

When the stress is being managed, we are then treating the organic traumatic brain injury symptoms. In subsequent chapters we will review a simple color-coded monitoring system that will visually reveal to the client and family how well their stress is being managed.

We are preserving the family's pre-injury roles and protecting the family unit itself. The secondary losses are being reduced and the client is mitigating his/her circumstances.

SUMMARY

In summary, stress plays a role in our lives. It can present as positive or negative and will exact a physiological response. The literature recognizes the impact of change as it relates to stress; the greater the change is, the greater is the stress. We have seen in Chapter 5 that the body's response to stress may also be confused with traumatic brain injury symptoms. This can be confusing for the clinical team who are making every effort to design a therapeutic program that will reap positive rewards for the client and family.

Changes in family roles further complicate the situation as these new family dynamics in themselves create more change for the client, making it harder to integrate the cognitive stimuli.

A traumatic brain injury happens not only to the client but also to the family. In relationship to the *rainbow effect* formula the absence of color in the loss stage visually represents the amount of change experienced by the client and, indirectly, by the family.

The clinical team advocates to the funder to put supports in place both for the client and family members.

The impact of role changes cannot be underestimated and must be identified before we move to the **intervention** stage of the formula. Chapter 7 will review what happens to a family if the stress is not managed and role changes occur.

In the next chapter we will explore the author's theory of the traumatically induced dysfunctional family.

CHAPTER 7

The Traumatically-Induced Dysfunctional Family Theory

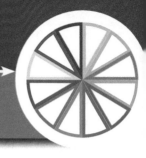

TOTAL SUM   –   DIAGNOSIS (LOSS)   +   INTERVENTION   =   RESIDUAL LOSS

 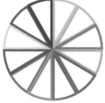

INTRODUCTION

In this chapter we will explore by case example the family system, how the family system operated before the loved one's traumatic brain injury, and how it is impacted by the recovery process, in particular when the survivor returns home. We will integrate our knowledge that the change exacted to the family system because of a family member's brain injury has produced stress and that any member of the family including the survivor may be exhibiting stress symptoms. We will review family systems and propose that the family is at risk and may begin to create a new dysfunctional dynamic, further complicating and jeopardizing the client's therapeutic outcome as well as the family unit.

SYSTEMS IN GENERAL

In society we require systems for order, effectiveness, rules, feedback, safety, security, homeostasis, and performance. At a larger scale we have government systems—firstly, at a federal level and then by territory, region, province, or state.

In business corporations, systems also exist, with managers providing support, feedback, and structure for the working employees.

Sporting teams also have a hierarchy and a system of order with clear expectations, roles, and protocols.

Schools have systems set out with the expectation of providing the organizational structure to foster a healthy learning environment. The school district provides the protocols and framework with clear expectations and definitions of jobs. The principal is the local authority in each school, further implementing the expected structure. The teachers serve as a role model and provide structure, routine, and order in the classroom.

Without systems, the previously mentioned scenarios would be in a state of chaos. We therefore recognize the value and importance of systems that provide a concrete place to function and be in relationship with others, facilitating performance and growth. Each of these scenarios provides a level of security, consistency, predictability, nurture, feedback, boundaries, and homeostasis.

FAMILY SYSTEMS

The family is no different. The family will have a system with rules, boundaries, expectations, values, beliefs, morals, method of communicating, structure, and roles. The family system and each member's role will also be affected by birth order, gender, age, culture, personalities, finances, responsibilities, health, and duties.

The family system is a place to express ourselves through interaction and co-operation by giving and receiving feedback. It is a place to grow, develop, and be in relationships. There are as many family systems as there are personalities. Family systems come in several varieties; within these varieties there will be cultural influences, financial implications, geographical implications, and societal norms. The number of persons in a family varies as does the number of parents. Some parents are single, widowed, divorced, blended, or same sex; some families house an older generation of parents, while some children are living with foster parents. The dynamics can become complex.

Within the family system there will be a subset of characteristics. One would hope that each family system is a healthy place that is loving, supportive, predictable, and safe. However, in reality we are imperfect beings; when we are grouped together in a living environment, our imperfections will come to light. To some degree all family systems will have a negative effect on the individual members at various intervals.

One only has to watch the news to recognize the reality that some family systems are faced with greater challenges. Some examples of systems that exact a greater negative impact on family members are shown in Table 7.1.

Within the context of the family who has experienced a member's traumatic brain injury, research has found that the TBI

Table 7.1 High-Risk Family Systems

Sex abuse—A family where sex abuse has occurred or is occurring
Legal issues—A family where a member or members are incarcerated or in conflict with the law
Unmet basic needs—A family where the basic needs of food, clothing, or shelter are not met
Psychiatric conditions—A family where a member has an untreated psychiatric condition
Physical or emotional neglect—A family where there is physical and/or emotional neglect
Serious and long-term illness—Where a family member is seriously ill with long-term effects
Addiction—A family that is devastated by a member's addiction to gambling, alcohol, drugs, sex, or food
Violence—A family where violence is prevalent or where the system has been impacted by external violence

survivor could be better served if the family was screened for pre-existing medical and psychiatric histories.

"The current findings indicate that caregivers of persons with moderate and severe TBI should be screened regarding their pre-injury medical and psychiatric histories early after injury to aid rehabilitation staff in identifying caregivers who are at risk for developing distress in the post acute period" [51, p. 151].

Professionals in the fields of clinical psychology and social work are highly trained in family systems and the dynamics that accompany them.

"The social work profession more than any other health care profession has historically recognized the importance of assessing the individual in the context of his or her family environment" [52, p. 194].

"Family systems theory grew out of the biologically based general systems theory. General systems theory focuses on how the parts of a system interact with one another. In general systems theory, an individual cell is one example of a system and in family systems theory the family is essentially its own system" [52, p. 195].

In the early 1960s, many family systems models were studied. "All the family therapy models share the basic principle of family systems theory that is that the individual cannot be fully understood or successfully treated without first understanding how the individual functions in his or her family system" [52, p. 196]. The intensive history taking as it relates to the *rainbow effect* allows the clinician to gain insight into the family system if carefully executed.

It is important as clinicians that we are cognizant of the fact that the family had a life before their loved one sustained a traumatic brain injury. The slate was not blank. Lives were busy—filled with expectations, routines, conflicts, successes, challenges, values, rules, and schedules. Some families with a TBI survivor may have had a very healthy family system prior to the loved one's injury, while others may be experiencing greater challenges as listed in Table 7.1. Let us take the time to study a family case history.

Case History: The Taylor Family Members' Roles Pre-Injury

The Taylor family is a close-knit family:

Tom, the dad, is a first-generation Canadian; his family hailed from Eastern Europe. His family of origin was not financially well off; sometimes they were in want of just their basic needs of food, clothing, and shelter. Tom never wants to see his own family suffer poverty and hunger the way he had to as a child. Tom works hard spending many long hours at the office. Traditional family roles and values are what feel comfortable and hold importance for Tom. Tom married Sally in part because she was willing to be a stay-at-home mom. He values and appreciates her domesticity. Tom is not one who emotes but Sally compensates with her sensitivity, compassion, and ability to nurture. They work well as a team.

Tom is a very serious man, and he is clearly the disciplinarian in the Taylor family. He can come across as a bit gruff and abrupt but his motivations arise out of wanting the best for his family. He takes his role as a father very seriously. Tom is not one who openly expresses his feelings, but rather shows his love by providing for and taking care of his family.

Sally was born and raised in a large city, and as a child she loved visiting her uncle and aunt on their farm in rural Quebec. She enjoyed cooking, baking, cleaning, ironing, and helping her aunt care for her little cousins. Sally vowed that when she grew up she wanted to be a stay-at-home mom; her desire to care for others has been an intrinsic part of her character since she was a child. Sally met Tom when she was 20; she appreciated how secure he made her feel. Sally felt that Tom had wisdom beyond his years. Despite being only 23, Tom was mature. He took his job as an insurance salesman very seriously. After Tom graduated from college he created a life plan for himself, setting financial goals and career milestones. Sally liked that about Tom and she felt that he was the perfect man for her; she could actualize her dream of being a mother, and Tom indicated that he would be more than supportive if she stayed home.

Sally recognized that Tom was serious but she felt certain that once they had saved a bit of money he would relax more and she would make every effort to create a happy home.

James was the first Taylor child to be born, and he was the apple of Sally's eye. She loved to tend to him and nurture him. James was an easy-going child who enjoyed staying close to his mom. As he grew up she was his biggest fan. The addition of a new family member further deepened Tom's resolve to work hard and provide for his family. Rather than spending much time with James, Tom worked even harder to build up a college fund for him.

As James grew up he developed a love of sports and had a large social circle. As the eldest, he enjoyed roughhousing with younger brothers Paul and Marc. Sally enjoyed attending James's football and baseball games. At some level, for James this compensated for the fact that his dad was always working and took little interest in his athletic acumen. James was now 18 and planning on attending college at some point, but he really wanted to travel first. Now that he was a young man he tended to butt heads with his dad's old-fashioned work ethic. James would have appreciated his dad coaching his football rather than working so hard. He wished that his dad would have some fun.

Paul was the second child to be welcomed into the Taylor family. He was a rambunctious toddler and youngster, always into things. It seemed that when it came to Paul that "no" seemed to be in the equation. Paul's favorite activity was to follow James around. He idolized James and loved hanging out with him. James was a good older brother to Paul, always including him in activities. Paul enjoyed his video games and took little interest in sports; after all, what was the point, with Mom making such a fuss over James's accomplishments? He could compete in the arena of academics. Despite a healthy dose of sibling rivalry, James and Paul loved and respected each other.

The Taylor clan was blessed with a third boy, Marc, 2 years after Paul's birth. Life was busy and Marc was a happy, funny child, entertaining the family with his antics. However, beneath the gregarious exterior was a soft, sensitive soul. Marc felt things deeply. He loved tagging along with his two older brothers but felt that he was a bit of a nuisance because of the age difference. As a youth Marc worked at the school support program mentoring younger handicapped children. He was close to his dad, helping out wherever he could around the house. Marc appreciated how hard his dad worked and was eager to get a job himself so he could contribute to his own college fund.

Case Example, including Injury

There was a terrible blizzard; the news reports were encouraging everyone to stay home, unless they had something urgent to do. Dinner was as boisterous as ever in the Taylor house. Tom was irritated by James's carefree attitude. A discussion over James's plan for university had erupted to a crescendo over dinner. James wanted to take a year off and travel Europe. Tom, who had worked hard all of his life, believed such a plan was frivolous. Sally knew that James would find his way, but Tom was not so sure. In an effort to direct him, Tom had laid the law down—that it was university in the fall or James was out on his own.

James had a squash game at 8:00 that was "urgent," he told his mom with a chuckle, fearless as ever. Sally laughed and looked at her brawny, confident son; surely he could handle this weather. "O.K., Jimmy, drive carefully. Love ya; be careful," she said. James replied, "You too; see you later. Dinner was great, by the way."

A phone call to the Taylor home was received at 9 p.m. There has been an accident and James has been critically injured. Shock and disbelief set in. Sally cried in horror, "No, not James! Oh, I never should have let him go! What was I thinking? It's all my fault! What kind of a mother am I?" James had sustained a traumatic brain injury. His Glasgow coma score was 7. His prognosis was guarded.

Tom immediately felt guilty that their last words were harsh; he also struggled with anger, thinking, "I told him not to go out in this weather." He did not know what to say to Sally. Paul was left in charge at home and Tom and Sally raced to the hospital.

Paul did not know what to think. Mom and Dad sure seemed upset and Dad seemed angry. Feeling helpless and somewhat deserted ("Why can't I go to the hospital with them?"), he heads to his room and gets lost in his video game, thinking, "James is invincible and always gets himself out of tough situations—he'll be fine; I'll bring him in my portable DVD so he can watch the game on Sunday." Young Marc retreated into his room, tears streaming down his face, but no one noticed. This would be the last time for several months that anyone really noticed that he had withdrawn and shut down.

James was in ICU and not responding to his parents at all. The situation remained the same for days. A new routine set in, and Sally stayed at the hospital virtually around the clock during the initial days, as did Tom. Unable to tolerate the desperateness of the situation Tom returned to his old routine and escaped into work, visiting James in the evenings.

Paul and Marc found it incredibly upsetting to visit James. Paul came by almost every day; normally tough and rambunctious, he felt helpless and confused. Marc sat by quietly looking at a brother that he no longer recognized. Days and weeks passed while Sally sat bedside; she was exhausted and had not been eating or sleeping much.

A distance is developing between Sally and Tom. Deep down, Sally blames Tom for arguing with James. Perhaps James was upset, preoccupied from the dinner conversation about university. Maybe that was why the accident happened— after all, he was an excellent driver. Why could Tom not back off about university? James was a good kid who would have figured it out. Now what did his future hold?

Sally, who had a special bond with her firstborn, rarely left his side in ICU. Her normal duties of meal preparation, cleaning, ironing, paying bills, and providing order to the household went unattended.

She decided that the younger boys and Tom could take care of themselves for once. For the first time, she began to resent all the work she did at home and how little they helped. She was emotionally exhausted and had nothing left to give them.

Tom was devastated and retreated into his world of work, letting destiny take its course. If he allowed himself to feel anything too much, a floodgate of emotion would erupt. He would have liked to be closer to James, and now it might never happen. The thought was overwhelming. He thought, "I'll just work hard; after all, we will need money to pay for his care. I'll let Sally do the hand holding; she's better at that." Tom did not realize that he had shut Sally and the younger boys out.

Sally felt it best if Paul and Marc stayed with her folks. This allowed Sally the opportunity to focus on James, protecting the younger boys from seeing him in a comatose state. She did not realize that Paul and Marc were beginning to feel abandoned by their parents. "Mom totally forgot my birthday," thought Paul. "I know James is really sick but she didn't even wish me happy birthday." For the first time Paul began to couple his grief with feelings of resentment. This was also causing him to feel guilt and shame—how could he feel like this when James was fighting for his life?

Young Marc had developed dark circles under his eyes and did not talk much, but no one had noticed. Both Sally and Tom were grateful that Marc was one of those kids who did not demand much. Little did they know that Marc felt lost. James had been his anchor; as the youngest it seemed to him that his parents were busy but James always had time for him. Marc was slipping into a depression;

he had grown thin and fatigued he spent most of his time in his room. Everyone thought he was coping much better than Paul, who had become quite verbal about the fact that he was getting tired of the world revolving around James.

The sleepless nights, fatigue, worry, and grief took their toll. As time passed, the family took in the reality of the situation; the tracheotomy, tubes, catheter, and non-responsiveness were horrifying. As James's eyes began to flicker, they saw a blank expression. New grief set in that he would not just wake up, like in the movies; the grief, however, was coupled with hope.

The harsh reality that James was not recognizing them was devastating. The doctors informed them that, depending on many factors, recovery would continue but might be slow; speech might be slurred, inappropriate, or nonexistent and physical movement impaired. James might not recognize his family members or, worse yet, might be uttering foul or angry words at those very people who had been standing guard as he recovered. A myriad of symptoms began to emerge, and reality slowly set in. James was no longer viewed as the person he once was. The long road of recovery began and so did the shift in family roles.

In this case, Sally shifted her role from mother, wife, and lover—nurturer of her husband and three sons—to advocate for and supporter of James. The family no longer had home-cooked meals, clean clothes on a regular basis, a clean house, or emotional support. This role shift had caused Tom, Marc, and Paul to feel abandoned and disorganized. Because of these feelings of abandonment, these three family members were facing a moral dilemma: They all realized that James was in terrible shape, but feelings of resentment and bitterness, coupled with guilt and shame, began to infiltrate their psyches.

Tom, who was ill prepared to cope with deep emotional loss, had taken to drinking alcohol nightly. In self-medicating, he was able to compartmentalize his feelings that life was now out of control.

With Tom's focus shifting from work to worry, his client service had declined and the family's financial situation was insidiously impacted. Sally was backlogged on paying bills and attending to the bank accounts and she was unaware of this new impending financial crisis.

Paul was tired of the focus always being on James. He surely loved him, but could his mom come home for just one night and make a meal? Dad got more critical the more he drank. Paul longed for the days of fun and laughter around the dinner table.

Marc's teacher had noticed a decline in Marc's performance; he seemed to be tired and apathetic. She was aware of the older brother's injury and, in an effort to help Marc, she placed a call to the Taylor house. She had made the decision that Marc needed professional help; she feared for his mental health. The teacher's phone call would further exacerbate the stress and concern for Tom and Sally. Life seemed to be spiraling out of control for the Taylor family.

As the family strove to cope with the impact of James's traumatic brain injury, their roles slowly and insidiously started to change. While in crisis, many assumptions are commonly made without the family communicating to each other. Sally assumed that Tom could take care of himself and that he would start to engage in more domestic tasks at home while she spent most of her time at the hospital. Sally had no idea how vulnerable Tom felt; he had never been an emotional person and did not have the skill set to engage in her domestic chores.

She was unaware that she did most of the emotional work in her relationship with Tom. Now that she was spread so thin, Tom was decompensating—self-medicating by drinking as his guilt over the argument with James consumed him.

Another assumption that can commonly be made is that the family members' needs changed as a result of the traumatic brain injury.

In fact, each family member's needs had remained the same. Tom needed Sally's support more now than ever. Marc and Paul were grieving the loss of their older brother and were frightened. They needed to be nurtured and supported. They needed the familiarity of home-cooked meals and an orderly environment. They were young and wanted to feel as though their lives counted for something as well. They had not fully matured emotionally and began to resent James's causing them to feel conflicted emotionally. The parents were understandably sidetracked with James's condition; the younger boys' needs were neglected and the activities that were important for them to engage in could go unattended. If this went on for any length of time, the younger boys could skip essential developmental milestones.

The younger boys still were expected to perform at school—that had not changed. But the loss of support, encouragement, and order that Sally used to provide was negatively impacting the performance of Marc and Paul academically.

The fact that Tom was drinking at night was also new and worrisome for the boys as they trod lightly to avoid conflict.

The literature reveals that family systems are complicated. What appears consistently is that the family system desires a place of sameness or homeostasis:

When one person in a family begins to change his or her behavior, the change will affect the entire family system. It is helpful to think of a family system as a mobile: When one part in a hanging mobile moves, this affects all parts of the mobile but in different ways, and each part adjusts to maintain balance in the system. [52, p. 197]

In the event that a parent is injured and the children are very young, another dynamic exists. "Any long-term separation will have a negative impact on the child's ability to attach, regulate affect, and can lead to a trauma response of numbing or hyperarousal" [52, p. 199].

Another situation that can occur is when a parent is injured and the child becomes a caregiver or assumes the role of parenting. This is a real risk for single-parent families where the parent who has custody is injured, "when the caretaker is unable to meet the developmental needs of the child, and the child begins to parent themselves [*sic*] and perhaps younger siblings earlier than developmentally appropriate. In a phenomenon called 'reversal of dependence needs' the child actually begins to parent the parent" [52, p. 200].

In a reversal of dependence needs, the parent's needs are placed before the child's. This sets the child up for a potential lifetime of inability to set healthy boundaries in relationships and make the important triad connections between thoughts, feelings and behaviors. It creates a lack of self-awareness and sometimes an over awareness of others' needs. [52, p. 200].

The research further reveals that:

A TBI has a greater impact on partners than on parents. The relation between partners becomes less stable and the stress experienced is greater…Partners voice more health and psychological complaints, score higher on depression scales and face crisis situations more often than parents. Parental stress is greater when it involves children living at home rather than grown-up children living away from home. [21, p. 1006]

"Children find it especially difficult in the event of parental trauma. Young children lose a parent and have to compete with the affected parent for the attention of the healthy parent. Older children living away from home are torn between their own family and that of their parents" [21, p. 1006].

"Siblings have lower self-concept, behavior problems, symptoms of depression and their relationship with the child with traumatic brain injury becomes more negative than before the injury" [21, p. 1006].

"Younger families with several young children are the most vulnerable. If in addition, there are financial problems and there is little social support, the stress is so great that it becomes impossible to function normally" [21, p. 1007].

The family members not involved in primary care distance themselves from the patient. The ability of children to cope is influenced above all by the gender of the affected parent and signs of depression from the unaffected parent. If the father suffers the injury, they present more "acting out" behavior. If, in addition, the mother displays symptoms of depression, behavioral problems among children rise significantly. The injury's severity has less of a bearing on how children behave. [21, p. 1006]

"Surprisingly, family members cope better with out-patient rehabilitation than with residential treatment even when the severity of the injury is the same" [21, p. 1008].

"Models of long-term support and care that alleviate sources of burden on relatives are urgently needed" [21, p. 1009].

Risk Factors for the Family Dealing with Traumatic Brain Injury

1. The change in health for the client results in unexpected changes for the family members.
2. In the acute stages the family has been traumatized, and their lives and the roles they played out in the family system may change for a period of time as the client's health is stabilized.
3. Other members of the family will begin to take on roles and responsibilities that are unfamiliar to them as a result of a family member being injured (Figures 7.1 and 7.2).
4. Family members may not have the skill or the emotional capacity or maturity to engage in the new roles effectively.
5. The family's finances may be affected, making it difficult to meet basic needs.
6. Each family member is having his or her own emotional response to the loved one's TBI.
7. The family members will begin to exhibit changes in behaviors and emotional responses to other family members as the family's rules and roles shift from their normal state of homeostasis.

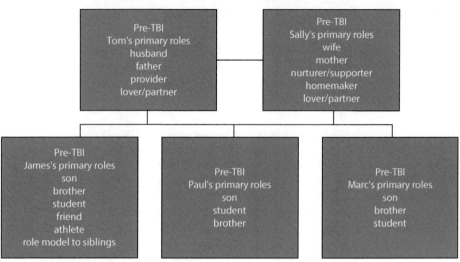

Figure 7.1 Family role mobile: Taylor family pre-injury.

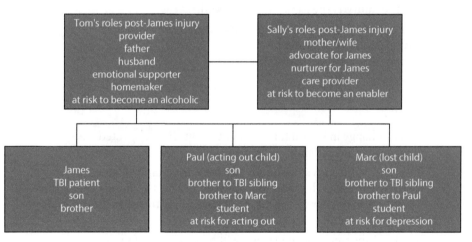

Figure 7.2 Family role mobile: Taylor family post-injury.

8. Change = stress and the family is at risk of experiencing stress symptoms (Table 5.2).

9. As indicated in the literature review, the family system has been well studied as it pertains to those family systems at high risk (Table 7.1).

Sharon Wegscheider-Cruse and Claudia Black have identified certain family roles.

"Arguably the most prevalent of these classifications is that written about by Wegscheider-Cruse, in which family members fall into five well-defined and generally nonoverlapping roles: enabler, hero, lost child, mascot, and scapegoat" [53, p. 535].

"The clinical characteristics of adults from families with an alcohol-dependent parent were similar to those from families experiencing other dysfunction" [53, p. 539].

These roles provide a framework understanding that there may be role shifts when a family experiences dysfunction and when family role changes have not been treated. For the purposes of the *rainbow effect*, the author observed in her clinical practice that these same roles that were observed in high-risk families began to emerge in the family that had been traumatized by a family member's TBI. The author has adopted the roles and descriptions listed in Table 7.2 and applied them to the TBI family:

Table 7.2 Family Roles

Sharon Wegscheider-Cruse	Claudia Black, PhD
The enabler	The codependent
"The enabler's primary role is to insulate a [family member] from the aversive consequences of his or her actions, thereby preserving the maladaptive patterns" (p. 536).	
The family hero	The responsible child
"The role of the hero is believed to be commonly played by the oldest child, who is capable of taking on greater responsibility for the well-being of the family early on. They are thought to neglect other areas of their lives (self-care, relationships, etc.)…They may feel overwhelmed as if the entire family is dependent on them to fulfil their role" (p. 536).	
The lost child	The adjuster
"The lost child is the one whose needs and wants are overlooked by the rest of the family in their attempts to cope"…Within the home, he or she may be withdrawn, having learned to disappear into the background of the family. This behaviour is reinforced by other members of the family, all of whom are too busy in their own roles to deal with the needs of yet another child. The lost child may be involved in fantasy (often through reading or television)" (p. 537).	
The mascot	The placator
"The child who falls into the role of the mascot (commonly thought to be the youngest) plays the part of a distracter from the problems within the family. It is his or her job to be cute, funny, and outgoing: Other family members can easily become swept up in the mascot's personality so as not to focus on the problem at hand" (p. 537).	
The scapegoat	The acting out child
"It is believed that as their behavior begins to deteriorate the scapegoat is blamed for many of the problems of the family, and they learn they cannot succeed in the eyes of their siblings or parents…The effects of these patterns of behavior later in life often manifest as legal problems, poor academic and vocational performance, and drug or alcohol use" (p. 537).	

Source: Vernig, P. M. 2011. *Substance Use and Misuse* 46 (4): 535–542.

In the author's clinical practice it was common, if not predictable, to witness family members taking on certain new behavioral characteristics after a loved one's TBI. It would be familiar to see a family member deny the brain injured person's TBI symptoms, giving unrealistic praise for a task that was done incorrectly and thus encouraging the client to make the same cognitive mistake in the future. This kind of unrealistic praise is foreign to the injured person's brain, thus making it difficult for learning.

Case 2

Bob sustained a TBI with a Glasgow coma score of 9. He was an avid chef and, historically, it was his job to cook the Christmas turkey. Ethel, his wife, was so happy to see Bob home that despite the findings in the occupational therapist's hospital cooking assessment that Bob had difficulty in cooking because of agnosia, in her denial, she encouraged Bob to cook the family turkey. Their entire family would be attending the dinner. The two teenage girls, Cindy and Karen, were excited that things had returned to normal. They invited Jack and Kevin, their boyfriends, for dinner. Bob put the turkey in the oven at noon. By 3:00 everyone could smell some type of burnt plastic odor. They scoured the house for the source, which ultimately led to the oven. In their surprise Bob had covered the turkey with Saran Wrap instead of tin foil. The turkey was ruined. Ethel continued to praise Bob for his efforts. Bob was grateful for the praise but he could not understand what had happened. In light of Ethel's praise Bob was further confused by the angry and hurt facial expressions on Cindy and Karen. Cindy retreated to her room in tears, and Karen glared at Bob and said that she and Kevin were going to Kevin's house for a "real" Christmas. Bob lashed out at Karen, telling her that if she had not had her loud music on, then he could have concentrated and this would not have happened.

In this case Ethel became an enabler, which in turn set Bob up for failure. He was confused, depressed about the turkey incident, and became afraid to try new things as he embarked on his therapy regime. Cindy became the lost child and in the future she decided to marry Jack at age 17 just to get away from the chaos. Karen became the scapegoat. Getting tired of everything being her fault, she ultimately ended up acting out and had problems with the law.

The research has revealed information regarding the quality of life for caregivers of persons with a severe head injury. "Reportedly, quality of life for the caregiver group was poor compared with healthy and chronic-disease groups" [50, pp. 375].

"With regard to quality of life, this investigation identified a decline in family members' quality of life after injury relative to pre-injury satisfaction" [50, p. 383].

Whenever a family experiences a trauma, the family unit reacts in some way to the crisis. There is no way to avoid the crisis, which has already happened. However, what can be managed is the toll it takes on the family system.

We have already provided the family with education on how change will negatively impact the survivor upon his return home (Table 5.1 in Chapter 5). The goal of minimizing the change is twofold: We want to control the change so that, when the client returns home, things are as familiar as they can possibly be—thus positioning the client's cognitive capacity to reidentify with life as before and thereby capitalize on the brain's capacity to relearn old familiar information.

The second goal is to preserve the family unit, protect the pre-injury roles and relationships, and provide a familiar climate of interaction for the client's community rehabilitation program. We need to continue to educate the family on the risk factors, educating them on how behaviors and feelings translate into outcomes. The impact of the change that has occurred to the family system as a result of the family member's traumatic brain injury is not to be left unattended.

"The importance of appreciating long-term family needs and other life quality issues should not be underestimated" [50, p. 383].

"Increased use of escape-avoidance as a coping strategy was associated with increased perceived burden and emotional distress" [51, p. 151].

As indicated in the preceding case examples, family members will experience feelings in response to the brain injury experience, as will the client. If the family member's feelings are negative, this in no way reduces or negates the family's love for one another; it is simply a response to stress. What is important is to identify the feelings. Behaviors are often indicative of feelings and emotion. How these emotions and feelings are managed will impact the outcome not just therapeutically for the client but also for the family unit's sustainability as a whole. Codes of silence can begin to infiltrate the family and lack of disclosure outside the family unit can occur.

Conditional love can occur on the part of the "walking wounded." At times they can pretend that they are okay in an effort to receive love from other family members. The brain-injured person is frequently confused because he or she hears words and praise being uttered (intended encouragement), but can sense through nonverbal communication that something is wrong. By the same token, living with a brain-injured person can be very frustrating and the TBI survivor can often be on the receiving end of any family member's frustration. It is the health care team's responsibility to educate the family and significant others on the best approach for giving feedback as the client embarks on the task of cognitive retraining in the home and community.

Table 7.3 is a list of common feelings and behaviors experienced by family members. In this example the outcome list is applicable to a situation where intervention was not provided.

Table 7.3 Feelings, Behaviors, and Outcomes without Intervention

Feelings	Behaviors	Outcomes
Gratitude for the TBI survivor	Dependency	Role reversal
Grief	Co-dependency	Crisis living
Panic	Enabling	Family breakdown
Fear	False praise	Confusion
Anxiety	Unrealistic expectations	Somatic complaints
Loss of control/doubt	Overprotection	Health problems
Regret	Covering up	Loss of self
Anger	Compensating for	Unsure of role
Sadness	Silence	Inability to express feelings
Loss	Acting out	Loss of life balance
Pain	Withdrawal	Lack of honesty
Guilt	Passivity	Push/pull in relationships
Denial	Aggression	Broken trust
Shame	Passive aggressive	Fixing
Low feelings of self-esteem	Depression	Abandonment
Loss of direction	Self-sabotage	Strained social situations
Depression	Blame self/others	Self-medicating, drugs, alcohol
Hopelessness	Stop expressing emotion	Divorce
Abandonment	Give conditional love	Illness
Resentment	Lack of insight	Loss of hope
Bitterness	Avoidance	Lost compass
Feeling trapped	Verbalization of resentment	Relationship breakdown

Outcomes with intervention: "Caregivers would greatly benefit from community or web-based family/caregiver support group programs, long-term case management services, ongoing family therapy, and assistance with daily household and family responsibilities" [50, p. 384].

IDEAL CONDITIONS FOR BEST CLINICAL OUTCOMES

1. A well co-ordinated hospital discharge meeting, including the hospital team, client, family, funder, and a member of the community team, who will become the case manager, is held.

2. A client day-pass and a home visit should be conducted with an occupational therapist prior to discharge.

3. All home safety issues, including renovations and vehicle modifications, should be completed prior to the client's discharge from hospital.

4. Funding and volunteers should be secured for the community portion of the rehabilitation plan (Chapters 13 and 14).

5. Education and recruitment of volunteers to assist with respite and attendant assistance outside the community program (Chapter 14) takes place.

6. Education on traumatic brain injury and risk factors for the family is provided.

7. Family supports, such as the following, should be in place:
   a. Home care for client
   b. Homemaker services, house cleaning, and meal preparation
   c. Child care
   d. Yard care
   e. Transportation to appointments and to rehabilitation activities
   f. Tutorial assistance for children
   g. Counseling for family
   h. Individual counseling for family members
   i. Couple counseling
   j. Client counseling
   k. A full community clinical team in place (Figure 3.7 in Chapter 3)

l. Advocacy for funding to meet the family's basic needs (Chapter 13)

   m. Introduction of client and family to local brain injury associations and support groups

OUTCOMES WITH CLINICAL INTERVENTION

1. Preservation of the dignity and motivation of the injured party and his or her loved ones

2. Maintenance of a home environment that is familiar to the client, setting him or her up for success

3. Provision of a safe place for the client to work on cognitive remediation

4. Preservation of family roles:

   a. The family unit stays together.

   b. The family members continue with their lives—school, work, etc.—for best outcomes.

   c. Family provides support to client as they continue with life with as much normalcy as possible.

5. Respect paid to the client and family members regarding the impact the stress has had on them in relation to their shared experience

6. Insight into the reality of the situation

7. Preservation of realistic hope

8. A strengthening of relationships accompanied by a deep respect of the shared core values

9. Each family member, including the TBI client, is involved in practicing a balanced lifestyle, maintaining insight, implementing stress reduction and energy conservation techniques, and accessing support

10. A family well versed on how to give feedback to the TBI survivor

SUMMARY

In this chapter we have explored the family system. We have reviewed examples of high-risk family systems. It is clear that the family unit of a brain-injured person is now at risk for dysfunction as a result of the family's trauma. We have seen in the case studies that the TAYLOR family had a full life before the incident of their loved one's traumatic brain injury. The literature review reveals the risks of role reversal for family members.

The case histories in this chapter give a practical example of the toll that a trauma such as a TBI can insidiously take on the family and how, despite the desire to assist in the loved one's recovery, maladaptive coping mechanisms can infiltrate the family relationships silently, moving them to dysfunction.

We have discussed the inherent inter-relationship of how feelings and behaviors such as giving unrealistic praise can impact the therapeutic outcome for the client and sustainability of the family unit.

We have reviewed the ideal conditions for the client's return home, putting supports in place to move on to our next stage of the *Lefaivre Rainbow Effect:* the **intervention** stage.

CHAPTER 8

Intervention

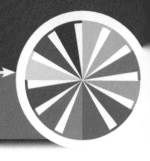

TOTAL SUM	–	DIAGNOSIS (LOSS)	+	INTERVENTION	=	RESIDUAL LOSS
				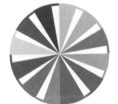		

INTRODUCTION

This is the exciting chapter—the one where we actually begin the intervention, the cognitive retraining. Each step taken to arrive at the stage of intervention has been carefully and skillfully managed so as to set the intervention stage up for success. Let us review how we reached this point.

SETTING THE STAGE FOR THE INTERVENTION

1. An extensive interview has revealed the client's pre-injury profile, which will serve as the template for the intervention.
2. Information has been gathered in each segment of the pie.
3. All medical assessments and reports have been completed in a timely fashion and have been reviewed by each member of the team.
4. The clinical reports will examine the diagnostic and functional losses realized by the client.
5. The impact of the client's losses on the family will be managed through advocating for funds or recruiting volunteers, allowing for service provision to reduce their stress and maintain their pre-injury lives.

6. The family and significant others will have received education and will have been provided written information to take home.

7. The client and family will be educated on the importance of keeping "life as usual," in particular as it relates to their pre-injury roles.

8. The client and family have been introduced to support systems such as their local brain injury associations.

ASSUMPTIONS

The following assumptions will be taken into consideration as we embark on the road to recovery with our clients:

1. Old information (meaning pre-injury likes, hobbies, activities, occupation, and interests), should be the framework upon which the therapy is designed. This old information appears to be more easily integrated by the injured brain, possibly because of the memory component.

2. Specifically chosen, well-matched one-to-one workers under the direction of the professional team are the most cost-effective personnel to provide the intensive repetition of activity to facilitate relearning or remediation of a task.

3. The one-to-one workers should be individually selected for each client, matching age, interest, and gender, and should be trained specifically regarding each individual client's condition.

4. We assume that the brain has the capacity to relearn or learn a task in a new and different way.

5. If there is structural damage that is permanent (the author is calling this lesional damage), then another part of the brain can take over components of this task learning in a new way.

6. If there is damage causing intermittent cognitive transmission of information (the author is calling this functional damage), then through repetition the brain has the capacity to relearn.

7. The environment can be adapted to promote new learning.

8. Therapeutic aids, adaptations, modifications, therapeutic devices, and augmentative communication systems can facilitate relearning.

There are many wonderful anatomy and physiology books on the market. The general structure and functions of the brain have been widely researched and well documented. I encourage the reader to find a well-versed and reputable anatomy text that outlines the associated functional features of the brain and how these characteristics translate to cognition, emotion, and behavior. You may also choose to visit the suggested reading section at the end of this book.

The literature is clear that the brain and its structures are interconnected. Because of this interconnection any given aspect of a cognitive, emotional, or behavioral task may be influenced by several areas of the brain. For the purpose of having a discussion on cognitive retraining, the author has included a cursory outline of some of the basic anatomical features of the brain as well as the resulting function.

It is important for the clinician to be able to anticipate and then analyze a client's performance based on the information provided on the etiology of the brain trauma; in doing so the clinician will have the advantage of radiologic imaging which may have shown areas of brain damage as well as neuropsychological assessments revealing areas of defect. Despite these diagnostic measures, when it comes to actual performance the outcome may be unanticipated, not only because of the brain damage but also because of the environmental stimuli.

THE BRAIN—A BRIEF OVERVIEW

The brain is an amazing and complicated structure. Everything we think, feel, imagine, and act upon and our movements, personality, intellect, and performance are managed by our brain (see Figure 8.1 and Table 8.1). The brain is a relatively small structure given the enormous job it has to perform.

The brain is fragile and is protected by three connective tissue membranes, also known as meninges: the dura mater, the arachnoid mater, and the pia mater. The brain is also cushioned by cerebrospinal fluid, which nourishes and protects the brain. And of course the brain is encased by the skull.

As community clinicians we will have been issued all of the available diagnostic and medical reports to date. It is important that we can translate these scientific reports into what it will mean for the client functionally. Given the nature of each specific brain injury, the clinical team will be able to anticipate the problem areas for the client. It is to this end that a brief description of certain areas of the brain and the related function have been included.

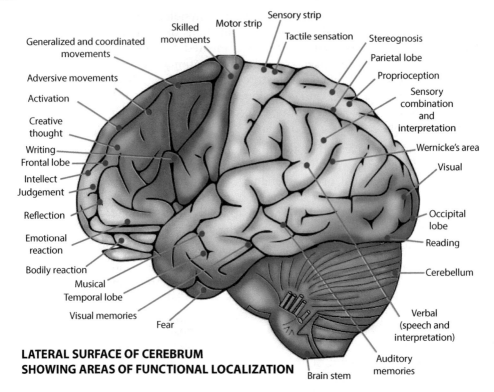

Generalized and coordinated movements

Adversive movements

Activation

Creative thought

Writing

Frontal lobe

Intellect

Judgement

Reflection

Emotional reaction

Bodily reaction

Musical

Temporal lobe

Visual memories

Fear

Skilled movements

Motor strip

Sensory strip

Tactile sensation

Stereognosis

Parietal lobe

Proprioception

Sensory combination and interpretation

Wernicke's area

Visual

Occipital lobe

Reading

Cerebellum

Verbal (speech and interpretation)

Auditory memories

Brain stem

**LATERAL SURFACE OF CEREBRUM
SHOWING AREAS OF FUNCTIONAL LOCALIZATION**

Figure 8.1 Brain function diagram.

Cerebrum

The right and left hemispheres comprise the cerebrum. It is believed that sight, perception, aspects of memory, thought, sensation, movement, and other forms of conscious behavior are processed here. The cerebrum can use past experiences or memories to strategize future decisions.

Cerebral Cortex

This area is of a higher function, allowing us to think and reason. It is this area that impacts our conscious decision making and planning.

Cerebellum

The cerebellum is the part of the brain that deals with unconscious coordination and balance—the "gymnast" of the brain. As another part of the brain initiates movement, this part of the brain assists in the execution. It also influences posture. The cerebellum assesses the position of the body in relation to sensory stimuli.

Table 8.1 Brain Function Table

	Function
Frontal lobe	• Voluntary movement • Problem solving • Personality and emotion • Initiation and judgment • Receptive speech center (Broca's area) • Memory • Sexual behavior • Planning • Behavior • Concentration • Impulse control • Thought
Parietal lobe	• Movement • Touch • Pain • Temperature • Somatic sensation • Orientation to space • Sensory processing and integration • Integration of sensory information from different lobes • Spatial processing • Memory • Interprets language and words
Occipital lobe	• Visual processing • Discrimination of movement • Color recognition
Temporal lobe	• Expressive language • Sequencing • Memory • Audition • Visual perception • Language processing • Vestibular and equilibrium processing • Personality
Cerebellum	• Balance and coordination
Brain stem	• Autonomic functions • Attention • Short-term memory
Limbic system	• Regulates emotion

Prefrontal Cortex

This area helps regulate emotions. This rational part of the brain controls impulses and self-control and participates in higher functions such as reasoning and judgment.

Brain Stem

The brain stem's activities, such as breathing, blood pressure and heart rate, sneezing, coughing, and hiccupping, occur without conscious awareness of these functions; they are automatic.

Wernicke's Area

This area of the brain is involved with receptive language; this is where we process our understanding of what someone else is saying to us.

Broca's Area

This area is thought to be involved in speech generation, involving the muscle movement required to form speech sounds, including the throat, tongue, and lips.

Limbic System

The limbic system deals with emotion and may be referred to as the "emotional" brain. This area deals with basic emotions such as fear, pain, pleasure, sexual excitement, anger, sadness, and much more. The structures of the brain interact closely with each other. In the case of the limbic system, there is a close relationship with the cerebral cortex. This allows the brain to process not just emotion but also the thought accompanying the emotion. Some memory is also processed in the limbic system; it is thought that areas within the limbic system take on new memories (short term) and convert them into long-term memories.

The limbic system has several parts, including:

1. The hippocampus is thought to participate in memory and learning.
2. The amygdala is thought to be in association with feelings of fear and aggression; it also appears to be linked to olfactory senses.
3. The hypothalamus is thought to influence hunger, thirst and body temperature as well as the ability to retain and learn new information. It is also thought to influence sleep cycles and, in concert with other areas of the brain,

is involved with emotion such as fear, aggression, sexual behavior, and other basic drives. This area also triggers a hormonal response from other areas of the brain such as the pituitary gland.

4. The thalamus relays sensory data; some of this information is autonomic, participating in arousal, memory, and awareness.

Cranial Nerves

Our clients will present with a myriad of symptoms as we observe their challenges with certain aspects of task performance in the community. It is important to be able to describe the client's challenge to the specialist in the respective area, such as the neurologist or physiatrist. To this end, a brief overview of the cranial nerves is also included to remind the clinician of symptoms that would be related to nerve damage.

There are 12 pairs of cranial nerves; within them are sensory, motor, and autonomic nerves:

1. Olfactory sensory nerve: smell transmitting olfactory stimuli

2. Optic sensory nerve: transmitting visual stimuli

3. Oculomotor nerve: supplies four of the six muscles that move the eyeball

4. Trochlear nerve: supplies a muscle that moves the eyeball

5. Trigeminal nerve: carries sensation from areas of the face and moves the muscles used for chewing

6. Abducens nerve: supplies a muscle that controls the eyeball in one direction

7. Facial nerve: feeds the muscle that allows us to make facial expressions

8. Vestibulocochlear nerve: the sensory nerve that transmits information pertaining to hearing and balance

9. Glossopharyngeal nerve: impacts taste derived from the tongue and impacts the pharynx in relation to swallowing

10. Vagus nerve: supplies several organs, including the thorax and abdomen, and impacts heart rate

11. Accessory nerve: supplies structures in the throat and some neck muscles and is involved in the control of the head, neck, and voice

12. Hypoglossal nerve: supplies the muscles of the tongue and controls movement of the tongue

LIMBIC SYSTEM

Case Example 1

Bob is a high-energy 20-year-old who loves his sports. He finds himself in a confrontation with Jack in a disagreement about the outcome of a football game where, in Jack's opinion, a referee made a bad call. The discussion escalates, reaching a crescendo when Jack makes a critical statement about Bob's knowledge of football rules. Bob sees red when he hears this insult and experiences the emotions of anger and agitation. The limbic system introduces thought to this scenario; Bob can reason how to express himself appropriately in this situation.

One can see that if the limbic system (Figure 8.2) has been damaged, then the ability to make good choices controlling emotions as well as the accompanying behavior may be impaired. Without intervention and education, those closest to the TBI client may find this deficit extremely difficult to live with. Not surprisingly, persons with this problem may find themselves in trouble, at times facing legal consequences. In the case of mild and sometimes moderate traumatic brain injury, little if any attention may have been paid to the client's increasing difficulty in social situations. It is not uncommon to hear that a loved one "is just not the same" after a fall. There are cases where clients may not have gone to emergency or, if they did, they were not admitted to hospital. In these cases the client is returned home without the education and support that is necessary to assist him or her to recover and to assist loved ones in becoming aware of why the behavior changes have occurred. This may be part of the reason for the increase in TBI cases being seen in the criminal justice system and homeless organizations. Bearing in mind that second and third brain injuries have a greater probability of occurrence after the first, if the initial brain injury goes unattended and the client and family are not educated, the outcome can be grim.

Mild to moderate TBI cases can frequently fly under the radar of appropriate intervention, particularly if there is no third-party liability or physical impairment to raise awareness to the situation. In these cases, without a diagnosis and appropriate intervention, the client will often report feelings of being misunderstood and can go on to live a life of social, occupational, and relational impairment and desperation. This is why, in the final chapter of the book, the author suggests that it would be prudent to screen for TBI wherever social maladaptation is observed in an individual in educational, prison, and homeless settings. The frequently coined term "the walking wounded" is aptly placed on this very unique and commonly misunderstood population.

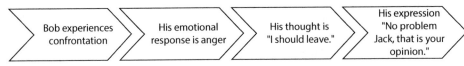

Figure 8.2 Limbic system: introducing thought to emotion.

MEMORY

> ### Case Example 2: Olfactory and Emotional Memories
>
> It is Thanksgiving; Sarah has been away at university and is returning home to her parents' house for the weekend. Just the very thought of Thanksgiving brings up happy memories for Sarah. As the day approaches she can imagine the smell of turkey and the warm feelings of seeing her aunts, uncles, and grandparents. Thanksgiving has always been a happy time for her as the family relaxes with good food and then long walks with her beloved grandpa. As Sarah arrives at the house she opens the door as wafting smells of roasting turkey and cranberry aromas tantalize her senses. She immediately begins to relax, feeling safe and loved as she goes to the kitchen to hug her mother. This example serves to exemplify how senses and emotion also participate in imprinting the memory. This is why the total sum section in the *Lefaivre Rainbow Effect* is so important. We, the health care providers, need to understand what has created memory for our clients. We can use the extensive history to better understand emotional and sensory triggers.

Obviously negative memories associated with sensory triggers should be avoided:

> ### Case Example 3: Negative Memories Associated with Olfactory Smells
>
> Anne was assaulted one day in Central Park. Ever since that day, the smell of freshly cut grass triggers a negative emotional reaction. This is important information; as we begin cognitive retraining we will be stimulating the brain including sensory and olfactory senses. The history taking is important, segregating out bad memories from good memories. Good memories and happy occasions associated with smell, taste, and touch will serve as invaluable information for the community clinical team. Bad memories will associate negative triggers and should be avoided.

Case Example 4: Tactile and Auditory Memories

Johnny is an only child; he would have loved a brother or sister but his mom and dad were busy professionals and only wanted one child. Johnny has a nanny whom he quite likes but she does not want to play much. Johnny spends a great deal of time with Mittens, his cat. Mittens follows Johnny around everywhere as though he were a young puppy. At night as his parents are working late again, Johnny sheds a tear of loneliness and derives comfort from petting Mittens. Mittens reciprocates with a warm lick and purrs Johnny to sleep. To this day, as an adult John finds comfort in petting animals and the purr of a cat will lull him to sleep anytime. This example shows how a tactile stimulus is involved in the creation of a memory, which produces an emotion. Any part of this experience—the smell of a cat, the tactile stimulation of fur, the sound of a cat purring—further imprints the memory.

Case Example 5: Auditory and Emotional Memory

Mary is a young nurse who was raised in a family where her father was mentally ill. Because of her father's illness, his emotions were not in check. Without provocation, at any given time Mary's dad could go on a tirade; he would raise his voice and yell for extended periods of time. Mary felt fear and uncertainty coupled with frustration and anger at the injustice of her father's verbal assaults. To this day, even as an adult if Mary is in the presence of someone who raises his or her voice she begins to panic, experiencing the same reaction that she did as a child when her father would rage.

SENSORY OVERLOAD: ANALOGY OF A BREAKER BOX

Let us think of the brain as the master breaker box in a house. If you look at the panel in the breaker box, there is an array of complex wires that come from the central panel and are distributed to various regions throughout the house. Each electrical outlet has its source of power delegated to a specific area despite that it originated from the master panel in the breaker box.

Case Example 6: Breaker Box Analogy—Sensory Overload

Mary and Jack have a large family of five children Mary spends a great deal of her day cooking, cleaning, and doing laundry. Mary has always loved the house that they built before their children were born, but she does get frustrated with one mysterious aspect of the home's electrical wiring. Mary can be cooking in the kitchen and have the coffee pot plugged in, the toaster turned on, and the dishwasher running. Nine times out of ten when this daily routine happens it occurs uneventfully. But, periodically, the breaker is tripped up. Mary and her husband have had several electricians in to examine the situation, to no avail. What is confusing for the couple is that as periodic as this experience is, it also happens with a certain amount of regularity. If they review the past year, the breaker has tripped at least a dozen times. This is frustrating and unnerving for the family as the breaker sometimes blows at the most inopportune times. Last year Mary was in the final stages of making Christmas dinner; the turkey was not quite cooked and the electricity went out yet again. After this event Jack decided that they would create a variety of circumstances that, by experience, they knew seemed to trigger this electrical short. They plugged in the toaster, ran the coffee maker, and turned on the dishwasher, but nothing happened. They then added in the electric can opener—again, nothing. They plugged in the blender—again, nothing. Then they thought maybe there was a load of laundry running each time the breaker blew, so they turned on the washing machine— again to no avail. As they sat down to have a cup of coffee and mull over the mystery of the breaker box, their daughter Sandy turned on the vacuum to clean her room, and the breaker blew.

This scenario is very similar to what happens with brain-injured clients. They can find themselves in a situation where they can successfully complete a given task and it is completed with accuracy and precision. This would indicate that the areas of the brain required to carry out this task are intact and functioning well. The same task can be attempted on a different day under similar circumstances and yet be met with failure. There is some dimension—whether it is **fatigue,** increased **environmental stimuli,** or **emotional overload**—that causes the clients on some days to be unable to execute a task successfully that in the past they could complete with ease. As the community health care team, we need to be keenly aware that the home and community are not controlled environments. There are other people living in the home, creating activity, noise, and emotional responses. The family will need to be aware that in creating external stimuli, inasmuch as we want to make every attempt to keep life as usual, adjustments may need to be made to set the client up for success.

> ## Case Example 7: Receptive Language—Sensory Overload
>
> Amy sustained a traumatic brain injury 5 months ago; it is known that the Wernicke's area in her brain sustained some damage. Amy has been working with the speech pathologist and is making headway in the area of receptive language in a clinical office environment. Rhyming and using word associations are proving to be helpful therapeutic tools. It has, however, been frustrating for Amy to try to comprehend what people are saying to her when she is at home. She is getting much better when she is talking to a person one on one; however, at home her younger teenage brother continues to play music in his room while her father is watching football on TV in the living room. These heightened auditory stimuli are causing Amy to become discouraged and confused as she attempts to understand what her mother is telling her in the kitchen. Amy becomes agitated and retreats to the basement. Her mother misunderstands Amy's silence and withdrawal and goes downstairs to suggest to Amy that she come to the living room and relax with her father and watch the game.

This is a realistic example of how one symptom in a myriad of eclectic brain functions can cause havoc. In this case, the family required education on Amy's receptive language problem. Amy's younger brother now uses a head set; Amy's dad has moved the TV further away from the main living area and kitchen to the basement and he turns the volume down. In addition, the family has been educated on speaking with Amy face to face; this additional visual cue, where Amy can assess facial expressions and body language, will assist in improving her auditory comprehension.

As Amy moves toward a vocational plan, she will be aware that receptive language can be a tricky point for her. When choosing a career, she will select an occupation where she can work in a quiet environment. When communicating, she will orchestrate personal face-to-face meetings, face time, or Skype as a better choice for her than the telephone, where there is no additional visual information.

Sensory overload is a common occurrence for the traumatically brain injured. For the health care professional, it can be difficult to sort out what is causing the sensory overload. The preceding example reviewed that auditory stimuli can result in sensory overload for someone with receptive language difficulties.

When **sensory overload** occurs for a TBI client, the resulting **behavior changes** can be confusing for those around them. It is not uncommon for a brain-injured person to have **crying spells,**

outbursts, verbal frustration, agitation, anxiety, depression, anger, loss of confidence, and withdrawal. The confusing aspect is that these might be **symptoms of the TBI** but they can also be **symptoms of sensory overload.** This is why it is so important to understand and observe what activities the client was engaging in before these symptoms occurred. If these symptoms are intermittent, then the clinician must unravel the work that the client's brain had engaged in prior to the exhibition of symptoms. Let us look at another example of sensory overload.

Case Example 8: Visual Sensory Overload

Barbra, who suffered a moderate brain injury 2 months ago, has been working on meal preparation. She has advanced to the point that she can now, with consistency, attend to all aspects of preparing a four-step simple meal. She is excited to show her visiting sister how she has progressed and is planning on making dinner for her tonight. Molly, her sister, has been visiting Barbra for a week. One day they discussed how nice it would be to freshen up Barbra's old kitchen. For fun, they looked at wallpaper and Barbra fell in love with a country print that was peppered with ripe cherries.

Barbra was out during the day, so Molly thought this was a wonderful time to surprise Barbra. She went to work putting up the cherry wallpaper in an effort to surprise Barbra; she was surprised with how many cherries there were once two walls were covered. It was, however, cheerful and gave the kitchen the facelift it needed.

When Barbra returned home after a restful day, she attempted to make dinner and could not proceed; she was overwhelmed and felt discouraged. She could not remember where the pots and pans were and she missed ingredients. Barbra was confused and agitated. When analyzed, this was a task that Barbra had successfully completed several times before. What was different this time? The wallpaper was all they could think of. After 2 weeks of unsuccessful attempts at meal preparation, they decided to take down the wallpaper and—voila—Barbra immediately felt calmer and was able to focus and become more organized in her thinking. Barbra was once again able to prepare a simple four-step meal. This is a wonderful example of how the increased visual stimuli negatively impacted Barbra's memory, sequencing, and organizational performance, making her success limited. The confusion of Barbra's intermittent success in cooking was solved. Barbra had success when there were limited visual stimuli and failure when there were increased visual stimuli.

SOME CAUSES OF SENSORY OVERLOAD

1. **Fatigue:** brain-injured clients will frequently be fatigued; this can cause sensory overload. It is important to grade the therapeutic goals into small, measurable steps, slowly increasing the client's physical and cognitive stamina. It is also important to understand the best time of day to engage in activities requiring cognitive, physical, and emotional energy. Sleep disturbance also needs to be addressed by the appropriate professional.
2. An increase of **visual stimuli** can cause sensory overload.
3. An increase of **auditory stimuli** can cause sensory overload.
4. Too much **physical activity** resulting in fatigue can cause sensory overload.
5. **Emotional** interactions can cause sensory overload.
6. **Pain** such as persistent headaches can limit the client's energy, predisposing him or her to sensory overload. (See additional resource material, Family Handouts Sensory Overload at http://www.crcpress.com/product/isbn/9781482228243.)

ENERGY CONSERVATION (See additional resource material, Family Handouts Energy Conservation at http://www.crcpress.com/product/isbn/9781482228243.)

Fatigue

Fatigue can be a problem for a person who has sustained a traumatic brain injury. It is important to manage and conserve energy to avoid sensory overload.

Let us assume that we have 100 units of energy a day. Let us think of our units of energy as money that we will withdraw from our bank account. There is $100 in the bank daily to be spent on expending energy, engaging in activity, or engaging in rest and relaxation, which will save energy. So we have $100 dollars each day to spend on the energy that we expend. If our client has a disrupted sleep, he may have spent $25 during the night. For someone with a TBI that is just relearning to dress, make the bed, and brush teeth, it may cost $45 in energy even before breakfast. Breakfast may take another $10 in energy; attending a physical therapy appointment may take another $30 of energy. In this case, even before the afternoon, this client has gone over the daily allotment of energy expenditure and is now in an overdraft position, which is synonymous with sensory overload (Table 8.2).

Table 8.2 Energy Conservation Banking Analogy

Bank account	Debit	Deposit
		$100
Disrupted sleep	$25	
Morning preparation	$45	
Breakfast	$10	
Physical therapy	$30	
Total	−$10	

Just like a bank account, when the account is overdrawn, there will be penalties and fees.

This day positions the client to experience sensory overload. If the client continues day after day expending more energy output than his or her body can afford, then he or she will continue to be in a mode of sensory overload, thus negatively impacting the therapeutic plan. If we think again of our energy in monetary terms, going over budget consistently will ultimately cause bankruptcy. If a client is consistently being overstimulated in any of the previously mentioned areas—**fatigue, visual, auditory, physical, emotional or pain**—then he or she also will be bankrupt of energy and unable to benefit fully from the therapeutic plan. The more serious implication is when there has been ongoing sensory overload, which can lead to depression, fatigue, hopelessness, and, in some cases, suicidal ideation.

Visual Energy Conservation

Organization and structure are of key importance for the client who is engaging in cognitive remediation. It is highly suggested that the environments where the client will be living be orderly. It may even be prudent to engage a cleaning company to assist with providing order to the home. It is a balancing act for the team: They want the environment to be familiar to the client; however, an environment that is visually overstimulating will not be conducive to cognitive retraining. The organization of the home can be a project that the client and the rehabilitation worker engage in together to give the client a sense of ownership and control. The purpose is to have designated areas for frequently used items such as a purse, keys, or wallet. Items used in any room should be stored in that same room. In regard to clothing, it is a good idea to divide the clothes into sections such as for casual, work, exercise, and evening wear as well as seasonal use for spring, summer, winter, and fall. Above all else, clutter should be minimized to avoid visual and sensory overload.

Auditory Sensory Overload

It is a good idea to educate those sharing the same living space with the client that reducing auditory stimulation, at least in the early stages, is favorable. In the event that it is necessary to have music or the television turned on, be observant of changes in the brain-injured survivor's behavior and emotions. If the client resides in an area where there is a great deal of external noise, such as highway noise, honking cars, or trains passing, this may be an issue and, again, continued observations are in order.

All parties involved with the TBI client should be aware that even the slightest noise they may be inadvertently making, such as finger or pencil tapping or leg shaking, can have adverse effects on the client's ability to focus and integrate information. It is not recommended to have music or the radio playing in the clinician's office, particularly in the waiting room or the area where the client will be tested. It is important to be aware of environmental noises such as leaky faucets or ceiling fans that are not balanced; these items should be repaired to avoid sensory overload of the client. When speaking to the client, avoid rapid speech or giving too much information at one time. It is a useful habit to have the client paraphrase back and clarify his or her understanding of your meaning.

Physical Overload

As previously mentioned, the client may find himself or herself fatigued; disrupted sleep can also be a symptom of traumatic brain injury. As the clinical team sets physical goals, which are necessary to build endurance and increase stamina, it is imperative that all team members are aware of the other demands placed on the client so that an organized physical program can be integrated into the client's overall therapy plan without overloading and causing excess fatigue for the client. Ensure that the client paces himself or herself in clinical sessions and encourage the client to apprise you of feelings of fatigue or agitation. For the health care provider, break down your sessions into time frames that are easily managed for the client; ask if the client is fatigued. Focus the client on one task at a time. If you notice that the client is losing attention, ask what is going on for him or her and encourage the client to be honest about how he or she feels. This will assist the client to gain insight and understanding of the effect that the environment can and will have on his or her ability to function.

Emotional Overload

We have extensively reviewed the stressful situation the brain-injured client and family find themselves in. It is of paramount importance that the stress be managed for all family members as well as the client. Pre-injury roles should remain intact and protected. Ensure that the client has adequate support in place to facilitate his or her participation in the therapy plan. It is very common when emotions run high that cognitive retraining is compromised as the client is emotionally overloaded. In light of the increased incidence of family breakdown and burnout, it is easy to see how the family's inability to cope with the potential emotional outcome of the situation could compromise the client's ability to engage in cognitive retraining. Counseling should be made available to any and all family members who require assistance adjusting to the new circumstances they find themselves in.

Pain Can Lead to Sensory Overload

We have reviewed in the section on energy conservation that we have a limited number of units of energy a day to spend. Pain can exact a terrible toll on a person, couple that with the confusion spawned from the brain injury and it is a difficult combination that frequently leads to sensory overload. Pain can sabotage the best rehabilitation plan. The physiatrist and, in particular, the neurologist should be called in to problem solve the best means of eradicating the client's pain. In some cases, it may be appropriate to advocate that the client attend an intensive pain management program where the ever increasing strategies to manage pain can be implemented as the cognitive retraining commences, thus decreasing the risk of failure and frustration for the client.

Summary to Sensory Overload

In summary to our review of sensory overload, the brain can become overloaded with too much stimulation—not too dissimilarly to the breaker box analogy. When a variety of stimuli charge the brain to produce a reaction or result, we challenge all of these interconnections within the brain to work in union to produce the desired outcome. If, through this process, a part of the brain that has been damaged has received stimulation, we may observe suboptimal results. Or if there is simply too much stimulation, the brain (again, not unlike the breaker box in a house) may "trip" and the client will display symptoms of being overloaded—for example, fatigue, agitation, withdrawal, or anger that again results in suboptimal results. In extreme cases of ongoing sensory overload, the client may express thoughts of suicide and feelings of depression and hopelessness. It is important that family members living with the client receive education on all aspects and types of sensory overload.

In the realm of community rehabilitation we, the health care providers, will experience the unique opportunity to observe the client carry out tasks in real home, community, work, and play situations. We will commence our therapy plan with small, goal-directed steps that, on the scale of probabilities, will be met with clinical success. As we increase the complexity of the task, we may be surprised at areas of challenge experienced by the client. It is here that we will return to basic functional anatomy. Because several areas of the brain are involved with any given task at one time, as we increase the cognitive demands with multifocused stimuli we may see an unanticipated change in function. If we carefully review the sensory and cognitive input and behavioral output, we can make a link or connection to what has made the task unachievable. It is through careful observation and documentation that sensory overload can be carefully examined and avoided.

Lesional Damage

For the purpose of this discussion the author refers to permanent structural damage as lesional. Imagine a severed spinal cord; despite effort, intention, and willpower, the severed spinal cord will not be able to transmit the nerve impulse to exact the desired goal of mobility. In this case, it does not matter how many times the client repeats the intent to walk: It will not successfully be executed. Lesional damage as it pertains to traumatic brain injury would functionally and consistently—not intermittently—be met with an unsuccessful outcome.

In the case of lesional damage, where there is a consistent unsuccessful outcome, the clinician will quickly want to modify the task and/or the environment and challenge a different part of the brain to process the information in a new way, to ensure success for the client. An example of this would be instead of giving verbal instructions, give a visual, functional demonstration of how to carry out the task.

Functional Damage

Again, for the purpose of this discussion, the author refers to intermittent success as functional damage. In the case of functional damage, in some instances a task can be carried out with no adverse consequence; however, in another circumstance the same task will be met with failure. Because the task has been successfully accomplished before, we can surmise that the areas of the brain required to execute this task are intact; therefore, the cause of the intermittent performance will be assigned to sensory overload.

In the case of functional damage, the clinical team will carefully observe the circumstances that offer the client the opportunity to complete positive execution of the task. For the purpose of relearning, we will be careful to avoid sensory overload and replicate the positive circumstance to repeat successful completion of the task.

Repetition

When a client is embarking on the journey of relearning it is a bit like starting a car. The battery may not be fully charged, having been left to sit for several months. The keys are in the ignition and, on first attempt, the engine will not turn over, but after several sputtering attempts, the engine will eventually turn over and start running consistently. It is the same for the brain that is healing and relearning. In the early stages, Tom was just coming out of his coma and, much to the dismay of his wife, Amanda, he did not recognize her; however, after weeks of visiting Tom and clarifying who she was, Tom was able to identify Amanda as his wife. Let us refer back to the analogy of the burn (Table 5.1 in Chapter 5), where we suggest that natural healing in the beginning stages can be coupled with relearning. Tom's brain was naturally healing; however, with the use of reminders such as looking at wedding pictures and Amanda repeatedly introducing herself as his wife, Tom was able to recall and identify his spouse accurately.

These examples beget the question for the community clinicians: How do we know the measure of stimuli to introduce into a staged plan for the client to carry out?

Thus far in the process we know that old familiar positive stimuli will be easier for the client to remember and thus successfully carry out tasks. We will also know about structural damage in the brain from the MRI, CAT, PET, and SPECT scans and can set goals accordingly. We will be versed in the areas most impacted by the traumatic brain injury through study of the radiological and diagnostic reports and the neuropsychological assessment. To gingerly side step sensory overloading the client, the team will:

1. Assign an age, interest, and gender appropriate one-to one-rehabilitation worker who will carry out the team's program.

2. We will start with small directed goals based on previous positive experiences that are meaningful to the client and that the entire team agrees with and has input on. Just like the brain having many areas of expertise, so does the community clinical team; we need to draw upon the interrelationship of the professional expertise involved in any client's care.

3. The team will be educated on therapeutic strategies as suggested by each respective discipline pursuant to the client's unique symptoms. For instance, for expressive language difficulties the speech pathologist will set out the guidelines that will be followed by the family and the team. For re-entry into the work force the

occupational therapist, the vocational consultant, and the neuropsychologist will outline the intervention strategy.

4. We will be aware of any demands that may be placed on the client outside the clinical team.

5. We will be aware of individual appointments that the client is required to attend.

SETTING GOALS

A good goal will be meaningful to the client. We have handled this aspect by understanding the client well through the history-taking exercise and anticipating that what was revealed as meaningful in the past will be meaningful in the future, even if the goal needs to be adapted and the environment modified:

Goals should be **positive**—something the client will do rather than stop doing.

Goals should be **specific** with a time, place, and a duration attached so that they can be measured.

Goals should be **behavioral** rather than a feeling.

Positive: I will go for a walk.

Specific: I will go for a walk along the water's edge with Sally every Monday, Wednesday, and Friday at 10 a.m. for 30 minutes.

Behavior: Walking is a behavior that results in a feeling: "I feel energized, happy, like I'm getting stronger after I go for a walk." It is easier to measure a behavior than a feeling.

The goals that are selected in the initial stages of the community rehabilitation plan should be selected on the basis of the client's ability to achieve them successfully, as well as the client's priorities and the team's preference on which cognitive deficit to focus on first.

The clinical team ultimately will select goals from a few of the segments of the pie—in the initial stages, selecting goals with the least risk of failure, adverse social and emotional impact, and sensory overload, and with the highest probability of success. It is appropriate to select from three areas of the pie initially and then to increase the program to include all segments of the pie as the client continues to build a solid database of successfully executed skills.

The goal attainment scale (GAS) was first developed by Kiresuk and Sherman [54]. Goal attainment scaling is a general method for evaluating comprehensive community mental health programs; it was initially created for use in the mental health system in the United States.

Table 8.3 Goal Chart

A. Better than expected
B. Expected
C. Less than expected

Source: Lefaivre, C. 2013. Amended goal attainment scale.
Unpublished; used with permission.

The model of setting goals as used in the *Lefaivre Rainbow Effect* has been extensively modified for use with the traumatically brain injured. Given the unique nature of this approach, the **total sum** or the pre-injury self is one of the sources of information to select the goals from, based on pre-injury memories, successes, likes, and interests. The second source of information to assist in the selection of goals is the symptoms resulting from the traumatic brain injury. The third item influencing the selection of goals is the client's priorities.

Similarly to the original version of the goal attainment scale, there are graded levels of accomplishment. There are three possible levels of accomplishment. They are shown in Table 8.3.

1. The selected goals are meaningful to the client **total sum** based on life before the TBI.
2. The selected goals are targeted at remediating a cognitive deficit through repetition of the task.
3. The repetition is observed, cued, or demonstrated by a one-to-one rehabilitation worker.
4. The selected goals are suggested by the team; inclusive in the goals are rehabilitation strategies in cooperation and agreement with the client and family.
5. The selected goals are color coded based on the nature of the goal and pursuant to the color-coded pie segments (Figure 4.4 in Chapter 4).
6. The selected goals are tracked along with the other daily tasks that the client engages in, and all tasks are color coded by the worker to the color-coded segment of the pie to track the balance of the client's life.
7. The one-to-one worker will observe how the client strategizes to accomplish any given goal and will document through observation how successfully the goal was accomplished, as well as the therapeutic measures taken to accomplish the goal.
8. The one-to-one worker will be educated by the team on how to handle the situation if the client is having trouble accomplishing the goal and the worker will

know when and how to cue the client or suggest withdrawal from the task.

9. The written observations, as well as the color-coded weekly schedule and the goal sheets will be submitted to the case manager for review with the worker on a weekly basis.

10. The case manager will determine when the clinical team needs to revisit which new goals should be assigned as the client successfully, through repetition and modification, learns each given task.

11. The aim is to reduce any stress symptoms and to return the client to a life of balance and homeostasis. When the color-coded weekly schedule is in balance, we should see that the stress symptoms have been managed and that the relearning phase has been successfully executed. Thus, *the rainbow is in effect!*

As the program evolves, the goals become more challenging. The program can become more difficult by increasing the difficulty of the task, increasing the amount of time spent on the same task, or changing the task altogether to something more complex.

The program will be met with some success and some challenges. If the goal appears too hard, try getting the worker to engage in more repetitions of the task, or if the client appears tired or expresses fatigue, take a break and then revisit the task. If there are still suboptimal results, then have the worker demonstrate the task or provide cues for the client; the worker may also at this point introduce modifications or make a change to the environment as directed by the clinician. There is a delicate balance of motivating and continuing to motivate the client while challenging and inspiring him or her to try to accomplish new tasks—thus the imperative need for a solid therapeutic rapport with our clients. The client's trust in the clinical team at this stage is critical. One can see that if the clinical team changes, this would be detrimental to the client. As we know, failure can be a major deterrent; it is because of this that we choose goals that have meaning to the client. It is also the reason that the clinical team, especially in the early stages, chooses goals that have the least risk of adverse social consequences such as embarrassment or rejection.

We now have the program in place; the worker has been chosen, the initial goals have been set, and the worker will need to observe carefully how the client engages in the tasks assigned to him or her. It is uncomfortable to have the worker document written observations as the client is attempting tasks in real-life situations. The worker will be skilled in making observations without having the client feel like he or she is on display by documenting after the worker departs from the client. The worker will require clear guidelines from the clinical team regarding what to look for. To encourage ease, the worker may carry a memory card that can be dictated into in order to relay key words used later to document the observations. It is important that the worker only document the observation of how the client's brain strategizes a task and not interpret the behavior. The interpretation is the job of the professional clinical team. When making observations, the following should be included if observed.

OBSERVATIONS

1. How did the client approach the task?
2. Was the effort met with success the first time? If not, how many attempts were required until the task was successfully executed?
3. If the client did not experience success, what were the circumstances, including environmental stimuli?
4. Did the situation improve with cueing or the introduction of aids and adaptations?
5. How did the client emotionally respond to the attempt (e.g., joyful, sad, withdrawn, or discouraged)?
6. What else was going on during the last 2 days that the client verbally expressed may be influencing his or her performance?

Example of One-to-One Worker's Observation Notes

Physical

Jane was reluctant to walk at 9 a.m. daily; she complained of feeling fatigued and was nervous that her neighbors would see her. She did, however, walk all 3 days and in fact met a neighbor on Wednesday. When the neighbor gave Jane a warm embrace, she was eager to go out the next day in the hope that she would see her neighbor again. Jane indicated how much she liked her neighbor and thought that when she felt better she could ask the neighbor to have tea with her. Jane also went to the gym with her one-to-one worker; she expressed that she feels stronger and is enjoying going to the gym.

Cognitive

Jane continues to find reading an arduous chore. She has set aside time to read the paper; she does this early in the morning before the family rises. She states that she can concentrate better when she is alone. This week the current events have been more interesting and she says that this makes it easier to concentrate. Jane is going to ask the team if she can read magazines rather than the newspaper. Jane has been faithful to her task of memory training but she says that it is her least favorite thing to do. The family have been supporting Jane and often encourage her to engage in this task.

Functional

Jane expressed that she was excited to make a tuna salad for her two teenage girls; this was a favorite, she said. Jane was able to find and utilize the necessary utensils and bowls needed and was easily able to mix the ingredients and successfully prepare the tuna salad. She was absolutely thrilled to be able to prepare the food and feed her family. Jane expressed feelings of excitement about the next cooking venture: She would like to try making a homemade soup with four ingredients. Jane was highly motivated to return to her duties in the kitchen and she had already asked John for a ride to the grocery store and prepared a list of ingredients in advance. Jane has been using premade meals for lunches and dinner; however, this week she has prepared five meals from scratch using simple ingredients. Jane took some time to dust the living room; she says that it made her feel a little dizzy when she tilted her head back to reach the high spots.

Emotional

Jane had a busy weekend. She expressed that she was feeling very fatigued, Jane said that she enjoyed writing and reading the positive cards; however, today she appeared uninspired to write. When asked where her gratitude journal was she admitted that she had misplaced it during the weekend when there was so much commotion going on in the house. A specific shelf in her bedroom was labeled for her journal, to avoid misplacing it in the future. Jane expressed that the time to write in her journal could be better utilized if she did this in the early morning before her family rises. Jane did state that her husband gave her a hug and kiss after she was able to make the salad and he told her he was proud of her. Jane wrote this on one of her positive cards.

Work

Jane attended her volunteer placement and she enjoyed it. However, Jane does reminisce a great deal about her old job in an upscale clothing store. She would like to go visit her co-workers at some point in the future but feels it is too soon now. Jane is finding that attending her college course is building her confidence. The instructor has been helpful to Jane after class; he verbally dictates the homework expectations in Jane's memory card.

Spiritual

Jane is finding the use of positive cards very uplifting. It has become a habit in the household that, before dinner, the family says grace and names one positive thing that happened to them that day. Jane keeps a stack of recipe cards at the dinner table and she is now in the consistent habit of writing down these positive comments and rereading them before she goes to sleep. Jane is faithful in her daily prayer; she has expressed that she understands how precious life is. Jane's deep faith gives her a quiet peace. She is comfortable going to church with the family; it has become easier over time. Jane is used to educating other parishioners that she finds remembering names difficult. This group of people assists in reminding Jane of their names.

Relaxation

Jane continues to be very tired, especially on Mondays. The weekends are busy with the children's sports. Jane would like to discuss with the clinical team how she can better manage her energy. This past weekend Jane burst out in tears at Sunday dinner. She did not prepare the dinner (her husband did), but because of her fatigue she said that all of her losses were just too much to deal with. Jane desperately expresses a desire to be able to care for her family by preparing their meals. She says this is her primary goal at the moment. Jane is taking time to rest; she notices that life is easier if she takes time to rest. Jane soaked in the tub three times this week. She has very quiet music playing when she does this. She says she gets lost in the moment when she is engaging in this activity and she muses that life seems almost normal at this time.

Sexuality

Jane has confided in me that she and her husband Jack have not had sexual relations since she has returned home from the hospital; he assures her that he still loves her and finds her attractive but he is afraid that she is too fragile. The couple has decided to bring this up with the social worker upon their next visit. Jane says she feels increasingly nervous that she will lose Jack. Jane did get her hair cut and styled this week. She mentioned that she found this experience exhausting; the background music at the salon agitated her as did all the chatter. Jane has a friend who is a hair stylist and Jane suggested that, in the short term, perhaps she could ask her friend to come to her house and style her hair. She will discuss this with her occupational therapist this week.

Social

The couple is still very much nesting and keeping to themselves. The children and Jack spend a great deal of time with Jane. This week, for the first time, Jane said hello to a neighbor when she was taking her short walk. It was like an injection of life for Jane; she even mentioned that she would like to invite the neighbor for tea. Bob took Jane to visit her best friend; she enjoyed getting out but found the conversation tiring. Later in the week Jane and this same friend went to a movie; this appeared to be a better activity for Jane with less talking.

Family

Jane expressed that she was feeling very fatigued this week. She said that helping Amy with her homework was tiring. Jane is also expressing feelings of insecurity that she may be losing her daughter's respect. As a result Jane and her husband decided not to have the family meeting until they could discuss Jane's concern with the social worker and get some tips on how to help Amy understand Jane's condition better. Because of Jane's fatigue and coupled with her feelings of insecurity, the couple decided not to go out for their date night as planned but rather to rent a movie at home. Jane has said that she trusts the social worker and enjoys the counseling sessions. She will bring up her feelings of insecurity with the social worker next Wednesday.

Community

Jane went to the grocery store to shop for the four ingredients needed for the tuna salad. Jane and her husband report that Jane was able to find three of the ingredients with no assistance and that she was able to ask a store attendant for help with finding the fourth item. Jane did say that she met one of the girls' teachers in the store and was unable to recall her name, causing her embarrassment. Jane reported that she was very fatigued after the shopping. Jane and Bob went to the farmers market. Jane enjoyed this outing and stated that it was easier to go out with Bob in the event that she meets someone that she knows. Bob then cues Jane on the person's name. The family went to the zoo on the weekend. Jane felt good about going out with the girls.

Leisure

Jane went bowling this week; after three attempts at throwing the bowling ball she decided just to observe. Her balance was prohibiting her from engaging in the task to any degree of success. Jane will discuss this with her physical therapist. Jane expresses that she misses swimming. I informed her that I would bring this up with the team to see if we could integrate swimming into the program. Jane and Bob went for a bike ride in a quiet forested area this past weekend. Jane absolutely loved getting out. She found that she could balance on the bike and enjoyed the peace of the forest. The couple plan to go again next weekend.

The Team Will Modify the Goals

Because Jane has been successful in the preparation of a simple four-step meal several times, she will prepare five meals this week including her desired homemade soup.

The social worker will have been contacted by the case manager to be informed of the husband's concern that his wife is too fragile for sexual relations The social worker will see the husband alone as well as with Jane. The social worker will also plan to meet with Amy to assist her in understanding her mother's condition and to listen to her concerns.

Jane's desire to reunite with her co-workers will be explored, Jane and the clinicians agree that visiting her co-workers at the mall would likely result in failure because of all of the sensory stimuli. The case manager will spend time with Jane exploring how best to handle the well wishes and questions that a visit from the co-workers may create and to explore alternate venues for meeting with her colleagues.

The issue of fatigue after the weekend will be discussed at a family meeting, where the two daughters will be educated that at the moment their mom will be able to attend only one of their games over the weekend. The energy conservation model referring to units of energy as money will be used to help with their understanding.

Jane has expressed an interest to the worker about starting to scrapbook. The occupational therapist will meet with Jane to explore other creative ventures that entail only four steps. The occupational therapist will modify a task that is similar to scrap booking such as labeling pictures in albums as a start.

Jane has expressed an interest in swimming; the physical therapist will attend the pool with Jane and the worker and design a swimming program that will be introduced into the program in 2 weeks' time.

COGNITIVE RETRAINING STRATEGIES

When the therapy is complete, 4 to 6 years into the recovery process, we should be able to see goal attainment scales that are color coded in each area of the pie segments as represented in Tables 8.4, 8.6, 8.7, and 8.8, showing balance and managed stress. The weekly schedule should be a representation of the goals as well as daily life; the visual picture of the weekly schedule is one of a rainbow of color (Tables 8.5 and 8.9). The balance is present and a semblance of homeostasis has been established creating a new normal; the stress is managed and at this point the *Lefaivre Rainbow Effect* has been implemented. The areas that are represented by white in the life pie (Figure 8.3) are

Table 8.4 Weekly Goal Sheet at Start of Therapy

Name: _____   Date: _____

Possible attainment level	Goal 1 Physical	Goal 2 Functional	Goal 3 Emotional	Goal 4	Goal 5
Better than expected	Walk 30 meters to end of driveway to pick up paper at 9 a.m. Tuesday, Thursday, Saturday, and Monday	Make a grocery list on Saturday at 11 a.m. Grocery shop Sunday at 3 p.m. Ask John for a ride to the grocery store on Monday	Write three positive cards every day; read them daily at 8 p.m. Write in journal daily at 7 p.m. Ask husband on Tues. at 7 p.m. to cite a positive gain you made this month		
Expected	Walk 30 meters to the end of driveway to pick up paper at 9 a.m. Tuesday, Thursday, and Saturday	List the four ingredients used in a tuna salad, Monday, 3 p.m. Ask John for a ride to the grocery store on Monday	Write three positive cards every day and read them daily at 8 p.m. Write in journal daily at 7 p.m.		
Less than expected	Walk 30 meters to the end of driveway to pick up paper on Monday at 9 a.m.	Look through recipe books for a tuna salad recipe on Saturday at 3 p.m. (15 min)	Write in journal daily at 7 p.m.		

Table 8.5 Weekly Schedule at Start of Therapy

Name: _____ Date: _____

	MONDAY	TUESDAY	WEDNESDAY	THURSDAY	FRIDAY	SATURDAY	SUNDAY	
								8:00 AM
		Walk 30 meters to pick up paper		Walk 30 meters to pick up paper		Walk 30 meters to pick up paper		9:00 AM
								10:00AM
		Ask John to drive me to the store	Read recipe list for salad ingredients			Make Grocery List		11:00 AM
								12:00 Noon
								1:00 PM
	Write 3 positive cards and read		Write 3 positive cards and read		Write 3 positive cards and read		Write 3 positive cards and read	2:00 PM
							Grocery Shop	3:00 PM
								4:00 PM
								5:00 PM
								6:00 PM
	Write in journal for 10 minutes	Write in journal for 10 minutes	Write in journal for 10 minutes	Write in journal for 10 minutes	Write in journal for 10 minutes	Write in journal for 10 minutes	Write in journal for 10 minutes	7:00 PM
								8:00 PM
								9:00 PM

Table 8.6 Weekly Goal Sheet at End of Therapy

Name: _____ Date: _____

Possible attainment level	Goal 1 Cognitive	Goal 2 Emotional	Goal 3 Work	Goal 4 Spiritual	Goal 5 Relaxation
Exceeded expectations	Read paper daily for 15 minutes at 9 a.m. Memory training on the computer for 20 minutes at 1 p.m. daily Discuss the news with husband for 20 minutes at 8 p.m.	Write and read three positive cards daily at 9 p.m. except Saturday Write in journal daily for 15 minutes at 1 p.m.	Volunteer at church 2 hours on Monday, Wednesday, and Friday, 3–6 p.m. Take college course at 11 a.m. Tuesday and Thursday (1 hour)	Pray daily 30 minutes, 7 a.m. Make a list of five things I am grateful for on Sunday at 4 p.m. Attend church on Sunday at 11 a.m.	Soak in the tub 30 minutes daily at 10 p.m. Listen to relaxing music 20 minutes, 7 p.m. Rest Tuesday, Wednesday, Thursday, and Sunday for 10 minutes at 10 a.m.
Expected	Read paper Monday, Tuesday, Wednesday, Friday, and Saturday at 9 a.m. for 15 minutes Memory training on the computer for 20 minutes Monday, Wednesday, and Saturday at 1 p.m.	Write three positive cards and read on Monday, Tuesday, Friday, and Sunday at 9 p.m. Write in journal for 15 minutes Monday, Wednesday, Thursday, Saturday, and Sunday at 1 p.m.	Volunteer at church for 2 hours Monday and Wednesday, 3–5 p.m. Take college course on Thursday at 11 a.m. (1 hour)	Pray Monday, Wednesday, Friday, and Saturday for 30 minutes at 7 a.m. Make a list of three things I am grateful for on Sunday at 4 p.m. Attend church Sunday at 11.a.m.	Soak in tub Monday, Tuesday, Wednesday, Friday, and Saturday for 30 minutes at 10 p.m. Listen to music on Tuesday, Thursday, and Sunday for. 20 minutes at 7 p.m. Rest on Tuesday and wednesday at 10 a.m. for 1 hour
Less than expected	Watch the news daily and discuss with husband for 20 minutes at 8 p.m.	Write three positive cards and read Monday and Friday at 1 p.m. Write in journal Monday and Friday at 9 p.m.	Take college course for 1 hour on Thursday at 11 a.m.	Attend church Sunday at 11 a.m.	Soak in tub Monday and Friday for 30 minutes at 10 p.m. Listen to music on Monday for 20 minutes at 7 p.m.

Table 8.7 Weekly Goal Sheet at End of Therapy

Name: _____ Date: _____

Possible attainment level	Goal 1 Social	Goal 2 Physical	Goal 3 Family	Goal 4 Community	Goal 5 Functional
Exceeded expectations	Visit friend Tuesday, Thursday, and Saturday from 3 to 4 p.m. Go to dinner and a movie with friend on Wednesday at 8 p.m.	Go to gym Monday, Wednesday, and Friday with Jane for 1.5 hours at 11 a.m. Walk Tuesday, Thursday, and Sunday for 1 hour at 8 a.m.	Help Amy with homework Monday, Wednesday, Friday, and Saturday at 7 p.m. for 1 hour Have date with husband on Saturday from 7 to 9 p.m. Have a family meeting Tuesday at 8 p.m.	Go to farmer's market Saturday at 10 a.m. with Bob for 1 hour Go to the zoo Sunday at 2 p.m. for 2 hours with children	Make simple dinner daily at 5 p.m. Make breakfast and lunch daily at 8 a.m. and 12 p.m. Wash floors and clean bathrooms at 10 a.m on Monday. Dust Friday at 10 a.m.
Expected	Visit friend on Tuesday and Thursday from 3 to 4 p.m. Go to movie with a friend at 8 p.m. on Wednesday	Go to gym with Jane for 1 hour on Monday, Wednesday, and Friday at 11 a.m. Walk Tuesday and Thursday for 45 minutes at 7 a.m. (Saturday at 6 a.m.)	Help Amy with homework on Monday, Wednesday, and Friday at 7 p.m. for 1 hour Have date with husband from 7 to 9 p.m. on Saturday	Go to farmer's market at 10 a.m. on Saturday with Bob for 45 minutes Go to the zoo with children for 2 hours on Sunday at 2 p.m.	Make dinner Tuesday, Thursday, Friday, and Saturday at 5 p.m. Make breakfast and lunch daily at 8 a.m. and 12 p.m. Dust on Friday at 10 a.m. Wash floors at 10 a.m. on Monday
Less than expected	Visit friend on Tuesday from 3 to 4 p.m.	Go to gym for 30 minutes on Monday, Wednesday, and Friday at 11 a.m. Walk Tuesday for 45 minutes at 8 a.m.	Help Amy with homework Wednesday and Friday at 7 p.m. for 1 hour	Go to farmer's market with Bob on Saturday for 30 minutes	Make a simple dinner Tuesday, Thursday, Friday, and Saturday at 5 p.m. Make lunch Monday, Wednesday, and Friday at 12 p.m. Dust on Friday at 10 a.m.

Table 8.8 Weekly Goal Sheet at End of Therapy

Name: _____   Date: _____

Possible attainment level	Goal 1		Goal 2		Goal 3	Goal 4	Goal 5
	Leisure		Sexuality				
Exceeded expectations	Go bowling at 7 p.m. on Monday for 2 hours Ride bike Saturday at 3 p.m. for 2 hours with Bob		Attend session with sexuality counselor at 8 p.m. on Tuesday and Thursday Talk with husband about setting date nights at 8 p.m. Sunday Have legs waxed and hair styled on Friday at 2 p.m.				
Expected	Go bowling at 7 p.m. on Monday for 1 hour Ride bike Saturday at 3 p.m. for 2 hours with Bob		Attend sexuality sessions Tuesday and Thursday at 8 p.m. Set up date night for 8 p.m. on Sunday Date night Saturday From 7 to 9 p.m. Get hair styled on Friday at 2 p.m.				
Less than expected	Go bowling at 7 p.m. on Monday for 30 minutes Ride bike with Bob on Saturday at 3 p.m. for 30 minutes		Set up date night with husband at 8 p.m. on Sunday				

Table 8.9 Weekly Schedule at End of Therapy

Name: _____ Date: _____

Monday	Tuesday	Wednesday	Thursday	Friday	Saturday	Sunday	
					Walk		6:00 a.m.
Pray	Walk	Pray	Walk	Pray	Pray	Pray	7:00 a.m.
Breakfast	Breakfast	Breakfast	Breakfast	Breakfast	Breakfast	Breakfast	8:00 a.m.
Read paper (15 min)	Read paper (15 min)	Read paper (15 min)		Read paper (15 min)	Read paper (15 min)		9:00 a.m.
	Rest	Rest	Rest	Dust house	Farmer's market		10:00 a.m.
Gym		Gym	College course	Gym		Church	11:00 a.m.
Lunch	Lunch	Lunch	Lunch	Lunch	Lunch	Lunch	12:00 noon
Write in journal	Write in journal	Write in journal	Write in journal	Write in journal	Write in journal	Write in journal	1:00 p.m.
Computer		Computer		Hairstyle	Computer	Zoo with kids	2:00 p.m.
Volunteer church		Volunteer church		Hairstyle	Ride bike	Zoo with kids	3:00 p.m.
Volunteer church	Visit friend	Volunteer church	Visit friend	Hairstyle	Ride bike	Gratitude journal	4:00 p.m.
Volunteer church	Make dinner	Volunteer church	Make dinner	Make dinner	Make dinner		5:00 p.m.
Eat dinner	Eat dinner	Eat dinner	Eat dinner	Eat dinner	Eat dinner	Eat dinner	6:00 p.m.

Continued

Table 8.9 (*Continued*) Weekly Schedule at End of Therapy

Name: _____   Date: _____

Monday	Tuesday	Wednesday	Thursday	Friday	Saturday	Sunday	
Bowling	Listen to music	Homework	Listen to music	Homework	Date night	Listen to music	7:00 p.m.
	Sex counseling	Movie/friend	Sex counseling		Date night	Set up dates	8:00 p.m.
Three positive cards	Three positive cards	Movie/friend	Three positive cards	Three positive cards	Date night	Three positive cards	9:00 p.m.
Soak in tub	Soak in tub	Movie/friend		Soak in tub	Soak in tub		10:00 p.m.

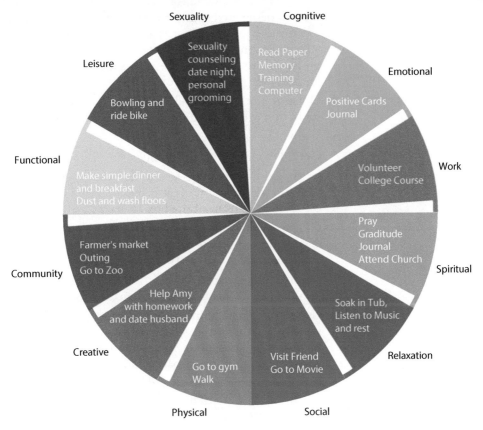

Figure 8.3 Intervention pie.

the losses that have not been restored. These areas represent the symptoms that will require lifelong management.

USEFUL THERAPEUTIC HINTS

Organization

Organization is paramount to assist in memory function, attention, and concentration and to avoid sensory overload. The author suggests that the organization is done with the client and, if necessary, with a house cleaning company and the one-to-one worker. The home needs to be cleaned and organized but **not reorganized** in such a manner that the client cannot recognize where things are. The following hints may be helpful:

1. Make sure that items used in a given room are in that room.
2. Each item should have a designated spot; labels are helpful.

147

3. Make a designated spot for frequently used items such as car and house keys, purse, and wallet. As well, create a list indicating where these items are placed. It should be logical; for instance, the keys should have a place immediately inside the door.

4. Organize clothes seasonally and for occasions (i.e., work, sport, casual, dressy and spring, summer, fall, and winter).

5. Use a personal organizer.

6. Get rid of clutter; it can visually overload a client.

7. Use boxes to store items so that they can be stacked. Be sure to take a picture of and label each item; glue the picture to the front of the box for easy identification.

8. Organize drawers, cupboards, and closets—again, decreasing the visual stimulation with use of storage containers that are labeled both in writing and pictorially.

9. Organize storage areas; label and allocate bins to specific supplies (e.g., "Christmas decorations, outdoor/indoor").

10. Use pictures on the inside of cupboard doors to show visually what is in this space and what it may be used for. In the case of agnosia, it is useful to have a picture of where the item is in use, particularly in the kitchen.

11. Label items such as bleach and laundry soap for correct identification. For instance, no. 1 is laundry soap, no. 2 is fabric softener, and red is a bleach label, such as "Do not touch; ask Bob first." Numbers, colors, or arrows can be useful in the case of agnosia.

12. Label the dials on the washer and dryer with numbers or colors or steps.

13. Have an inventory done of the freezer and tape a list with pictures onto the lid. When an item is taken out of the freezer, it is taken off the list.

14. Purchase an auto shut-off iron, kettle, tea kettle, and coffee pot.

15. Purchase two-handed equipment for safety.

16. Purchase smoke and carbon monoxide alarms.

17. Fix leaky faucets and unbalanced ceiling fans.

Provide Structure

1. Schedules should be created and posted where they are visible, such as on the refrigerator.

2. Routines should be consistent and predictable.

3. List the activities of daily living and post in the appropriate rooms; this is particularly useful when short-term

memory is an issue. For instance, make a list in the bathroom listing the steps necessary to take a shower and to brush teeth. When the task is completed, it should be ticked off for that day and that time.

Memory Strategies

1. If severe memory issues are present, create a posted list for meals that have been eaten, as well as a chart tracking medications taken and the times that it was taken. Have the worker and client tick off when the client has completed the task.

2. Use blister packs for medications.

3. Set timers to remind the client of medication times, either on a phone, computer, or watch.

4. Ensure that appointment times are clearly labeled on the schedule on the fridge and in the electronic calendar or phone.

5. On a calendar, highlight important dates and times (e.g., insurance and taxes due dates, anniversaries, birthdays, and appointments).

6. Allow ample time to get to appointments to reduce agitating the client by rushing.

7. Set up ringer reminders in advance of the appointment, allowing time to get to the appointment.

8. Ensure that professional offices call the day before and the morning of the scheduled appointment to remind the client of the appointment.

9. At the end of an appointment have the clinician enter into the client's phone or daytimer the next appointment or have him or her voice-record instructions on a dictaphone or memory card.

10. In the case of bill payment, set up with the worker automatic withdrawal where possible or, in advance of the client's skill development, assign bill payment to another person.

11. Use a dictaphone, verbal memory card, daytimer, or personal digital assistant to assist with memory.

12. If the client cannot locate his or her car, use the fob car alarm to locate the vehicle.

13. It is helpful to program frequently used numbers into an autodial phone. Post a chart within visual proximity to the phone. Indicate the number to enter for each person and include a picture of the person who will be called.

Communication

1. Educate family members on the effect of auditory noise for the TBI loved one. It is recommended for family members to use headsets if possible when listening to music or listening to something auditory on computers, as well as turning the volume on the television down or placing the television in another room.

2. Make a rule in the early days that only one person speaks at a time.

3. Paraphrase.

4. Clarify.

5. If word finding is difficult for the client, rhyming or word association may help trigger the desired response.

6. The client can be prompted with, "This word sounds like_____."

7. The client can be prompted with, "You use this item to _____" and then demonstrating the use.

8. "This word sounds starts with the *Rrrr* sound."

Emotional Affect

1. In the case of impaired emotional affect have the client ask for feedback from a trusted source as to the appropriateness of his or her facial expressions. Use pictures that show emotional expressions to help identify emotions and have the client identify which picture reflects what he or she is feeling; have the client practice the appropriate facial expressions in a mirror.

2. If the client is presenting as agitated or in a state of aggression, make a sliding scale of voice tones. For instance, whispering is 1 and yelling is 10. Have the client ask trusted sources, including the family, one-to-one worker and professionals, how the tone of his or her voice reflects the level of emotion felt. Have all parties give appropriate feedback. Educate the client on reducing the volume and tone of voice to reflect the emotion he or she feels. It is a good idea to apply numbers to the sliding scale.

3. Have the client keep a journal; documenting his or her level of energy over the course of the day from this sensory overload can be analyzed.

4. Have the client with the worker identify physical, mental, input, and output as it relates to the banking analogy as a system to manage and conserve energy.

5. Have the client identify the feelings and behaviors that precede sensory overload.

Emotional Mood

1. Use positive cards. Have the client write each accomplishment, joy, pleasure, and what they are grateful for on a recipe card—one thought per card. The client should continue to add and read daily, imprinting new memories in the memory bank.

2. Have the client keep a gratitude journal; this is a wonderful precursor to assist the client to embrace the "new me."

3. Encourage the client to communicate feelings and ask for help if required.

4. If the client is feeling down, ask him or her, "If you were feeling good, what would you be doing?"

5. Have the client make a list of what makes him or her feel good, add to positive cards and gratitude journal, and continue to track successes—particularly in these areas that have special meaning for the client.

Problem Solving

1. Use advantage/disadvantage lists as well as pro and con lists.

2. If returning to school use recorders, ask the instructor if you can take the exam in a quiet room to reduce stimuli.

3. If returning to school or work, start slowly with reduced hours and a reduced course load.

4. If studying, choose a quiet place with limited visual and auditory noise.

Energy Conservation

1. In the initial stages using homemakers, pre-prepared meals, meals on wheels, or store-bought deli meals may reduce the demand on the client, conserving energy for other tasks.

2. In the early stages, recruit volunteers for various tasks not paid for by a third funder such as meal preparation,

going for a walk, calling family members to report in, driving, visiting, or providing respite. Have the client journal his or her level of energy over the course of the day so that this sensory overload related to fatigue can be analyzed.

Community Integration

(See suggested websites at the end of the book.)

1. Source out specialized programs at colleges, recreation centers, sporting activity, and support groups at brain injury associations.

Transportation

1. In the event of the inability to drive, use the handi-dart or a taxi pass, recruit volunteer drivers, or purchase a therapeutic bus pass.

Sensory Overload

1. When symptoms, such as headache, behavior outbursts, confusion, and reduced concentration, attention, and memory occur, analyze what the stimuli were for the client at least 24 hours before. Document when the change occurred. Reconstruct the overall stimuli occurring at that time. At another time recreate the goal, reducing the extraneous stimuli. When success occurs, document the environmental and emotional expectations for the client. In the future, avoid the stimulus or the combination of stimuli that has created the sensory overload and educate the client and family.

Stereognosis

This is the ability to perceive the size, shape, and texture of objects by means of touch. When a client has difficulty in this area, it can be extremely frustrating and tiring. Just think of how many times you reach for a coffee cup without looking or search in your purse for your car keys. An individual with this symptom can become easily tired because he or she uses extra units of energy to identify objects visually. It is helpful to introduce tactile touch into the therapy regime. A game can be set up: Take a large bucket and, on different days, fill it with various tactile items—for instance, rice, cotton balls, beans, or marbles. Hide commonly used items, such as keys, comb, hair brush, spoon, lipstick, etc., in the bucket in the midst of the tactile items. The goal is for the client to identify the item by touch without visual input.

Proprioception

Is the ability to identify our body's position in space independent of vision? People with difficulty in this area may have balance and coordination issues. They may appear accident prone and clumsy. It is helpful to have the one-to-one worker engage in different tasks with the client with the client's eyes closed. For instance, the client and worker can go for a walk; the client will close his or her eyes and the worker will ensure that he or she has provided support and taken safety precautions by firmly gripping the client's arm. They will walk slowly. To upgrade the task, the client can place his or her head in various positions simultaneously while walking. To upgrade the exercise even more, the worker can take the client to places where the terrain is uneven such as a beach or a gravel lane. This work can also be done on an exercise ball, with the client in a seated position and the therapist providing support. The worker can have the client close his or her eyes and attempt to touch his or her nose with an index finger, alternating left to right—first slowly and then rapidly. The therapist can place his or her arms in a certain position and then ask the client to replicate this position with eyes closed. The client then opens his or her eyes and can then visually correct body position.

Agnosia

Apperceptive Visual Agnosia

This is the ability to assemble pieces of an image into something that is a usable whole. If a client has problems in this area, he or she may have difficulty comprehending how objects relate to one another. This can prove to be a challenge when the client attempts to engage in multilevel tasks. Cooking is a good example. There are several steps and many objects used to prepare a meal. It is helpful to have the worker cue the client as to the desired outcome and then review the steps to execute the task successfully. It is important to start off with single-step tasks and then upgrade to more complex tasks. On a recreational level, putting puzzles together can be useful. The clinician can also create a pictorial board depicting several objects, and the client can create a story about what the objects are used for. Eventually, the client can create the pictorial board, depicting a sequence of objects, and then verbalize what they are used for.

Associative Visual Agnosia

Clients who have problems in this area will have difficulty remembering information associated with the object—for instance, the name or the use of the object. The worker can display objects one at a time; the worker will demonstrate what the object is used for, and then the client will be asked to verbalize what the object is used for. This exercise will advance to the point that the objects can all be laid out on a table. The worker will then give a cue to the use of one of the objects and the client will need to identify the associated object. As the worker spends time with the client, it can become a game to identify objects and their use. The worker can provide clues, letting the client know if he or she is hot or cold in the verdict of the objects' use.

Prosopagnosia

Clients who have difficulty in this area will have a hard time recognizing people's faces. Family members should be educated on how to cue the client gracefully, adding in information about how the client knows this person and triggering associated memories. If written comprehension is intact, the use of name tags in the early days can be helpful. Looking at photos and recreating the scenario surrounding the memory of the persons in the photos can be fun and helpful. First, the worker or family member can tell the story, and on another day, prompt the client with clues to retell the story.

Phonagnosia

Clients experiencing difficulty in this area will have problems identifying voices. Once again, a game can be set up. A recorder can be used to record familiar family, friends', and clinicians' voices. This can become a game with points attached. The worker again can give clues with associated memory—for instance, "This voice belongs to a woman that you have had lunch with this month."

Apraxia

Clients with problems in this area will have difficulty performing voluntary and skillful movement when using one or more body parts. It is helpful to have the worker engage in repetitive physical exercises requiring the client to engage in purposeful movement. This can start with throwing a softball or a beach ball and advance to kicking the ball while sitting. This can advance to virtually any sporting activity.

Constructional Apraxia

Clients who are having difficulty in this area will display problems with building or drawing. It can be helpful to engage in recreational tasks such as building models, completing puzzles, or sewing. Be sure to start with very simple tasks to avoid failure. The clinician will refer back to the client's history, which will present other familiar activities that can be introduced to produce the required stimulus. For instance, if the client was a gardener, this task would then be incorporated into the therapy regime as a vehicle for cognitive retraining.

Ideokinetic Apraxia

With this condition clients will have difficulty carrying out simple tasks. When this presents as a problem, simple tasks should be repeatedly approached with the worker using repetition, including visual demonstration and auditory cueing. Tasks that have meaning for the client will measure a better outcome.

Dyspraxia

Clients who have difficulty in this area will display problems with thinking out, planning out, and executing movements or tasks. Exercises can be designed starting with single-step tasks and advance to more complex tasks. For instance, once again using the example of gardening, the worker can assist the client to make a plan for the garden. A picture can be drawn up, and colors and varieties of plants will be listed. They will then go to the greenhouse; the client will find the items on the lists. On another day the plan that was initially drawn by the client will be executed as the client makes decisions of where to place the plants to make the drawing come to life. A footnote is that it is common to have family members "do for" the client. (It is difficult to watch a loved one struggle.) Education should be provided so that in a controlled, graded way the client can learn to problem solve again.

Ataxia

Clients who are experiencing this problem can have difficulty ambulating. They may appear intoxicated. The associated ridicule can be very hard. It is important to assist the client to have a well prepared rebuttal if he or she is misinterpreted as being intoxicated. Activity such as working at a pottery wheel can stabilize the client's movement because the object is moving rather than the client. The physical therapist will prepare a physical regime to improve coordination that can be carried out by the worker.

Dysarthria

In this case the muscles of the face and mouth have become weak and move slowly or perhaps not at all. Some symptoms can be slurred speech, drooling, mumbling, speaking slowly, and abnormal intonation. It can be helpful to encourage the client to speak slowly and to pause frequently. The client should be encouraged to clarify with the listener if he or she is being understood. Energy conservation is important as fatigue will worsen the symptoms. Alternate means of communicating can be introduced, such as computer or electronic equipment, alphabet boards, or gesturing. Loved ones should be educated to reduce distraction and background noise. Paraphrase and clarify, pay attention, and watch the client speak or ask the client to write the message.

Benign Positional Vertigo

Clients who have this condition may be prone to sudden sensations of spinning and dizziness when turning or moving their heads. This can result in falls and general accident proneness as well as nausea. This problem originates in the otolith organ in the inner ear. The otolith organ contains tiny crystals; if these crystals are dislodged, the client will become more sensitive to head movements. This can be manually treated by a neurologist or a specially trained physical therapist.

Hemianopsia

When a client has this condition, he or she will not see objects in half of the visual field in one or both eyes. Safety is of prime importance when this condition is present. It is not recommended that the client drive. The clinical team will assist the client in compensating for the loss in the affected visual field, educating the client to be cognizant to turning the head and or upper torso completely. It is important that the client maneuvers through their environment slowly and cautiously.

Right- and Left-Side Neglect

Clients who experience either right- or left-side neglect should be encouraged to keep their hands within their visual field. It is helpful to have the client take ownership over the limb that is neglected. It is important to educate loved ones and encourage them to have the client cross his or her midline when engaging in upper extremity activity. For instance, at the dinner table pass the food items in such a way as to force the client to cross over his or her midline with the affected hand.

Depth Perception

Clients who are experiencing difficulty with depth perception will have problems judging the distance between objects. How this translates into function once again will be reflected as clumsiness, awkwardness, and accident proneness. It is helpful to choose activities that the client enjoyed prior to the brain injury. For instance, for a young male interested in sports, the clinician can start with having the client sit and then the clinician will roll a soccer ball, encouraging the client to kick the ball back; this should alternate left and right. When this is consistently executed, have the client stand and kick the ball. The task can now involve a stationary object and having the client connect to the object, such as hitting a golf ball. Then advance to ping pong, gradually escalating to a fast moving object such as racquet ball. In the early days, clients should exercise caution when ambulating—particularly when stepping off curbs. The use of sharp objects such as knives should be cautiously approached until depth perception can be reintegrated.

SUMMARY

In summary, to the intervention we have set the stage for the intervention by being thorough with the **total sum** and **loss** sections of the *Lefaivre Rainbow Effect*. We have made the assumption that the brain can relearn on its own or with adaptation and environmental changes. The clinical team will have an understanding of anatomy and the general etiology of the client's TBI, anticipating the challenges that the client will face. The team will be cognizant of the client's susceptibility to sensory overload as we reflect on the breaker box analogy. The team will ensure that a system of energy conservation is in place. The one-to-one worker will keenly observe when and how the brain processes stimuli revealing lesional or functional clues. Positive, specific, and behavioral goals will be set using a color-coded goal scale and weekly schedule. When tasks from each section of the life pie are reflected in the color-coded weekly schedule balance, perhaps a difference balance has been restored and a new place of homeostastis has been achieved. We will assume that the stress has been managed and that the organic traumatic brain injury symptoms are being addressed. The display of color on the weekly schedule will reflect that the rainbow or the balance is in effect—thus the *rainbow effect*.

CHAPTER 9

Residual Loss Cost-of-Future-Care Analysis

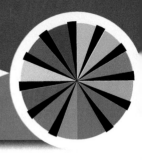

TOTAL SUM	–	DIAGNOSIS (LOSS)	+	INTERVENTION	=	RESIDUAL LOSS

   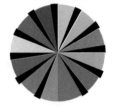

INTRODUCTION

We are now at the **residual loss** stage of the formula. We, the health care team, have worked our way through the *Lefaivre Rainbow Effect* and made a commitment to the client for the 4- to 6-year therapeutic process.

In review,

1. We have unveiled the client's pre-injury life, habits, joys, accomplishments, and sorrows by conducting an extensive history and have used this to build and design the unique treatment model for the client.

2. We have educated the family and reduced the impact of stress on the family, maintaining their pre-injury roles, by advocating for assistance.

3. We have reduced the impact of stress on the client, minimizing secondary losses, and we have devised a treatment regime that is goal directed and meaningful to the client.

4. We, the health care providers, have documented all of our interactions, assessments, and appointments in a report format admissible to the legal requirements of an expert witness.

We are now in the final stages of care for the client. It will be agreed upon by the health care/legal/insurance team that we have reached the stage of residual loss. This is the stage where the deficits that remain will most likely be permanent. They can be dealt with by utilizing aids and adaptations and through relearning and modification to the environment; however, most of the symptoms at this stage will remain permanent. It is at this stage that all health care clinicians will write their final reports. These reports can be extensive, including the original tests and assessment findings, diagnoses, prognoses, interventions and treatment regimes, clinical milestones, setbacks, and successes. The black sections in the life pie in Figure 9.1 reflect the areas and percentages of deficit that remain even after therapeutic intervention. The black segments indicate the residual loss.

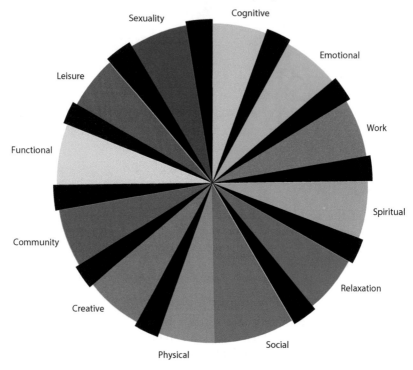

Figure 9.1 Residual loss pie.

Within these last reports each health care provider will render his or her final opinion; inclusive in these opinions can be recommendations for future care requirements or anticipated financial costs required to maintain the stability of the treatment outcome. It is within these reports that the legal counsel will find the prognosis for the client, specifically as it relates to the client's ability to return to his or her own occupation, be successfully retrained, and engage in competitive employment. The reports and the opinions of the experts help to establish wage loss and future wage loss, to determine any future care costs that may be incurred, and to assist the brain-injured survivor over the long term. In preparing a cost-of-future-care analysis, the diagnosis and prognosis should be included—particularly as it relates to future costs. Include supporting opinions, indicating whether the client has the capacity to live independently and, if so, whether there are any present or future costs necessary to ensure success and safety.

It is within these reports and the accompanying expert witness testimony that a monetary reward will be established for the client's losses in the case of third-party liability.

The importance of the cost of future care lies in the foundation that the entire team will have contributed to the findings. One person will be assigned to the writing of this report. It is frequently the occupational therapist because of the functional aspect of his or her care, but it can also be another member of the team—quite typically the clinician who has assumed the role of case manager.

The cost of future care is a document that extensively reviews the medical literature on the client, highlighting areas where costs have been incurred, where they will continue to be incurred, and any anticipated costs yet to be determined. In the chapter on litigation we will review the importance of appropriate record keeping and report writing. The cost of future care is unique in that it not only cites the author's professional opinion from his or her own discipline's perspective, but also incorporates the team's findings, even highlighting discrepancies in medical opinions. It is very important that this report is thorough and well written and prepared by a skilled professional. The report needs to be unbiased and neutral, neither advocating nor minimizing the client's loss. It is a fact-based report based on the professional team's opinions. It is imperative that this report be written only when the residual loss is determined and not before. If it is prepared too early in the recovery process, then all losses have yet to become apparent.

A novice lawyer may request a report of this nature early on (within 1–2 years of the recovery process). It is the responsibility of the clinician to educate the lawyer on the prematurity of this request from a clinical perspective.

PREPARING A COST-OF-FUTURE-CARE ANALYSIS

The following is useful to guide the clinician in preparing the cost-of-future-care:

Preparing a Cost-of-Future-Care Analysis

Date _____

Referral source _____

Referral address _____

Prepared by _____

Dear _____

Re: client name _____

Date of injury _____

My file # _____

Your file # _____

Thank you for your request dated Aug. 15, 2014. Pursuant to this request I have visited Mr. A and his wife in their home environment on the following dates [include an appendix for dates, time, and length of duration of the visit]. The purpose of my involvement in this case is to provide a cost-of-future-care analysis as requested by _____ indicating any future needs and associated costs that the client may have as a result of the motor vehicle accident of May 5, 2009.

Professional Qualifications

I am a _____ (list professional credentials)

I am a graduate of _____ (cite universities and faculty attended)

I am registered with _____ (state/provincial licensing board or college)

Professional associations, local, and national: _____

Professional position currently held: _____

I have _____ years of experience in _____

Enclosed is my curriculum vitae (include current position and responsibilities and an appendix along with the other team members' curriculum vitae)

Review of Medical Literature (including Any Pictures and Videos)

Prior to commencing my assessment I perused and made study of the following medical reports:

Dr. Jones, MD (Oct. 6, 2010)

Mountain General Hospital discharge summary (Oct. 26, 2010)

Dr. Morgan, MD (Feb. 23, 2012)

[Review each medical report and summarize—for example]:

I understand from reviewing Dr. Jones's reports that the client's pre-existing diagnosis is as follows:

1. Hyperthyroidism
2. Coronary artery disease with angina and previous inferior infarctions

3. Peripheral vascular disease with left subclavian steel with bypass graft as well as bypass surgery to the right leg

4. Acid reflux treated with Pariet 20 mcg

I understand that the diagnosis related to the injuries at the time of the accident on May 05, 2009, is as follows:

1. Left pulmonary contusion with resultant pneumonia
2. Left renal contusion with transient microscopic hematuria
3. Fractured inferior pubic ramus left pelvis
4. Spleen contusion
5. Closed head injury
6. Left acromioclavicular sprain and rotator cuff tendonitis

Mountain General Hospital (Aug. 26, 2009)

Review same as preceding example:

Dr. Morgan, Feb. 23, 2012

Review same as preceding example:

[Repeat this format for each medical report.]

[Now is the time to insert your own assessment.]

History

List assessments, dates, time, length of assessment, your findings, and the functional implications. Weave in the other health care professional findings as they correspond to yours. Culminate with your own professional opinion.

In writing your report:

1. The first section is based on your own professional expertise.
2. The second section is the accrual of the team's anticipated costs for the client.
3. The third section is the actual accrual of cost estimates from two or three sources establishing a table of costs incurred already, one time initial costs, and then replacement costs.

When you are sourcing out the costs of the recommended item, be sure also to get the anticipated life span of the purchase. If, for instance, the cost of a raised toilet seat is $100 and it has a life span of 4 years, state this in the report. You will see in Appendix 9A at the end of this chapter that there is a column for the initial purchase and a second column for the yearly replacement value. In this case $100 would be written in the initial purchase column. The yearly replacement value is $25 for a 4-year life span on a $100 purchase. It cannot be emphasized enough that the clinician must be very thorough. The reason for getting the three estimates is that costs can vary greatly; in order to get your report admitted, three quotes give a cross-section. Then take the mean average for use in your costing table. Be sure to cite your quote source in a bibliography. It is also important to note in your assumption section whether you have included relevant taxes. The cost of future care will then be sent to an actuary/economist who will build in inflation rates and expected life span of the client, indexing the figures accordingly.

It is important that this report be neutral as well as specific. It should be written in such a way that it answers any potential questions. If the report can be admitted without expert testimony, then it has been well written.

Let us take a moment to review important points to remember:

1. Ensure that your history is indicative of the client's pre-injury life.

2. Ensure that your assessments have been well supported and that your treatment regime is well documented.

3. Ensure that there is treatment evidence to support that the stress has been managed and the costs are directly related to the traumatic brain injury in question.

4. Ensure that you have rendered an opinion from your professional perspective.

5. Ensure that pre-existing conditions have been separated out of the costs.

6. Ensure that if this cost of future care represents a second or third TBI, that the costs are clearly related to the causation of the injury in question.

7. Enclose relevant quotes related to costs that are written in other medical reports.

8. If you feel that a cost has been missed, then with the referral source's permission, call the related professional in question and clarify whether the questioned cost should be included. Then cite the conversation in your report, including the date.

9. In writing the report, ensure that you are very clear about where you saw the client: For instance, "During my visit on May 12, 2010, I visited the client in his home environment for the purpose of assessing the safety of his staircase in relation to his increasing mobility issues"—or— "During my visit with the client on Aug. 5, 2011, I saw him in his volunteer work placement to assess the ergonomic factors relating to his rotator cuff injury."

10. Making a statement such as "he describes his parents as having influenced him in his later years" raises a question of whether

this is positive or negative. A vague or extraneous statement may necessitate that the expert testify by allowing him or her the opportunity to clarify.

11. It is important to be thorough. During the history taking you found out that the client quit school in grade 10; if the follow-up questions were not asked, then it leaves a blank that is open to interpretation: Could he have been a malingerer back then? Was he a problem student? Did his family move or was it because his dad passed away? All of these unanswered questions leave the report and the professional open to scrutiny, supporting the importance of the extensive history even in this later stage of service delivery.

12. When costing out items for the home and workplace it is important to be able to paint a picture for the judge and jury. Better yet, include pictures in your report or even a video. It is easy for the defense to pick holes in a report where a home or work assessment was not conducted—for example, "The client lives on an acreage." Or the clinician could better frame the situation by describing that the client lives on a 10-acre wheat farm. He is 30 miles away from the nearest town and 5 miles away from the nearest neighbor. The road entering the property is not paved; with heavy snowfall, access to the home will be compromised as the client used to use a tractor to remove the snow 5 months of the year and is now incapable of doing so. Then insert a medical quote supporting this position.

13. Make sure that when you proof your report you read it with a critical eye looking for discrepancies in suggested costs. For instance, in my previous clinical report I said that the client is now independent in all areas of activities of daily living. In my final cost-of-future-care report, I include homemaker service. Why is this if the client is totally independent? Even one discrepancy can weaken the report, negatively impacting its usefulness and monetary settlement for the client.

14. When reporting on your testing results, ensure that the outcome of each test and assessment is woven together with all test results producing a practical analysis. For example, "The client was unable to complete the lift, push, pull section of a work assessment." Indicate what that means for his function at home and at work and what service or adaptation can be put in place to improve his function.

15. Be careful to diagnose if you are licensed to do so—as in the case of a doctor—or, conversely, do not diagnose if you are not licensed to do so. For example, all the health care providers are well aware of the client's left visual hemianopsia, but

to state that he has this condition without referencing the diagnostician can be a problem.

16. In the event that an undesirable situation of the family providing care has occurred, it is important to indicate this and cost out the service that the family member is currently providing in the cost of future care. For example, "The client's mother attends to the client's personal care and grooming needs, including dressing, brushing teeth, toileting, and making meals." For the purposes of the cost of future care, the clinician would cost out the price of an attendant, and possibly a homemaker, based on the assumption that the mother may not, in the long term, be available to assist her son.

17. Insert medical quotes to support the team's as well as your own findings.

There will be instances where there are varying professional opinions. When there are differing opinions by the experts retained by the referral source, make sure that this gets resolved in your own mind. It requires that you get permission from the referral source to speak to any other medical expert that he or she has retained. Once you have received clarification on the reasons for the discrepancy of the opinions, rationalize an appropriate explanation for the difference. Under no circumstance should you approach other experts without permission when working for plaintiff or defense counsel.

Summary and Recommendations

The summary will include your own professional opinion and also the opinions of any other clinician that has worked therapeutically with the client. When opinions that impact a future cost are made by clinicians, make sure to include the opinion and the projected cost. Some examples of areas requiring a cost assessment include:

1. Services to continue to alleviate stress and secondary losses
2. Professional services
3. Aids and adaptations
4. Equipment
5. Medications
6. Home renovations
7. Vehicle modification, transportation, driver education
8. Employability and retraining
9. Residential services
10. Pain clinics
11. Specialized neuro-behavioral programs
12. Assistance to allow the client to live independently

13. Any prognosis, including future anticipated surgeries and costs

14. Any degenerative processes anticipated (such as arthritis) also included

15. Costs "yet to be determined"—as is the case with a young child. Identify the potential need for future tutorial assistance once in school.

Make sure that you provide a solid professional opinion, including projected future needs for the client from your own discipline's perspective, before you go on to amalgamate the costs outlined by the team.

Assumptions

It is important to make assumptions in your cost-of-future-care analysis because this is an area that will be under scrutiny if you are called to court to defend your report. It is a good idea to have a supporting quote from the medical reports to support your assumptions. Assumptions can read something like this: I assume that:

1. The client will need assistance for the remainder of his life. "This client will continue to need assistance for the duration of his life; he will require 24-hour care"—Dr. Jones, Oct. 6, 2010.

2. The injuries sustained in the motor vehicle accident will not impact the expectant life span of the client. "Mr. Adams's expectant life span has not been impacted by the motor vehicle accident of May 5, 2009"—Dr. Malone, April 7, 2010.

3. Mr. Adams will continue to work part time (make quotation).

4. Mr. Adams will continue to be married to Mrs. Adams (make quotation).

5. Mr. Adams will continue to reside in his home (make quotation).

6. Mr. Adams will have at least two knee surgeries requiring care in the next 5 years (make quotation).

7. These costs include all applicable taxes

If there are symptoms from a pre-existing condition or a previous brain injury, they should be covered in your assumptions as well.

There may be situations where two or three scenarios could apply. For example:

1. Scenario 1: Mr. Adams continues to live in the family home with his wife and adult child and will continue to require additional services.

2. Scenario 2: Mrs. Adams is no longer living in the family home and the adult child moves out to attend university. Full-time multi-level support is required.

3. Scenario 3: Mr. Adams moves to a family care home.

HELPFUL HINTS FOR PREPARING A COST-OF-FUTURE-CARE ANALYSIS

1. Create a table of contents for the report. It is recommended that you list the table of contents in chronological order from most recent to oldest. It is important that the letter of referral is also listed and dated.

2. It is important to review all the medical information. Read the medical reports thoroughly. Ensure that you have all available medical consultations. Highlight anything that indicates:

    ◆ Cost
    ◆ Etiology
    ◆ Level of performance
    ◆ Anticipated level of performance in the future
    ◆ Diagnoses and prognoses including primary and secondary losses
    ◆ Employability and future employability
    ◆ Impingement of ability to engage in activities of daily living
    ◆ Future surgeries
    ◆ Future degeneration
    ◆ Support currently provided by family members (cost these out as well)

3. I would recommend that you dictate or type as you review the medical reports and highlight any quote requiring a cost assessment and flag for future cross-reference with other medical reports to corroborate. It is important when you are proofing your report to ensure that you have quoted medical reports verbatim.

4. After reviewing all medical reports as well as your own file, start to dictate or word process.

5. State the reason for your report.

6. List your qualifications.

7. List where you trained.

8. List your work experience.

9. State any limitations (such as missing medical reports).

10. State the length of time that you have been involved with the client.

11. State the time, dates, and locations when you assessed the client and who was present at the time.

12. If you have discrepancies in medical quotes, do not eliminate those quotes but rather put them into context and then, at the end, indicate what your opinion is to

make sense of that situation. If there are differing medical opinions and you feel the individuals do not have adequate information, seek permission from the referral source to contact these medical professionals, make arrangements for them to receive any missing information, and ask for an addendum to their reports. If you are being asked to do a cost of future care and you feel that the client has not improved to the point where you can assess residual loss, then it is within your parameters to suggest to the referral source that it is too soon to determine future costs and that it would make sense to adjourn the trial.

13. Move on to your own history and involvement with the case. Integrate medical quotes, especially diagnoses and prognosis corroborating information from all other clinical team members.

14. Then create a list of assumptions, stating the parameters under which you wrote the report. If possible, include a quote from the medical reports that supports each assumption.

15. Get three quotes for each item that you are costing out. Use the mean average. Record the source of the quotes in a comprehensive bibliography.

16. Ensure that the math is accurate when you are calculating.

17. Ensure that you state if tax is included or excluded.

18. Ensure that you include previously purchased items, indicating with an * (asterisk), whether they were reimbursed or not.

19. Ensure that all costs are listed in logical groups such as professional services, equipment, medications, etc.

20. Ensure that all costs are listed in the appropriate column— "Initial Costs and Recurring Costs"—as well as anticipated future costs. Ensure that all columns are totaled.

21. If it is time to do a cost of future care and the client's circumstances are likely to change (e.g., his wife is in poor health and may not live long), it may be appropriate upon discussion with the referral source to provide one, two, or three scenarios allowing for the eventuality of variables. Ensure that the reason for the multiple scenarios is clearly stated.

22. Ensure that you are stating your own opinion and that you are not only citing other clinician's opinions and regurgitating information.

23. It is best to send out your report only once as a final report. Do not send out a rough draft, which may lead the court to surmise that your opinion has changed.

Each client's case is unique. There is not one brain injury that is identical to another. Therefore, every cost-of-future-care analysis will be as unique as our clients are. It is important not to leave a stone unturned when it comes to preparing this report. The client, family, and clinical team have worked very hard to ensure that the client's timely intervention has reduced or eliminated maladaptive coping mechanisms based on unadjusted stress symptoms. We have preserved the family unit, assisting in any way to provide supports so that the family unit survives and thrives. At this final point in the active rehabilitation process, the medical reports resulting in a final cost-of-future-care analysis will make every effort to ensure that available funds will be awarded to ensure the ongoing efficacy and maintenance of the gains made by the client. The template in Appendix 9A will prompt the professional constructing the cost-of-future-care report to look at any potentiality of future needs that may occur for the client as a result of the injuries sustained (see Table 9.1).

Table 9.1 Common Areas to Consider in a Cost-of-Future-Care Analysis

Home renovations
• Bathroom/kitchen renovations to lower counter tops • Install grab bars in shower • Install ramps and widen doorways • Install bath and bed lifts • Remove carpet and install hardwood or laminate • Renovate shower or bath stall for accessibility • Wheel chair ramps • Raised toilet seats
Equipment
• Automatic shut-off kettle • Automatic shut-off coffee maker • Lightweight pots and pans with double handles • Augmentative communication systems • Memory card • Dictaphone • Audio recorder • iPad • iPhone • Voice-activated computer • Voice-activation electrical system to turn lights, blinds on/off • Auditory easy listener for assistance in vocational retraining • Orthotics/prosthetics • One-handed equipment

Table 9.1 (*Continued*) Common Areas to Consider in a Cost-of-Future-Care Analysis

Professional services

- Neuropsychologist
- Psychologist
- Occupational therapy
- Physical therapy
- Speech therapy
- Counseling
- One-to-one rehabilitation worker
- Aid/life skills worker
- Attendant care
- Massage therapy
- Cleaning services
- Homemakers
- Meal preparation
- Handyman services
- Yard care/snow removal
- Personal trainer
- Daycare assistance
- Case manager
- Sexual counselor
- Financial advisor

Residential services

- Residential care facility
- Group home
- Pain clinic
- Transportation costs
- Neurobehavioral program

Medications

- Prescriptions

Education/vocational

- Retraining
- Job coach
- Job placement
- Tutorial assistance
- Supplies/dictaphone/auditory recorder
- Specialized computer equipment
- Attendance at traumatic brain injury conference/travel/accommodation/meals

Continued

Table 9.1 (*Continued*) Common Areas to Consider in a Cost-of-Future-Care Analysis

Recreation
• Gym/recreation membership • Hobby classes • Exercise equipment
Transportation
• Vehicle modification lift • Handicap bus pass • Handicap parking pass • Taxi • Handi-dart • Driver simulation test • Driving lessons
Anticipated future surgical costs
• Supplies • Home care • Nursing care • Meals on wheels

SUMMARY

In summary, the cost-of-future-care report is the final stage of the *Lefaivre Rainbow Effect* formula. It is the last area of service to the client. It is the culmination of the entire journey with the client and family. If all of the stages have been followed, the cost of future care will truly reflect the organic residual loss—those impairments that will now become part of the new fabric of the client's and family's lives.

The clinical team will have facilitated the therapeutic process, the client will have mitigated his/her losses to the best of his/her potential, and the "new normal" has now become that place of homeostasis. The gains that have been made are in large part because the client and family have been positioned for success by all stakeholders involved.

The family unit has been protected, minimizing the extraneous secondary loss that can complicate the litigation process. The client's stress has been managed and a system for monitoring and managing ongoing stress is in place. To maintain this level of recovery, the therapeutic system that has been so effective and the services that have supported the client and family may need to remain in place or to be reintroduced periodically over the client's life. Further to this, any changes related to the injury for the future will need to be anticipated, such as arthritic changes prohibiting mobility or future surgeries related to the accident.

The picture that will remain for the client should be clear. The very important role of determining and costing out resources, supplies, and equipment will be the final therapeutic aspect of the community rehabilitation program. Each professional clinician will render a final opinion as to accomplishments, ongoing areas of challenge, and anticipated future needs of the client. The health care provider who writes the cost of future care brings the team's opinions together in one report with all recommendations having been cost out. This report will be given to an actuary, who will index it, culminating in a settlement of the claim.

In some cases, the funds may be made in a lump settlement to the client or they may be structured; in either case, the clinical team will remain available to the client on an as-needed basis and will have left the client with a wealth of coping mechanisms and a modified skill set.

APPENDIX 9A: TEMPLATE FOR CREATING A COST-OF-FUTURE-CARE ANALYSIS

Date:
Referral source:
Referral source address:
Prepared by:
Dear _____
Re: client name:
Date of injury:
My file #:
Your file #:
Purpose of the report:
Dates, times, places of visits:
Professional qualifications:

Review medical literature:
    Dr. Jones, Mar. 7, 2010
    Dr. Andrews, Nov. 5, 2010
    Dr. Smith, Feb. 15, 2011

Continued

Pictures and videos:
Past medical history:
Current medical history:
Problems arising from the injury:
History:
Test and assessment results:
Final opinion:
Assumptions of the cost of future care:
Costs:
Bibliography of sources for quotes:

	Initial costs	Yearly replacement value
Home renovations		
Wheelchair ramp (projected life span: 10 years)	$1,900*	$190
Shower grab bar, 90° angle (one-time cost)	$63.75*	
Walk-in bathtub (lifetime warranty)	$6,300	
Bathroom renovation	$15,000*	
Widen the doorways for accessibility (seven doors × $876)	$6,132*	
Kitchen renovations Lower countertop Move wall and create wheelchair-accessible space	$23,000*	
Equipment		
Raised toilet seat (expected life span: 8 years)	$35*	$4.37
Timer (life span: 3 years)	$18*	$6
Electric can opener (life span: 7 years)	$32*	$4.57
Lightweight double-handled pots and pans (life span: 20 years)	$275.50	$13.77
Smoke detector (life span: 5 years)	$29.90*	$5.98
Automatic shut-off iron (life span: 7 years)	$78.99*	$11.28

Automatic shut-off kettle (life span: 7 years)	$39.98*	$5.71
Fire extinguisher (replace every 3 years)	$32	$10.66
Exercise bike (in place of gym membership) (life span: 15 years)	$879	$58.60
Modified wheelchair van (life span 8.5 years)	$54,995	$6,470
Professional services		
Clinical psychologist: 10 hours for 1 year $175 per hour	$1750*	
Occupational therapist: $120 per hour × 10 hours per year (for 3 years) Thereafter as needed	$1200	$1,200 (for additional 2 years) Cost undetermined
Case manager: $100 per hour, 2 hours per month (for 5 years)	$2,400	$2,400 (for additional 4 years)
One-to-one rehabilitation worker: $35 per hour × 10 hours a month for 1 year $35 per hour × 10 hours per month for an additional 2 years $35 per hour × 5 hours per month for an additional 2 years	$4,200	$4,200 (for additional 2 years) $2,100 (for additional 2 years)
Additional services		
Homemaker: 8 hours a week for life at $22 per hour	$9,152*	$9,152
Spring and fall cleaning: 10 hours at $22 per hour × 2 times a year		$440
Child care: $21 per hour, 10 hours a week (for 7 years)	$10,920	$10,920 (for 7 years)
Snow removal for 6 months: $37 a week	$888	$888
Yard care: $37 a week for 6 months	$888	$888
Window cleaning spring and fall: $175 × 2 times a year		$350
Sleep disorders clinic	$3,275	
Travel: air plus tax	$476.2	
Cab return trip to airport	$76	

Continued

Residential Care		
Not appropriate for this client		
Medications		
Arthritis (name the medication): $50 per month for life	$600*	$600
Antiseizure medication: $67 per month for life	$804*	$804
Botox: one injection every 3 months for headaches (for life): $1,200 per injection	$3,600*	$3,600
Vocational/educational		
Vocational assessment: 10 hours at $120 per hour for 1 year	$1,200	$1,200
Vocational placement and support: four times over the client life span: $120 × 20 hours		$2,400 (four times over client's life span)
Attendance at brain injury conference for client and husband: $375 × 2 includes travel costs	$750	$750 (for life)
Recreation		
Pottery or other creative class: $125 × 30 years		$125 (30 years)
Handicapped recreation passes	$50	$50
Modified sports camp (for 10 years)		$450 (for 10 years)
Future unanticipated costs		
Arthritis, surgery		Undetermined at this time
Total	**$151,165.30**	**$49,422.94**

* Indicates items previously purchased by the family and not yet reimbursed.

Costs do not include provincial state/territory or federal taxes where applicable.

CHAPTER 10

Litigation

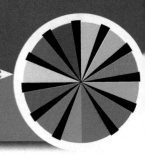

TOTAL SUM	−	DIAGNOSIS (LOSS)	+	INTERVENTION	=	RESIDUAL LOSS

   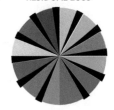

INTRODUCTION

This chapter on litigation requires an overview. As part of the author's clinical practice, she was required to testify in court in the province of British Columbia, Canada. With her 25+ years of clinical experience and attendance at legal and traumatic brain injury conferences and workshops, the knowledge accrued serves as the backbone to the content of this chapter. The caveat is that laws vary from country to country and jurisdiction to jurisdiction. The opinions offered in this chapter do not serve as advice or legal counsel, but rather as an overview challenging the professional clinician to understand the nature and responsibility of becoming an expert witness through the provision of medical legal reports. I highly encourage professionals reading this chapter to visit their professional organizations' websites to become familiar with their respective codes of conduct and ethics. I further recommend their visiting the applicable national bar associations for further legal information relevant to their region.

A further note: within the author's clinical practice an extensive in-house training program was provided to employees and contractors. Within the context of this training regime, personal injury lawyers read mock reports written by the clinicians and conducted workshops where the clinicians would be cross-examined by a skilled lawyer in a mock trial. This was an effective practice preparing the clinicians to be admitted as experts, particularly for the first time. In light of the fact that court transcripts are public record, the cross-examination of an expert becomes a permanent part of the clinician's curriculum vitae.

If a clinician is not admitted as an expert or if the report carried little weight, even one time, it may be difficult to be admitted again. It is common practice for a skilled lawyer to revisit previous court transcripts where the expert's weakness will be revealed and use this information to discredit the expert witness in the future. The lawyer will also become aware of opinions expressed in the past and will look for any discrepancies under cross-examination. An interesting quote was found:

Cross-examination of an expert is a battle, not a skirmish. It requires marshalling of resources, exhaustive preparation, keenness of mind, total concentration and an ability to react quickly. Armed with only hours of preparation, the advocate must confront, challenge and discredit someone whose lifetime work it has been to master the subject in issue. [56]

THE LITIGATION PROCESS

In the preceding chapters we have come to understand that there are a variety of scenarios where a TBI client may be in a position to file a claim against another party. For this to occur, there needs to be another party involved, and that party will have been determined as at least partially liable for the brain-injured survivor's losses. Let us review the process:

1. There has been an accident where a person (plaintiff) has been injured.

2. A second person contributed to some degree to this accident and bears some responsibility and accordingly is identified as the defendant.

3. A plaintiff lawyer will be retained to act on the part of the injured party; typically, this occurs very soon after the accident, possibly while the injured person is still in hospital.

4. The plaintiff lawyer will commence the action by filing the appropriate documentation within the relevant limitation period.

5. Ensure that you have discussions with the lawyer or referral source to determine what limitations, if any, exist in funding community rehabilitation during the interim period. Each case is different and there are many reasons why funding could be limited.

6. Despite the fact that the legal settlement is several years away and is primarily dictated by the pace of the rehabilitation program (typically 4–6 years), the plaintiff's medical and rehabilitation requirements need

to be attended to and worked out on a regular basis with the referral source.

7. In countries such as Canada, where a socialized medical system is in place, the emergency, intensive care unit, acute care, and hospital rehabilitation costs are generally covered by government funding. In other countries these may be out-of-pocket expenses to the family or a copay system may be in place.

8. When the plaintiff is discharged from the hospital rehabilitation system, there may be fewer government funded professional resources available for long-term community follow-up. It is common that professionals providing community rehabilitation will provide service on a private fee-for-service basis. The payment for these services can come from a variety of sources, with each funder having its own agenda. It is important to note that any clinical record provided by any professional can be used in the court proceedings and may be used as evidence in trial.

9. The clinician may wear several hats; the best way is always to conduct yourself professionally and compose all your notes and reports with the knowledge that sooner or later both sides to the legal equation will be reading them. Only put in writing what you would be prepared to have the world see. In this day and age it means no kidding in e-mails; be professional at all times.

The medical team is ultimately relied upon for the opinions they give in good faith based on the developed rehabilitation evidence over the period of the rehabilitation process, which is generally in a traumatic brain injury case over 4 or 6 years. The medical team should never vary from this, though the referral sources may be different, such as:

- Plaintiff
- Defense
- Rehabilitation coordinator
- Adjuster
- Tort adjuster

The clinician's notes and reports should be consistent across the board. The expert's opinion should not vary under cross-examination. It is imperative to render an opinion that is not influenced by the referral source but rather is a professional opinion. Never try to make a case that is not supported by the developed evidence. The clinician's value is in being able to identify the client's problems, to document accordingly, and to be able to support his or her opinion under cross-examination and not waver or become biased.

THE EXPERT WITNESS

An expert witness is someone who has been retained to render a neutral, unbiased opinion based on developed evidence. Quite commonly, medical experts preface their opinion with a phrase that reads something like this: "I am aware that, as an expert, my duty is to assist the court and not to be an advocate for any party. I have prepared this report in conformity with that duty and will abide by that duty if I am called upon to provide oral or written testimony."

A medical expert may have a choice in whether he or she provides expert witness testimony; for instance, a clinician may choose to accept a referral to prepare a cost-of-future-care report for the defense counsel—well aware that he or she may be called to testify to defend the report.

In another instance a health care provider who has been providing treatment to the client may be subpoenaed to give testimony. Any member of the clinical team may become an expert witness; it is because of this that we must understand how to document properly throughout the rehabilitation process to ensure that, in the eventuality of the records being subpoenaed to court, the professional is prepared. One cannot go back in time and rewrite, destroy, or alter records.

The issue of commitment, which has been previously discussed, is another contentious point. If the clinician who originally assessed the client is no longer working with the client or unavailable to give testimony, the continuity of the claim and the evidence is disrupted. This can negatively impact all parties involved, including the TBI client, and alter the settlement outcome, thus further emphasizing the ethical importance of commitment of the clinicians for the duration of the claim.

The expert witness has been called to testify to answer a specific question. It is important for the professional not to deviate from his/her area of expertise. Neither should he or she minimize, embellish, or negate facts. The expert witness must render an opinion based on sufficiently developed evidence.

IMPORTANT POINTS TO REMEMBER FOR THE EXPERT WITNESS

1. Prepare reports anticipating that they may be called to trial. The reports should be professional, accurate, unbiased, thorough, valid, reliable, and objective.

2. Stay within your professional expertise when preparing all documentation.

3. Ensure that you continue with ongoing education; your currency will be under scrutiny.

4. Make sure that you are registered with all relevant licensing bodies and professional associations.

5. Ensure that any testing procedures are updated and current.

6. Ensure that your record keeping is in order and that dates, times, and length of session are accurately recorded. Bear in mind that accounting records reflecting invoices for your time can also be subpoenaed; therefore, consistency is of paramount importance.

7. Ensure that you have made a commitment to the duration of the case in question.

8. Ensure that you have a letter of referral clearly outlining why you are involved in the case.

9. Be sure that you have a signed release of information from the client or the client's committee.

10. Be well versed on the roles of all parties, both within the clinical team and within the legal context of the case.

11. Ensure that you have available to you all medical and rehabilitation reports pertaining to the case prior to preparing your final report.

MEDICAL LEGAL REPORT WRITING

1. Ensure that you are providing an opinion from your professional frame of reference and that you have not been compromised in any way by the limitation of the funder.

2. Ensure that your assessment is complete and thorough.

3. It is advised to have a working file where there will be some handwritten notes such as when the client is being tested.

4. Keep copies of all draft reports; they are subject to trial cross-examination.

5. It is also advised that a master file be kept. This file should have all medical records from emergency through to community rehabilitation. These reports should be typed consultations including radiologic findings.

6. It is imperative that the initial request for service be made available. It is advised that this important document should be kept on the front of the master file.

When the referral is being made, you will receive partial written and, most likely, partial verbal instructions; you must have written or verbal instruction. Then you will repeat your understanding of the reason for the referral in your initial report. An outline of the instruction should be clear, so that in no way will it compromise your ethical obligation as a clinician to be thorough. It is here that the important aspect of a professional being limited by the funder will be noted and can put the professional health care provider at risk upon cross-examination—thus supporting the importance of the clinician educating and advocating to the funder so that a full and accurate assessment and treatment regime can be provided to the client as outlined in the *rainbow effect* formula. In light of the fact that the health care provider is being paid by a referral source that is most likely not medically trained, it is incumbent on the clinician to ensure that he or she is not compromising clinical and professional standards by the funder's request. This is why the clinical team needs to recognize the importance of educating the funder, particularly so that the client is positioned to mitigate their circumstances.

7. If you are unsure when writing a report, be careful that you use a word describing this—such as "it appears" or "I assume."

8. It is important to be unbiased in your report writing; at all costs avoid making comments using insensitive words and making a statement of claim—for instance, making a statement that the client "is an alcoholic" or that "the house is filthy." Rather, one could frame the same scenario as "the client disclosed that he had had a few beers before his appointment" or "upon conducting a home assessment the client made a comment that he did not have time to clean the house."

9. Be careful not to make value statements—such as "the client is very difficult"; rather, make a statement like, "the client finds it difficult to stay on task and the rehabilitation worker has observed on many occasions that the client appears frustrated when he is overloaded or fatigued." Another example could be, "I feel that the client is malingering." A better approach is "the client missed several appointments and fell behind in his therapy as a result."

10. It is important to be well prepared; a note on the file saying "dictated but not read" is never a good idea.

11. Ensure that accounting records are kept in separate files, bearing in mind that these also can be subpoenaed.

12. Steer clear of attempting to use legal jargon; this places the clinician outside his or her area of expertise.

13. If there are discrepancies in medical opinions, do not ignore these but rather clarify them and provide verbiage making sense of why there are differing opinions.

14. When quoting another professional in your report, ensure accuracy. It is never good form to criticize another practitioner's work.

15. Ensure that reports are accurate with no typographical errors.

MY TO-DO'S PREPARING TO GO TO COURT

Being called to testify in court may be stressful. Your referral source will not necessarily prepare you for the stress involved in providing your expert testimony at trial. There are several dynamics at play that can change your anticipated attendance at court, such as unanticipated adjournments, rescheduling of witnesses, or changes in appearance times at trial. Failure to review the expectations the referral source has of your testimony—resulting in endless hours of preparation, a good deal of which is simply wasted time—should be avoided. Remember that the referral source is not aware of your anxiety or stress and will generally be unaware that you are working overtime to prepare to give your testimony. Often this leads to disgruntlement by the referral source when your final account is rendered. The referral source may think that much of the time you have spent was not necessary. Make sure you clarify, clarify, clarify—asking the important questions of "When am I being called?" "What are the expectations and what type of preparation does the referral source suggest I engage in?"

Oftentimes it is difficult to get through to the lawyer. A strategy that often works is to explain that you take appearing in court very seriously and prepare in advance for testifying as an expert witness. Inform the lawyer that you are about to start to prepare and require his or her input on the extent of your preparation (Figure 10.1). Insist on telephone appointments ensuring that both parties will be prepared for the discussion.

EXPERT WITNESS TESTIMONY

The role of the clinician as an expert witness is crucial to the outcome of a client's case. This process ultimately defines the loss and awards the client with monies to purchase care for a lifetime of needs. If the cost of future care is not accepted or the general loss, wage loss, future wage loss, and employability questions remain

1. Finding out when I have been called to appear in court is of key importance. If I have been called early in the trial, the more likely it is that I will actually be called to testify and the more important my testimony seems to be. If I have been scheduled to appear toward the end of the trial, the less likely it is that I will actually be called. If I cannot get the lawyer to commit to when he might call me, I can use the strategy of discussing having him serve a subpoena to me so that I will know for certain.

2. Have I been subpoenaed to court?   Yes No

3. If no, have I contacted the lawyer to ask to be subpoenaed?   Yes No

4. Have I been requested to appear in court?   Yes No

5. When have I been subpoenaed/requested to appear?

    Day: _____

    Time: _____

    Location: _____

6. Is the court time definitive or is there a chance that it could be bumped? Several cases are scheduled for the same day, so many will settle in advance. As you get closer to the date, the lawyer will have some idea if his or her case has been bumped or has been assigned a definitive date.

    Definitive: Yes No

7. Finding out who has called me and who all the players are is of prime importance.

8. What is the name of the lawyer who has called me, his/her company, and location?

    _____

    What is his position, plaintiff or defense? _____

    Did I work for him in service delivery?   Yes No

    If no, who was the referral source (name, position, and location)?

    _____

9. What is the name of the lawyer on the other side, his/her company, and location?

    What is his/her position, plaintiff or defense? _____

    Did I work for him/her in service delivery?   Yes No

10. Has the referral source changed since the original referral was made?

    If yes, state names of all referral sources, the date when
    the referral changed, and the reason why.   Yes No

    Original referral source _____

    Current referral source _____

    When did the source change? _____

    Why? _____

Figure 10.1 My to-do's for court preparation.

11. What is the style of the lawyer who has called me?

_____

12. Finding out why I have been called to appear is also of key importance. If I am being called by my referral source, why is he or she doing this? What is his or her strategy?

Strategy: _____

13. If I am being called by opposing counsel, I need to know why I am being called. I need to ask my referral source to find out if it is because of my report or because of my experience. If someone from their side has critiqued my report, what areas of my report is counsel opposed to?

Who critiqued my report? State name and position:

_____

_____

14. What are the hot spots in my report that I need to be conscious of as outlined by counsel(s)?

_____

15. Reread my report in light of the hot spots identified by counsel.   Yes No

16. Ensure that the following items are clear in my report:

    a. Date of referral and a statement of service required are included.   Yes No

    b. All medical reports are listed.   Yes No

    c. All medical reports have been carefully reviewed.   Yes No

    d. If differing opinions are cited, list opinions and pages referenced in my report.

       I need to be clear as to how I have dealt with these differing opinions.

       Opinion 1: _____

       Page number: _____

       Opinion 2: _____

       Page number _____

    e. Videotapes referenced if applicable.   Yes No

    f. Dates, locations, and names of all present during visits with client are noted.   Yes No

    g. Professional qualifications are stated.   Yes No

       List any changes since the first report.

       _____

    h. My assessments are clear and I understand how and why I used them.   Yes No

       List assessments that were not done and reasons why:

       _____

Figure 10.1 (*Continued*) My to-do's for court preparation.

i.	The assumptions underpinning my opinion are clear.	Yes No
j.	List any medical diagnoses or prognoses used and give medical report reference: _____	
k.	Complete an accurate history (any changes since my report?)	Yes No
l.	My professional opinion is clearly and objectively stated. _____	Yes No
m.	There are at least two (preferably three) costs for each item that has been researched.	Yes No
n.	All references researched are listed.	Yes No

Note: Any questions that have been answered in the negative are potential hot spots and could be brought out in cross-examination.

17. Ask the referral source if any new medical information has come in on the file since my final report was written.

If yes, ask for approval to review and do an addendum report. Yes No

18. If anything has changed in my opinion, ask for approval to do an Addendum (remember I cannot change my original report.) Yes No

19. Update curriculum vitae and ensure referral source has updated copy. Yes No

20. Set up an appointment with the lawyer calling me to prepare. Yes No

Note: This should be scheduled for very close to the appearance date in case the file settles.

21. Prepare my file. Yes No

a.	Create an index or table of contents for material.	Yes No
b.	Tab the file according to the index or table of contents.	Yes No
c.	Ensure that dates, times, and length of consultations, are clear and available.	Yes No
d.	Ensure that material is listed in chronological order from most recent to oldest.	Yes No
e.	Ensure that documentation is clean.	Yes No
f.	Ensure that there is a letter of referral.	Yes No
g.	Ensure that there is a signed release of information from client.	Yes No
h.	Ensure that there is no accounting material in the clinical file.	Yes No
i.	Ensure that there is no misfiled information.	Yes No
j.	Ensure that videotapes/pictures (if they exist) are part of file	Yes No
k.	Ensure that there are curriculum vitae for the other health care professionals.	Yes No

22. Ensure that the master file is tabbed, indexed, and in the same order as the working file. Yes No

Figure 10.1 (*Continued*) My to-do's for court preparation.

unclear, the court will not have the required information to make an informed decision regarding how to award the client monies for the damages suffered. If the family has not had adequate support and thus are exhibiting breakdown, this can camouflage the actual situation of the TBI survivor. The defense can work the angle that the family breakdown is the problem rather than the client's brain injury.

At the point of settlement, most community care will be available through the private sector. The client will need to pay a fee for service after the settlement of the claim. It is imperative that the clinicians be admitted as expert witnesses each time they are called to court. It is important to note that expert witness testimony is part of the court-documented record, which is easily accessed as a public record online.

Let us examine the process of being admitted as an expert witness:

1. The first step is for the clinician to be accepted as an expert witness.

2. The party who has called you will make an attempt to have you admitted as an expert based on:

    a. Your qualifications

    b. Your experience and whether you have been admitted as an expert before. "In this area it is helpful to carefully and critically review the expert's previous writings including any other testimony and look for differences" [57, p. 12]

    c. The strength of your curriculum vitae

    d. Any publications you have had and the currency of the publication ("A meticulous review of the expert's qualifications including publications and presentations to diminish [or, if possible, destroy] their qualifications") [57, p. 13]

    e. Your commitment to ongoing education

    f. Being a member in good standing of your professional governing body

    g. Your consistency in service to the traumatically brain injured and your commitment to becoming a specialist; having had numerous jobs is not a positive in this case. One needs to be a specialist rather than a generalist.

The defense will make an attempt at [57, p. 11]:

- "Attacking qualifications and when
- Attacking underlying factual assumptions
- Exposing the opinion as a matter of judgment"

The defense will be well prepared, having reviewed any previous testimony given by the expert; if there were trouble spots in previous testimony, this, in itself, may be grounds to disqualify the expert.

The major underpinning will be to discredit the expert by challenging the work, opinion, and theory. Questions will be directed at discrepancies in medical opinions or discrepancies given in previously recorded testimony. The relevance of the report may be in question; if any omissions have been made, this is a setup for the defense. Information should never be omitted; rather it should be recognized.

The strategy may be to fluster the expert, resulting in the expert appearing disorganized. Commonly, the clinician is asked to read from the copious records—thus the need for a carefully indexed table of contents and bibliography.

If the **total sum stage** has not been completed or if the neuropsychological assessment has not been recruited, then the foundational tenants to rendering an opinion are disturbed, making it difficult to render convincing testimony.

"The expert opinion is only as strong as the underlying factual basis. Opinion evidence is worthless, and arguably irrelevant, if there is an absence of factual foundation for the opinion" [57, p. 10].

It is also important to note that many lawyers will hire a professional from the same discipline as the expert to poke holes in the report and assist the lawyer to prepare the cross-examination.

3. The clinician has now been admitted as an expert; at any time in the course of the testimony the expert may lose this standing. For instance, the expert's credentials may be accepted, but if the report is weak and unsubstantiated the judge or jury may not deem the report to be expert. If the clinician seems biased or the defense has been successful in proving that the assumptions that the opinion was based on are faulty, then the report and thus the expert can be rejected. If the clinician assumes the role of advocate rather than truth sayer, the court may see the clinician as biased. If the clinician steps out of the bounds of his or her professional expertise, this can also negatively impact admissibility as well as the weight given to the report. If the expert becomes agitated, he or she may appear not to be transparent.

4. The expert, once admitted, will render a professional opinion. This opinion and the report will serve to assist the judge and/or jury to make a decision regarding the monetary award for the client. The judge will determine the weight that he or she will place on the expert's testimony and report. The weight of the report will generally be declared in the judge's reason for judgment.

5. Helpful hints:

    a. Dress professionally.

    b. Be on time.

    c. Have your file tidy and organized.

    d. Understand how to address the court (e.g., my lord, my lady, your honor).

    e. Stay within the scope of your practice.

    f. Do not answer questions that have not been asked.

    g. Be clear on standards of practice within your profession.

    h. Deliver your opinion in a strong, clear voice using lay terms.

    i. Be accurate and transparent.

    j. If you do not know the answer, admit that you do not know the answer.

    k. Never engage with the cross-examining lawyer if he or she is attacking in approach.

    l. Never use vague words such as "maybe" or "kind of."

    m. Do not ramble.

    n. Do not make generalizations or be too rigid: "everyone thinks this"; "always" or "never."

    o. Offer a solid opinion about what has been written, pursuant to the medical reports, assessment of the client, and the client's therapeutic outcome.

    p. Make sure that you can answer questions on all of the assessments in terms of the circumstances in which they were administered, why they were administered, what the result was, and what the result means functionally.

    q. Body language should be confident and comfortable, not adversarial.

    r. Address the appropriate party in your response to questions; it may be the judge or the jury. Be clear before you take the stand.

    s. Do not personalize, thinking that this is a personal attack.

    t. Tell the truth.

SUMMARY

In summary, the realm of testifying in court as an expert witness can be daunting at best. It appears to be a bit of a chess game. The expert will serve himself or herself well by learning how the game works, as well as the roles of the significant players and the protocols. If the *rainbow effect* formula has been followed, then the expert will find himself or herself positioned well to give testimony.

The expert will play a significant role in declaring the reality of the client's situation. This is the last portion of providing a service to the brain-injured client and family. If we have done our job well assisting the client to mitigate his or her circumstances, if we have advocated for services to help the family, if we have reduced the financial stress for the client by directing the family to any and all financial resources, then all that is left is to render a final opinion from our professional perspective.

It is of paramount importance to be organized and prepared. All reporting over this 4- to 6-year period will have been prepared with the possibility of the expert being subpoenaed to testify in court.

It is in being an expert witness that the clinician stakes his or her professional credibility. One aims to be admitted as an expert and to have one's final opinion and resulting report carry heavy weight.

APPENDIX 10A: LITIGATION TERMS DEFINED

Actuary (Economist): Person who calculates the value of money for the expected life span of the client. He or she uses tables or indexes for inflation. He or she builds in taxes and inflation. This is the person who will calculate the wage loss and present value of the future wage loss and cost of future care.

Adjuster: An employee who works out of a claims center and is responsible for settling minor claims. There are claims adjusters, bodily injury the adjusters, and injury management coordinators.

Advance on Tort: Plaintiff lawyer negotiates with the major loss examiner or defense counsel for advances on the tort.

Arbitration: A forum in which each party and its counsel present its position before a neutral third party who renders a specific award. Arbitration uses a neutral third party to resolve disputes with an arbitrator experienced in the substantive law of the case. Arbitrators generally act similarly to a judge and make decisions about evidence and written opinions that can be binding or nonbinding.

Committee: A person who is responsible for an incompetent, injured person's estate, resources, etc. while the person is still living. For example, this person would be in charge of making decisions such as buying or selling a house or car for the injured person.

Competitively Employable: The question to remember regarding employability is not just whether the client can do the job but whether he or she would be hired over someone else to do that job.

Cost-of-Future-Care Analysis: The cost of future care should be calculated only when the client has mitigated his or her losses and reached a plateau in his or her rehabilitation. The analysis evaluates what costs a client will incur for the rest of his or her life in order to maintain the current level of function. This includes everything that all health professionals have recommended for the present and future care, as well as the doctor's prognosis.

Defendant: The person who is being sued by the plaintiff and who it is alleged is wholly or partially responsible for the plaintiff's injuries.

Head Office Claims: A department handling catastrophic claims.

Head Office Examiner: This is the person who manages the defense portion of the file including retaining defense counsel.

Independent Medical Evaluation (IME): This is conducted primarily for legal or quantifying purposes and generally does not mean treatment. It is privileged information.

Liability: Determines who is at fault for the accident partially or in the entirety.

Limits or Limits of the Policy: Limits is the amount of insurance held by the defendant's insurance policy that may or may not be sufficient to cover the costs of the plaintiff's claim.

Mediation: Mediation is a voluntary and confidential process under which an impartial person, the mediator, facilitates communication between the parties to promote reconciliation, settlement, or understanding among them. The parties try to negotiate a resolution of their differences on terms acceptable to all sides. The mediation process is nonbinding.

Mitigate: To make all reasonable efforts at reducing the losses.

Non-pecuniary Damages: Losses that you cannot see (such as loss of self-esteem, pain and suffering, etc.) which affect quality of living.

Own Occupation: The job that the client held prior to the injury.

Partial No-Fault Insurance System: A partial no-fault system provides for medical and rehabilitation needs of the client regardless of his liability. The litigation process can still take place.

Plaintiff: The person who has been injured and commences an action against the named defendant for damages sustained becomes the plaintiff.

Present-Day Value: The costs outlined in the cost of future care are costs in terms of present-day values. It is the actuaries' job to build in the index tab and inflation, etc.

Public Trustee: The ultimate guardian for the mentally incompetent citizen.

Reasons for Judgment: This is a document that the judge prepares to explain what his or her ruling on the case is and why he or she has ruled this way. This may include the weight he or she places on certain experts' testimony and reports.

Rehabilitation Coordinator: The person who is responsible for authorizing payment for rehabilitation from an injured party's rehabilitation benefits.

Statute of Limitation: This is the period of time when the person can sue for damages. When this time period has expired, he or she can no longer commence an action.

Tort: This is another term for the litigation process.

Underinsured Motorist Protection: Insurance you carry to cover you if the other person involved in a motor vehicle accident is not insured, or is underinsured.

Writ or NOCC (Notice of Civil Claim): This document will have various names based on jurisdiction. For instance, in British Columbia, Canada, the NOCC is the document by which legal proceedings are commenced, and sets out the details for what has given rise to the action. For example, the details of the accident, the client's injuries, and the losses sustained.

CHAPTER 11

Business Practices and Public Relations

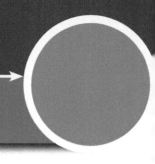

INTRODUCTION

Health care providers are medically trained individuals who by virtue of working with the traumatically brain injured may now find themselves in the realm of business.

There is every likelihood that the community clinicians will find themselves in the world of private practice, which is a fee-for-service business. This can be a challenge in that our professional training programs generally do not cover the topic of running your own business.

It has been reviewed in the preceding chapters that the brain-injured population requires commitment on behalf of the care provider. In the author's opinion it verges on unethical to be retained to work at a full-time job—for instance, in a hospital—while moonlighting in private practice (carrying one or two brain-injured cases to possibly augment income). As we have already cited, this situation is fraught with problems in regard to service delivery and availability, not to mention being admitted as an expert witness.

If one is to venture into the private business sector, then risks need to be taken.

Let us remove ourselves from the world of health care and reflect on an example from another business sector.

I go to my favorite restaurant; there is a long wait to get a table and they cannot seem to find my reservation. Once a table is available, the waiter takes 1 hour to place our orders. When the orders arrive, there is a mix-up with one meal: The order was gluten free and the meal arrived with a mound of wheat pasta. One steak was very rare, but the order was for medium well. Because the wait for the food had taken so long, the pasta was set aside and the rare steak was consumed with little satisfaction.

This sounds like a disaster; on the scale of probabilities, the patrons will not return to this restaurant and, moreover, they will tell anyone who will listen about the nightmarish experience, further compounding the terrible public relations for the establishment.

It is interesting to read about the psychology of service. Once goodwill is lost, it can take years to gain it back. The bottom line is that we do not want to lose goodwill in the first place.

The question then becomes how can we provide excellent service to our clients; promote our service through goodwill and word of mouth; maintain a business office; be admitted as an expert witness, with heavy weight placed on our work; incur the expense of running an office; and engage in some level of public relations so we continue to get more work.

Oftentimes a start-up clinician will go lightly on incurring the expense required to run a professional business, waiting until the revenues are high enough to support a professional setup financially.

Let us go back to our restaurant scenario. If we go to a restaurant where we have heard that the food is great, but when we enter the establishment it appears run-down, with mismatched dishes and tattered tablecloths, it gives an impression to the customer of not being sanitary just because it was so run-down. In this case the excellent food may not draw the customer back again.

The same thing can happen in business. If the clinician's clinical skills are wonderful but the referral source gets an answering machine each time he or she tries to reach the clinician, this may reduce how effective the referral source perceives the clinician's service to be.

Let us imagine that the referral source gets a phone call from the client's family. The family is upset that the home renovations are different from what they understood and the clinician organizing the renovations is at another full-time job and is unable to receive or return phone calls. This can impact the perceived and real professionalism of the clinician.

The old adage "dress for success" holds some merit. If we want to be taken seriously, then we have to be serious. If we want our clients to have good therapeutic outcomes, then we need to be available. If we want to get repeat referrals, then we need to be set up as a professional business.

One of the major pitfalls of being a sole private practitioner is access and availability. If the clinician is working with a client, then he or she is unavailable to answer the phone, do an intake for a new referral, or accept a crisis phone call from a client. How do we solve the many demands placed on the health care professional? Let us break the process down.

WHAT DOES A GOOD BUSINESS PROFILE LOOK LIKE?

1. The clinician has business cards and some type of pamphlet/website describing services, including hours of operation, new referral process, and rates.

2. The clinician will have a system set up so that a real person answers the phone.

3. The clinician will be available through pager, text, or beeper for emergencies.

4. The clinician will return phone calls and respond to e-mails and text in a time-efficient manner within 24 hours for non-emergencies.

5. New referrals can be seen within a very reasonable time.

6. Reports will be issued within a reasonable time after having seen the client.

7. A professional place of business will be established to see clients and conduct team meetings; this should be a comfortable environment for the client.

8. The place of business will be wheelchair accessible with ample parking.

9. There should be a system of feedback such as a customer satisfaction inventory (Table 11.2).

10. The clinician will use a time management system that allows for client crises and the spontaneous needs of a new referral—such as an unscheduled attendance at a discharge meeting tomorrow, the completion of home renovations for the client's discharge in 1 week, or a spontaneous call to testify in court as a medical expert (see Chapter 12).

11. The clinician will have an ongoing public relations plan to ensure that goodwill is kept and that repeat referrals continue.

12. The clinician will have a plan of service coverage when on vacation or leave.

ESTABLISHING A PROFESSIONAL PROFILE IN THE START-UP PHASE

Office Space

1. Share office space with other clinicians, sharing the rent and triple net costs.

2. If you are working alone, you can rent furnished professional office space by the day. This service will oftentimes include a professional receptionist. This type of space is valuable for a clinician that prefers a home office but also requires space to see the client and hold team meetings.

Telephone and Reception Service

1. Share office space with a person in the business of providing word processing services; a reduction in rent can be in exchange for answering the telephone for your practice. This allows for the brain-injured person to speak to a live person. Answering machines can be very confusing for someone who has suffered a brain injury.

2. Contract to a messaging service; if you are busy with a client, your phone can be rerouted to the messaging company where, again, the client can speak to a live person. In this case the messaging company would require you to train personnel on how to handle the brain-injured client's phone calls.

Developing a Partnership

1. Developing a partnership with another person of the same profession or with a group of health care providers from a variety of disciplines can offer the opportunity to work collaboratively as a team.

2. This situation has an up side: It provides the opportunity to have another clinician cover the primary clinician's cases when on vacation and allows for better availability to take on new referrals if any one clinician is fully booked.

3. The down side of a partnership is that there may be difficulties with standards of care or on mutually agreed upon business or financial objectives.

Creating a Company

1. In creating a company, the owner is taking a greater risk in that he or she can be deemed liable for the service provision of employees and contractors.

2. In this case, taking out adequate malpractice, liability, and general insurance is of paramount importance.

3. Provision of corporate standards of care, protocols and policies, and in-house training are the responsibility of the employer.

4. Maintaining continuity of care, completing random audits of cases to ensure quality and standards, hiring and firing as necessary add to the owner's roster of things to do.

5. The upside of this scenario is that several clinicians can be available for taking on work, so the management of the fruits of marketing can be successfully distributed. The referral source will also have a selection of clinicians

to choose from. This will most effectively allow the client to be matched with a clinician that is personality, race, gender, and language appropriate.

6. This scenario allows for vacation coverage and tight time lines.

7. The downside is that, typically, employees and contractors will not have the same level of commitment as the owner of the business. If one clinician falls short of excellence, this can impact negatively all of the other clinicians working within this company as well as the company itself. In reality, if one clinician within a company is testifying in court, he or she may end up in the position of defending other clinicians' previously rejected expert opinions. Therefore, the onus of responsibility ultimately falls to the owner for setting standards, including quality control measures, avoiding liability and malpractice exposure. The goodwill of the company can be positively or negatively impacted by each clinician's performance.

8. This scenario requires a full-fledged business plan with multilevels of standard controls such as billing practices, time lines of service delivery, time management, quality statistics, customer satisfaction surveys, scheduling, and marketing.

As health care providers, it is important to have balance in our own lives. Because we strive for balance we will be taking vacations and putting in reasonable hours at work. A clinical caseload of this nature will require professional coverage when the primary clinician is on vacation, even if just for a short period of time. It is the primary clinician's responsibility to organize the transference of the file to another suitable professional of the same discipline, to ensure quality and continuity of care.

It is important to remember that the referral source has retained a particular professional. By introducing a new clinician for vacation coverage, this new clinician will now gain valuable knowledge of the client's traumatic brain injury; this in turn could influence the legal flow of the case by introducing another potential expert. It is respectful and important to communicate any transference of a clinical case with the funder. It may also be appropriate to introduce the vacation relief clinician to the funder other team members, family, and client.

Prior to transferring the case, the primary clinician will complete a brief summary of the case to date. It will include clinical milestones, significant others, goals, hot spots, and political and funding issues. It is important to educate the new clinician by producing a list of current to do's on each case. The transfer tracking protocol in Table 11.1 has been useful in a clinical setting.

Table 11.1 Transfer Tracking Sheet

Client name: _____		Date: _____	
Transferring clinician: _____			
New in-charge clinician: _____			
1.	Approvals	Yes	Date
	a. Agreed to by referral source	_____	_____
	b. Agreed to by client	_____	_____
	c. Written notification sent to referral source	_____	_____
2.	Summary		
	a. Completed, including overview of client file (include clinical milestones, names and telephone numbers of care providers, hot spots, and political issues)	_____	_____
	b. Reviewed with new therapist verbally and in writing	_____	_____
3.	List of to-do's of immediate clinical issues		
	a. Completed	_____	_____
	b. Reviewed with new therapist	_____	_____
4.	Introductions	Date scheduled	Date held
	a. To referral source	_____	_____
	b. To client/family	_____	_____
	c. To team members	_____	_____
	_____	_____	_____
	_____	_____	_____
	_____	_____	_____
	_____	_____	_____
	_____	_____	_____
5.	Changes should be noted in billing invoices	_____	_____
6.	Final transfer summary issued to new clinician	_____	_____

ENHANCING YOUR IMAGE: PUBLIC RELATIONS

1. When starting up your health care business it is helpful to send out introductory announcements to referral sources. Include a business card and pamphlet about the service.

2. It can be helpful to offer a brief free workshop about your service; you can also offer to see a client pro bono, which will serve as an example of your work.

3. A website should be designed to include relevant information about the service provider including the languages in which the service can be provided, gender and experience of the clinical team, professional designation, and geographical areas serviced. The website should also include a user-friendly guide explaining how to make a referral.

4. Introduce yourself and drop off a curriculum vitae to people in the industry such as:

   - Neuropsychologists
   - Clinical psychologists
   - Physiatrists
   - Social workers at the hospital
   - Physical therapists
   - Speech and language pathologists
   - Hospital discharge case managers
   - Insurance claims centers (adjusters; try to meet the manager)
   - Insurance rehabilitation coordinators (try to meet the manager)
   - Workers' compensation coordinator
   - Local health authority brain injury programs
   - Private schools and public school authorities
   - Vocational rehabilitation services
   - Executive director of the brain injury association
   - Government employment counselors in your area
   - Personal injury lawyers specializing in traumatic brain injury
   - Major loss examiners
   - Victims assistance
   - Veterans affairs
   - Aboriginal affairs

5. Announcing the opening of your business with an open house can also be an effective means of getting to know referral sources and other clinical team members. The clinician can host an open house, and a brief PowerPoint presentation is an effective way to provide your information to guests. Have a guest book available with an option for guests to sign up for a complimentary quarterly company newsletter, which will include small excerpts focused on service, education, therapeutic tips, and resources for the TBI client. It is helpful to have a basket beside the guest book so that guests may leave their business cards.

6. Create a company newsletter including new information on the previously mentioned topics and circulate to interested parties.

7. Submit abstracts and poster presentations at respected brain injury and professional conferences.

8. Contribute articles to various recognized publications.

9. Have a professional booth at relevant brain injury conferences.

10. Keep a master record of all referral sources broken down by category.

11. Stay in touch with referral sources as clinical files are closing; make personal contact to see if any new files can be directed your way as your time opens up.

12. If you are traveling to see a client in a rural area, inform all of your referral sources of your visit to this area in the event that they have a client that needs to be seen in the same vicinity. This also allows you to be more cost effective to the funder by pro-rating travel costs.

13. Maintain a public profile, advertising online, as well as the yellow and white pages in the telephone directory.

14. Utilize holidays such as Christmas and Thanksgiving as an opportunity to reach out and connect with referral sources.

15. Keep mini personal notes on referral sources, pets, ages of children, interests, hobbies. When opportunities arise, such as at conferences, these can be used as points of conversation.

16. When attending conferences, do not travel in a group with co-workers; rather, make it an objective to meet new people in the field. It is easiest to approach an odd-numbered group (e.g., three or five) because it will be easier to join in the conversation with sidebars rather than interrupting.

17. The easiest and most cost-effective means of marketing is by creating and maintaining goodwill with present referral sources through positive work relationships, availability, and providing excellent clinical results. This offers the opportunity to create a reputation where others seeking service will hear of your good work.

18. In working with present referral sources you may be called to testify in court; in doing a good job, this provides an opportunity to have a public record of your work in transcript files.

19. Clients will be attending brain injury support groups and they will share stories of their service providers' excellent consistent client care. This will give reason for the client to recommend your service; conversely, if the client is not pleased with your service and this is verbalized and shared, it can jeopardize your reputation.

20. Be aware of your caseload and its time requirements; this allows you to project the demands on your time for the future.

21. Ensure that there is a plan for suitable backup service provision during your vacation or any period of absence.

22. Assess your available time to be able to take on new clients and provide excellent care (Table 12.7). You do not want to turn down work, but, by the same token, you cannot ethically take on too much work.

23. Follow the time management system as laid out in Chapter 12.

24. Complete the quality statistics to ensure the efficacy and cost effectiveness of your service in comparison to industry standards.

25. If there are no available industry standards, create corporate guidelines regarding parameters around time spent on any given task (Table 12.1) so that time billed for a specific service is equitable and consistent despite the selection of clinician.

26. Ensure that the job task list and the quality statistics build in quality control so that the parameters of performance are measured by the time it would take for an experienced clinician to complete the task.

27. Invite feedback from your referral sources through a customer satisfaction survey (Table 11.2).

28. Implement appropriate recommendations made by the referral source as indicated in the customer satisfaction survey.

Table 11.2 Customer Satisfaction Survey

Date: _____ Clinician: _____
Referral source: _____
We appreciate your taking the time to comment on the following:

Poor		Average					Excellent		

1. Relationship with client

1	2	3	4	5	6	7	8	9	10

2. Relationship with family

1	2	3	4	5	6	7	8	9	10

3. Assessment

1	2	3	4	5	6	7	8	9	10

4. Effectiveness of rehabilitation program

1	2	3	4	5	6	7	8	9	10

5. Cost

1	2	3	4	5	6	7	8	9	10

6. Report writing

1	2	3	4	5	6	7	8	9	10

7. Case management

1	2	3	4	5	6	7	8	9	10

8. Communication style

1	2	3	4	5	6	7	8	9	10

9: Relationship with referral source

1	2	3	4	5	6	7	8	9	10

10. Overall clinical skills

1	2	3	4	5	6	7	8	9	10

11. Overall performance

1	2	3	4	5	6	7	8	9	10

12. Expert witness testimony

1	2	3	4	5	6	7	8	9	10
Total									**120**

13. Will you refer again? _____ Yes _____ No

14. Comments: Recommendations

SUMMARY

In summary, health care providers may find that they wear several hats—those of clinician, case manager, and business person.

Because of the constraints in government funding, the long-term service delivery model in many countries is falling into the private domain. This poses a challenge to the health care provider who is trained in a medical or psychosocial field. In most university course curricula, business practice is not included outside the field of business.

The clinician will be required out of necessity to develop business skills to be successful in service delivery.

Because of this we have reviewed the need for a solid business plan. The clinician has several models of partnership to choose from: developing a true partnership, becoming an employer and either employing or contracting out to retained health care professionals, or working solo and retaining additional office and clerical services.

The goal is excellence in client care and service delivery, availability, and a system to deal cost effectively with emergencies and crises. A system of backup support is required when the primary care provider goes on vacation. Standards of practice and standards of care including policies and procedures will need to be established.

A marketing and public relations plan addressing the need to maintain areas of goodwill and a plan to maintain or expand the market will be as ongoing, as clinical service is.

Lastly, strict and careful examination of quality within the private service delivery sector needs to be inherent to any practice, whether it is a solo practitioner or a large corporation. Customer satisfaction inventories are an effective way to ensure feedback, which facilitates the clinician to maintain accountability.

The responsibility of carrying applicable malpractice, general, and liability insurance falls to the private practitioner.

This chapter positions us well to move forward to the time management system, where a practical application regarding use of time will give the clinician the necessary tools to put the previously mentioned quality control into practice.

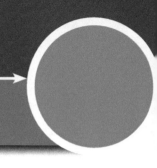

CHAPTER 12

Four-Week Time Management System

INTRODUCTION

This chapter will focus on the health care provider's method of time management. It may seem a bit odd or redundant at face value to include time management in a medical book focused on cognitive retraining for the traumatically brain injured. However, the author found in her practice that a time management system was critical for the provision of quality care and absolutely necessary from a business perspective.

In the early years it was a common occurrence for the clinical staff to become overloaded and burnt out if the unanticipated client crises were not built into their scheduling. Moreover, when unplanned clinical situations occurred the clinician was required to work more hours to address the client's need, but the billable time was lower because of the increased disorganization. Out of necessity the author developed a time management system specific to the industry of providing quality, cost-effective care to the traumatically brain injured.

Let us take a closer look at how the client's traumatic brain injury experience will impact the professional health care provider's ability to be an effective time manager.

As we review the traumatic brain injury experience, we will see a family that has been traumatized and is trying to get life back on track to resume normalcy, with peace and calm. We have reviewed in the intervention chapter how confusing all of this experience is for the survivor. We understand the risks for the client and family in association with stress and sensory overload. We understand that we must reduce or eliminate the stress for the client and family and most certainly we should not add to it. The aim is to prepare the home, the family, and the team to be in a position to provide time-sensitive, safe intervention responding to high-priority situations as they arise. There are several key scenarios that will necessitate immediate intervention. The clinician can build this likelihood into the schedule. The following will require immediate attention on the part of the health care provider.

When the client is about to be discharged back home to the family, there may be safety hazards in the environment that will require renovation or adaptation before the client returns home. Once the discharge date has been established, there will be a limited amount of time to make the necessary changes to the home environment.

The family has been traumatized by this life event; situations will arise, particularly in the early stages of the client's return home, requiring timely intervention. In these early days it is not appropriate to place a client on a wait list for an appointment at a much later date. Over time, the immediate need for clinical assistance will reduce dramatically. However, when a case is new, it is very important to have a system that will allow the clinician to be available as the needs arise. We can do this by anticipating the client's needs in advance.

Stress is a factor for the client and family and can create spontaneous emotional problems that need to be addressed as the situation occurs to protect the family system and the relationships within the system.

The ongoing litigation process will create time-sensitive demands at various intervals for the health care providers.

We understand the social and personal issues arising for the client and family, and we, the health care providers, have made every effort to reduce the stress for the client and family with an aim to keep order in their lives. It is inherent in this process that we also must have order in our clinical schedules to assist and not complicate the situation. In reality, health care providers are very busy people; the very nature of our clinical caseloads makes our schedules subject to change at any given moment as crises arise.

The reality is that we can utilize traditional time management systems, we can make lists, and we can set priorities, goals, and objectives but our schedules are not ours alone. Our clients are part of our daily schedule even if they do not have a scheduled appointment for that day. Each time we receive an unanticipated phone call, text, or e-mail during what we thought was going to be an organized, predictable day, it can disrupt our schedule. When this disruption occurs, it inevitably impacts the appointments we have scheduled for that day.

Typically, when schedules shift, the clinician will drop or postpone whatever is his or her least favorite task. Unfortunately, this is often report writing. If we refer back to the earlier chapters we will understand that, when one member of the clinical team lags behind in report writing, it impacts the entire team's ability to move forward in developing treatment regimes. Without any given discipline's report, the team's accuracy in the intervention plan is reduced. It is to this end that the task of report writing cannot be deferred because of another client's crisis. If we allow this to happen, we are now subjecting the client who did have a scheduled appointment to a pending crisis if his or her issues are not dealt with as well.

Another item that is prone to delay in the event of the clinician's schedule being disrupted is the return of phone calls. Let us imagine that a brain-injured client was discharged from hospital 3 weeks ago. The client displayed problems with identifying where his room was in the hospital, and wandering was an issue. Upon discharge, the client was oriented to time, place, person, and location; however, once home, his family noticed that he had regressed in this area and was leaving the house frequently and getting lost. The mother and father were spelling each other, taking days off work to ensure that their son was safe. Based on the client's improvement of orientation in hospital, the parents had assumed that their son would be better in a few days. The situation was not getting better and the family was now exhibiting stress symptoms, such as not sleeping, for worry. The client was acting out because of the restrictions placed on him. This problem was unanticipated by the clinical team.

The case manager had a fully booked day when this crisis phone call comes in from the family. It was clearly understood by the clinician that the call had to take priority, so something had to drop out of the day's schedule. The question was what? There is a snowball effect in this type of business. It is not a question of "if" a crisis will occur; rather, it is a question of "when" and "how many." If the clinical tasks dropped from the schedule are not dealt with, then they become crises very quickly.

Another area of concern for the clinician is ongoing work. In some cases 10 to 15 cases may be all that a given professional can take on and provide excellent service; this is particularly relevant if the clinician is actively involved in the community rehabilitation program. Because the treatment lasts for 4 to 6 years and the caseload is relatively small when one or two files close, it may leave a gap in the clinician's ability to earn a living. This requires that the clinician's attention not only be focused on the ongoing clinical needs of the clients listed on the caseload, as well as the anticipated crisis, but also on maintaining goodwill through public relations to ensure future referrals. It can be an ethical dilemma as to how many cases to take on. If a clinician takes on too many files, several things will happen.

Too many clients in a caseload result in:

1. The client may not get to see the professional in a timely fashion.
2. This may cause delays in purchasing wheelchairs, completing home renovations, providing education to family, or commencing clinical interventions.

3. If a client is wait listed it can cause a delay in other health care providers' ability to provide therapy given that input from each discipline is required.

4. It can increase the family's stress, putting the unit at risk and negatively impacting the client's clinical outcome.

5. If a professional has too many clients it may compromise his or her admissibility as an expert if disorganization and canceled appointments can be proven.

6. Under cross-examination, the focus can revert to the ethics of keeping clients on wait lists or the length of time a client waited in office to see the professional.

7. It can reduce the weight the judge assigns to the expert report and compromise credibility, impacting the clinician's reputation.

8. Possibly and most important, if a client is left waiting on a list or in a wait room, he or she may feel discarded and abandoned in a time of need, increasing feelings of fear and causing agitation.

9. By the time the client does get in to see the clinician, he or she may have sensory overload and be so agitated as not to reap benefit from the session. The clinician may need to answer questions in court regarding the impact of leaving the client in wait and the resulting cognitive and emotional sequelae.

10. The therapeutic relationship can be jeopardized.

11. The clinical outcome may be compromised.

THE PREMISE

This system has been designed to build in the variables associated with time management and the inevitable associated crises. The assumptions are that:

1. Each community clinician will establish how many clients is a full-time caseload.

2. A public relations and marketing plan is built into the schedule to maintain goodwill and assure repeat and new referrals.

3. Clients deserve and in fact require prompt attention once the referral is made.

4. The completion of home, vehicle, and work renovations should be a priority prior to the client's return to said environment.

5. In the event of a clinical crisis, immediate intervention should be made available.

6. Clients should not be left to wait more than 10 minutes in a waiting room, avoiding the cognitive overlay.

7. The variables of being subpoenaed to court, creating a lengthy report such as a cost-of-future-care analysis, attendance at discharge hospital meetings, and client crises need to be anticipated and provision made for in the time management system in the event that they occur.

8. A system of anticipating the clinical needs of all of the clients on a caseload over a 4-week period of time, projecting the amount of time required to complete the task, is necessary to ensure quality clinical care, maintain billable hours, and give appropriate insight into whether the caseload has room for new referrals.

This is a different type of time management system; it has worked well in clinical practice, in particular for those health care providers working with the traumatically brain injured in a non-salaried government position—namely, the community private-practice team. The community team members are juggling many balls at one time. They have caseloads where the clients are at different stages of recovery. Some clients may be in the initial stages of care. There will be an influx of service in the initial stages of treatment, assessments will be conducted by the various team members, home renovations will be completed, and education meetings with the client and family will be in process.

There will be other peak points in the continuum of service over the 4- to 6-year period of community clinical care. They are often seen:

1. At the initial assessment stage

2. In the early period, where there is relearning of life skills, and activities of daily living

3. At the introduction of community reintegration including social, recreation, and cognitive skills training

4. At the stage of return to work, including volunteering, pre-vocational, and job re-entry, including work-hardening programs.

5. When the residual loss is in the final stage where an increase of time is required to prepare a lifetime plan for the client and family.

There are peaks and valleys in the 4- to 6-year treatment regime. When there are peaks this is indicative of a greater percentage of time required by the clinical team to provide the necessary intervention, usually with the inclusion of a one-to-one rehabilitation worker. The flow of intervention may commonly look something like Figure 12.1.

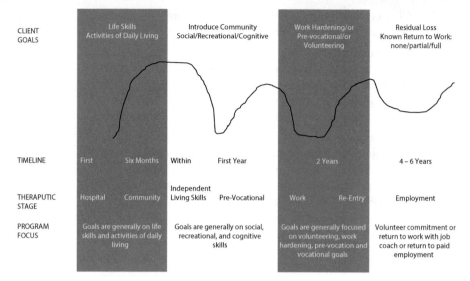

CLIENT GOALS	Life Skills Activities of Daily Living	Introduce Community Social/Recreational/Cognitive	Work Hardening/or Pre-vocational/or Volunteering	Residual Loss Known Return to Work: none/partial/full
TIMELINE	First Six Months	Within First Year	2 Years	4 – 6 Years
THERAPUTIC STAGE	Hospital Community	Independent Living Skills Pre-Vocational	Work Re-Entry	Employment
PROGRAM FOCUS	Goals are generally on life skills and activities of daily living	Goals are generally on social, recreational, and cognitive skills	Goals are generally focused on volunteering, work hardening, pre-vocation and vocational goals	Volunteer commitment or return to work with job coach or return to paid employment

Figure 12.1 The peaks and valleys in the rehabilitation process.

GOALS OF THE TIME MANAGEMENT SYSTEM

The purpose of the time management system is to organize oneself in such a way as to anticipate disruptions in daily schedules. Rather than the interruptions having a spiraling domino effect, this approach will tackle the unanticipated scheduling demands as routine. Time will have been set aside so that any crisis or unanticipated interruption can be handled in a calm, professional manner. This system provides organization for a clinical practice over a 4-week period; time will always be set aside for the inevitable variables. However, if by chance none occur in that given week, tasks from the next week will get bumped up. This is a prioritization method that is revolving as we engage in the ongoing therapeutic process with the client. This system improves client care, maintains order for the clinician (avoiding burnout), and improves customer satisfaction and billable hours. The ultimate goal of quality, cost-effective service is integral to this system of time management. The system of color coded prioratization is an organization tool that is effective and compatible with any calender system, whether paper or electronic.

THE PROCESS

1. The clinician will establish a system of best practice for service delivery to TBI clients. This means that there will be policies and procedures associated with service delivery.

2. The clinician will anticipate that clients will have unanticipated needs as they maneuver through the uncharted waters of rehabilitation. It is imperative that the clinician's practice is calm and organized to improve productivity and maintain quality.

3. A template for a billing schedule will be devised. This is important on many levels. Firstly, the referral source generally wants the clinician to quote the amount of time that will be required to carry out the task. There should be a certain structure to the quotation. In the author's experience, a list of tasks with an associated time frame is outlined based on the time that it would take for an experienced health care provider to complete each task with some allowance for variation in the client's condition. This then becomes the corporate standard. The person engaging in the intake procedure can refer to this job task list and will be able to give a more educated quote (Table 12.1). From this quote and the quality statistics (Table 12.7), a projection of required time can be estimated. This allows the clinician to plan and it also indicates if there is room to take on any new clients or if more effort needs to be expended in the arena of marketing and public relations.

4. This structure will reduce stress and confusion for the clinician, client, and family by creating an allowance for crisis, rather than reacting to the crisis. The availability of the clinician fosters a relationship of trust with the client.

5. The caseload will be managed in a timely, cost-effective manner.

6. This time management system allows for public relations building on goodwill and thus repeat referrals.

7. Organization reduces liability exposure.

This job task list is a sample. It does not reflect or endorse any specific assessment tools but rather serves as a template for each clinician from every discipline to view and then recreate as it relates to his or her practice.

HOW THE TIME MANAGEMENT SYSTEM WORKS

Method

1. A full client list is the basis for the planning (Table 12.2).

2. The client list should include names, location, referral source, referral contact, and phone number for quick reference.

Table 12.1 Example of Job Task List for an Occupational Therapist

1.	Received referral/verbal discussion of request	15 to 30 minutes
2.	Review of medical information (depends on how many medical reports there are to read)	Variable
3.	Phone consultation with medical professionals (depends on how many are involved and how complex the injury is)	Variable
4.	Phone consult or meetings with school, hospital staff, doctors, or other team members	1.00–1.5 hours
5.	Phone consultation with client (make appt., get directions)	5–15 minutes
Assessments		
1.	History	2–3 hours
2.	Functional home assessment:	
	a. Administration	1.5 hours
	b. Video	1.5 hours
	c. Interpretation	30–45 minutes
3.	Current complaints	30–45 minutes
4.	Current and previous daily schedules	30–45 minutes
5.	Balanced lifestyle sheet	30 minutes to 1 hour
6.	Assertiveness inventory:	
	a. Administration	15 minutes
	b. Interpretation	10 minutes
	c. Recommendations	15 minutes
7.	Leisure survey:	
	a. Administration	1 hour
	b. Interpretation	30 minutes
	c. Creative adaptation to program	1 hour
8.	Pre-vocational inventory	
	a. Community investigation	1 hour
	b. Implementation	1–2 hours

Table 12.1 (*Continued*) Example of Job Task List for an Occupational Therapist

9.	Adjustment rating scale	
	a. Administration	30 minutes
	b. Interpretation	15 minutes
10.	Dexterity tests:	
	a. Administration	45 minutes to 1 hour
	b. Interpretation	20 minutes
11.	Fine motor coordination test:	
	a. Administration	45 minutes
	b. Interpretation	15 minutes
12.	Work screening interview:	
	a. Administration	15 minutes
	b. Interpretation	15 minutes
13.	Aptitude inventory:	
	a. Administration	30 minutes
	b. Interpretation	15 minutes
14.	Career inventory:	
	a. Administration	30 minutes
	b. Interpretation	30 minutes
15.	Perceptual evaluation:	
	a. Administration	1 hour
	b. Interpretation	15 minutes
16.	Life events inventory:	
	a. Administration	45 minutes
	b. Interpretation	30 minutes
	c. Adaptive recommendations	15 minutes

Continued

Table 12.1 (*Continued*) Example of Job Task List for an Occupational Therapist

17.	Behavior rating scale:	
	a. Administration	30 minutes
	b. Interpretation	15 minutes
18.	Physical ability inventory:	
	a. Administration	30 minutes
	b. Work site evaluation	2 hours
	c. Video or pictures	Variable plus costs
	d. Meeting with employer	1 to 1.5 hours
	e. Review of job description	30 minutes
	f. Recommendation of adaptive equipment	15 minutes
19.	Summary and recommendations	30–90 minutes
	a. Review with client	1 hour
20.	Phone consultations	Variable
21.	Report writing—initial assessment	1 hour
22.	Cost-of-future-care analysis	Variable up to 40 hours
23.	Cost-of-future-care pricing	Variable
24.	Court preparation	Variable
25.	Court attendance	Variable
Ongoing rehabilitation consulting		
1.	Meeting with one-to-one rehabilitation workers	1–1.5 hours/week
2.	Review of one-to-one workers' documentation	20 minutes/week
3.	Organization of team meetings	1 hour
4.	Attendance at team meetings	1 hour
5.	Complete monthly dictation	30–45 minutes
6.	Community reintegration:	
	a. Design	Variable
	b. Implementation	Variable
	c. Follow-up	Variable

Table 12.2 Master Client List

Client	Client location	Client phone	Funding source	Referral contact	Referral phone	File status
Walter Dunbar	Vancouver	488-1112	Union—Vancouver	Kathryn Kosley	862-3333	Active
Harry Thetics	Surrey	599-1113	Insurance—Vernon	Maisie Malloy	850-0044	Active
George Peterson	West Vancouver	980-2538	Union—Vancouver	Tatiana Smith	231-1111	Active
Tom Minor	Burnaby	443-2223	Law Firm Inc.	Candy Ellery	453-9999	Active
Richard Wain	Abbotsford	855-3321	WCB—Vancouver	Kathryn Kosley	862-3333	Active
Charles Locke	Vancouver	221-4456	Law Firm Inc.	Peter James	231-1811	Closed 3
Gary McGeorge	Vancouver	435-2265	Insurance—Hope	Maisie Malloy	850-0044	Active
Portia Lavoire	Vancouver	681-2567	Insurance—Abbotsford	Maisie Malloy	850-0044	Active
Karl Koster	West Vancouver	980-3321	Insurance—Kelowna	Maisie Malloy	850-0044	Active
Jim Breen	Vancouver	323-7896	Insurance—Burnaby	Tatiana Smith	231-1111	Active
Jane Dour	Coquitlam	939-0099	Insurance—Abbotsford	Lorrie Gentry	850-0045	Active
Mary Hopkins	Coquitlam	465-7789	Employment agency	Randy Baggette	583-4444	Abeyance
Ethel Barnell	Hope	888-8888	Insurance—Hope	Tatiana Smith	231-1111	Pending
Russell White	West Vancouver	980-3253	Law Firm Inc.	Kathryn Kosley	862-3333	Closed 3

Total: 10 active, 1 abeyance, 1 pending, 2 closed.

Note: Client names and phone numbers are fictitious.

3. The client should be given a status. The status sections include:

   a. **Active:** This file will require active rehabilitation, ongoing intervention, and attendance at team meetings and may experience the occasional crisis. This type of traumatic brain injury case will require 10 to 14 hours a month on average during the peaks and 5 to 7 hours in the valleys (Figure 12.1).

   b. **Abeyance:** This means that the clinician is waiting for something—for example, a surgery to be completed, the client to be discharged from hospital, or the client to relocate to the clinician's area. An abeyanced file should only be left in this status for 3 months because the clinician is holding a spot for this person, planning around the eventuality that he or she will become an active client and will require the clinician's time. If the file stays in abeyance for too long with no sign of it becoming active, something may have changed and it may need to be moved to the closed section (for example, the client has decided against surgery or will not be moving to the clinician's area). In the case of an abeyanced file, the clinician should continue communication with the referral source so that he or she can be apprised of the ongoing status of the file. If it continues to be in abeyance with no logical reason, the clinician should inform the referral source that he or she will remove the client from the master list until it is closer to becoming active. When too many files are in abeyance, it impacts the clinician's ability to take on more work. This type of file can generate up to an hour a month for ongoing communication. Remember that the clinician does not commence billing until he or she has been retained and the file is active. Therefore, any time spent on the file is unbillable.

   c. **Closed:** The file has settled or closed and it should remain on the list for 3 months post-discharge. The reason for this is that disbursements will continue to come in and the master list should reflect the closure process so that the records are in sync with the accounting records. Even if the file has settled, a clinician may still be requested to produce records for payment. There is typically a lag in time from settlement to payment. However, if the case is designated as active rather than closed, it will skew the quality statistics. Therefore, label the file pursuant to the month by closed (1) closed (2) and closed (3).

d. **Pending:** A pending file is when a referral source has made an inquiry as to the clinician's availability; for instance, a TBI client will be discharged approximately 1 month from now and an inquiry has been made as to the clinician's availability, but no firm request for service has been issued. In this case projected time should be built into the 4-week schedule for follow-up with the contact person as to the necessity of the service. Similarly to the abeyanced file, this file is sitting in wait, so 1 hour a month for follow-up should be estimated; again, this is unbillable time. A file should not sit in pending for more than 4 months.

Review of Clinical Files

When a clinician receives a new referral, an assessment is completed. Once the teams' assessments are complete, their unified findings will translate into the therapeutic plan generating a list of to-do's for the case manager. At any point in time there will be items that require attention—some more pressing than others. The clinician who refers to the 4-week schedule will be able to anticipate his or her workload at any point and time. This knowledge will serve to help the health care provider understand his or her availability to take on new cases or to engage in public relations to generate more referrals. This system will also anticipate and intercept crises before they occur. It will also serve to cue the tardy clinician that procrastination issues are looming. Examples of tasks that could end up on a clinician's list of to-do's could include (in no particular order of importance):

1. Assess the client.
2. Make appointments.
3. Return phone calls, e-mails, or texts.
4. Educate family.
5. Recruit, hire, and educate one-to-one rehabilitation workers.
6. Meet weekly with one-to-one rehabilitation workers.

7. Design therapeutic intervention.
8. Reevaluate the therapy plan.
9. Set up a team meeting.
10. Attend a team meeting.
11. Write reports.
12. Call other team members.
13. Set up and follow through with appointments with the client and family.
14. Set up a community program.
15. Set up a sensory integration program.
16. Set up and follow through with counseling sessions.
17. Set up a return to work program.
18. Reassess the client.
19. Attend a hospital discharge meeting.
20. Set up home renovations.
21. Respond to client crises.
22. Attend court.
23. Meet with lawyer to prepare to testify.
24. Liaise with other team members.
25. Meet with the funder to advocate for funds.
26. Educate volunteers.
27. Meet with possible referral sources.
28. See a client pro bono.

At first glance, all of these varying tasks that are important to each and every client may seem daunting to manage; however, with the practical 4-week color-coded time management system, it is entirely manageable. Preparing a list of to-do's on each client file may seem like an onerous task; however, let us bear in mind that these are not all new files. As you receive new referrals, you will assess and establish your list of to-do's and insert these to-do's into your already existing weekly schedules. In regard to your active files, each week's tasks will arise and you simply keep a running list of to-do's, color code them, and insert them into the appropriate week. This can be easily executed when using a computerized or paper scheduling system. It takes little time to re-assess and prioritize at the beginning of the week. This system also requires the monthly completion of quality statistics, including your projected time at the beginning of the month. At the end of the month, the clinician will compare the projected time with the actual billed time and assess any diffrentials. This system in its color-coded manner will serve to cue the health care provider visually of any tendencies to procrastinate or, on the other hand, to anticipate interruptions or emergencies.

After reviewing your files you will compile a complete list of to-do's for each client; this list should include the estimated time required to complete each task. Ensure that you include all details. It is common to neglect to include those tasks that take 5 or 10 minutes; missing this detail is fraught with difficulty both in terms of organization and in terms of billing accurately for time spent. It is important to include each task. Each task should be given a realistic amount of time to complete. It is important to stay within industry standards; refer to the job task list that is applicable to each discipline's code of conduct and think of each task in terms of how likely it is to become a crisis if left unattended for 1 week, 2 weeks, 3 weeks, or 4 weeks.

The to-do's are time sensitive based on a color system for:

Week 1 (must be completed this week)

Week 2 (there is some flexibility to defer this task by 1 week; then it becomes a red the following week)

Week 3 (these tasks may be deferred for 1 week becoming a green the following week)

Week 4 (these tasks may be deferred for 1 week, becoming a blue the following week)

To better understand how the 4-week time management system works, brief hypothetical cases have been described. Let us review an example of a caseload assuming that 11 active files is a full caseload; inclusive in the time demands will be a built-in public relations plan. These cases are all at different stages in the rehabilitation process requiring various amounts of time and urgency.

It is important to note that these are not full case histories (meaning from start to finish), but rather are cases at various stages in one point in time in the case manager's work schedule. The case manager could represent any clinician. These cases are meant to be an illustration that we, the clinical team, are dealing with real lives. Each case will have priorities and it is in managing and anticipating the priorities and avoiding crises that the clinician will be positioned to provide excellent care.

Some of the cases are at the early stages of intervention and some are at the point of closure. These cases are current and the demands are real. The purpose of including the case histories is to illustrate the human complexity of the time demands on the clinician and the real risks associated with serving persons with traumatic brain injury and other catastrophic injuries. Each family's needs are varied and important. The author is using realistic case examples to humanize the business of time management. It is very easy to make lists of to-do's, set priorities, and draw up schedules; however, it is the content of what is in the schedule that outlines the risks for the client and family if the clinician's time is poorly managed. In the case of the traumatically brain-injured client and his or her family there is little if any room for disorganization or time lags in intervention. There are enough land mines surrounding the actual process of recovery without any member of the clinical team contributing negatively to the situation.

Each of the following case examples is written from the perspective of the case manager.

CASE HISTORIES AND TO-DO'S FOR TIME MANAGEMENT SYSTEM

Client 1: Walter Dunbar

Walter Dunbar is a 35-year-old single man who resides in a small town in rural Manitoba. At the time of his accident he had been living independently and was working at a meat-packing plant. His mother, Barbara, was a teacher and is now retired and his father, Jack, was a pig farmer; they are in their late 70s and in good health but have little emotional reserve. Walter has two siblings: a younger brother, Al, and an older sister, Jane, to both of whom he is close.

Walter completed grade 12, taking the industrial stream of courses. Walter admits that he was not an academic and was much better at using his hands. He enjoyed working with his father on the family farm and puttering with the farm equipment. He was happy in his job at the meat-packing plant.

Walter had always been very social, a sort of "man's man." There was not a great deal to do in the small rural community, so Walter and his buddies enjoyed spontaneous games of touch football and baseball; they also enjoyed hunting, fishing, and four-wheeling. The outdoors was where Walter was in his element. Of course, the town pub was a favorite hangout among Walter and his friends. In fact, his father worried when the boys got together and drank.

One evening Walter and his buddies were leaving the pub early after several drinks and decided that four-wheeling at night would be fun. They set out in the dark. Walter's balance was impaired due to the alcohol consumption and within minutes he fell off his vehicle and injured his pelvis. His buddy Mark could not hear Walter's cry for help over the noise of his four-wheeler and he appears to have inadvertently run directly over Walter's head. Mark knew he had hit something and turned around to witness Walter lying motionless.

Walter was seen in the emergency room. The neurological exam showed Walter to be in a coma, and the emergency physician classified his Glasgow coma score to be 6. Over the next 12 hours, the doctor reclassified his score to 8. Walter was intubated. The initial CAT scan showed a contusion or hemorrhage.

Walter was placed on a ventilator. He eventually needed a tracheotomy as he could not protect his own airway. A feeding tube was in place to maintain his nutrition. Walter remained in a coma for 10 days. His family sat vigil by his bedside. When Walter began to emerge from his coma, it was clear that he was in a great deal of pain. He appeared agitated and confused. He had no memory of the events that caused him to be in hospital. He had a 4-day post-traumatic amnesia. Walter's fractured pelvis had been surgically attended to. Once discharged from the intensive care unit, he spent 4½ weeks in the hospital rehabilitation center.

Walter was being discharged from hospital back to the care of his aging parents. His siblings were concerned with this plan but at the moment there was no other option. Walter wanted to go back to his own house but was told that neither this nor driving was an option. Walter had very limited insight into his condition. He had a left hemiparesis impacting his left dominant arm more than his left leg. Walter could ambulate with assistance upon discharge from hospital.

At the point of hospital discharge he continued to suffer:

1. There was pain from his fractured pelvis.
2. His ability to ambulate was compounded somewhat by his left hemiparesis.
3. Impairment was noted in his working memory, both short-term and long-term memory.
4. There was impairment of effectively working through multistep tasks.
5. There was impairment in the ability to problem solve when dealing with unfamiliar tasks.
6. He had difficulty with money management tasks.
7. He had difficulty with self-care due to the left hemiparesis.

8. He had difficulty with feeding as he was left-hand dominant.

9. He had difficulty with name recall.

10. He had difficulty with anger outbursts and agitation.

11. He had difficulty with impulse control.

12. There was flat emotional affect.

13. There was poor attention span.

Walter's prognosis for a full recovery was guarded. The hospital team agreed that keeping Walter in his familiar small town was the best option. Moving Walter to a larger center for placement in a group home seemed to have more disadvantages than advantages. The siblings were not in a position to take Walter into their own homes due to space limitations and work schedules. It was felt that returning Walter to his parent's home for the next few months would be the best environment for his healing, provided that supports could be put in place for the parents. Walter's parents, despite their age, wanted Walter with them.

For the purpose of this discussion, this case is already in process, with the community team assessing Walter's and the family's needs. The case manager sees the potential volatility in this situation and needs to find time to coordinate the community team and get supports in place for Walter and his parents. There is a sense of urgency to provide support for the family and commence rehabilitation for Walter.

Upon discharge from hospital, the physiatrist recommended a physical therapy program to improve Walter's hemiparesis and increase his tolerance for activity. The hospital occupational therapist has recommended a regime of activity of daily living exercises that should be carried out by a rehabilitation worker. A focus would be placed on independent living. The occupational therapist and the neuropsychologist have encouraged some introduction to pre-vocational tasks on the farm with the assistance of the rehabilitation worker.

Walter's siblings have been very helpful and supportive to both Walter and their parents; they are extremely concerned that Walter will be living with his fragile and emotionally distraught parents. Walter's mom is extremely nervous about having Walter at home. His sudden outbursts, which seem to be directed predominantly toward her, have created a tension and a particular kind of uncomfortable fear. The care team is well aware of Walter's anger and disinhibition issues. It has been very important to provide counseling for the parents and cognitive and emotional rehabilitation strategies for Walter. It was determined in hospital that Walter would need intense intervention as determined by the multidisciplinary team; the community clinical team has designed a therapeutic regime that will be carried out in the home and community by the one-to-one rehabilitation worker. The case manager is fast tracking getting this service in place, and the recruitment of a strong young male worker has commenced at the same time as the community team is assessing Walter.

As we know from the history, Walter was initially injured falling off his vehicle; the defense is taking the position that Walter may have sustained his traumatic brain injury at this point. However, it is also clear from his friend Mark's own admission that he recalls running over something and when he returned to the site he found Walter unconscious. He was certain then that he had run over Walter, but is now unsure.

This admission has commenced a legal action against Mark's insurance policy, which is compromised because of his alcohol consumption. The fact that Mark is not visiting Walter and that Walter does not understand why he has not come to his aid is further compounding Walter's feeling of loss.

Mark has been advised by his lawyers to have no contact with his best friend and Walter interprets Mark's absence as rejection and feels depressed as a result.

Walter's insurance policy is also compromised because of his alcohol consumption. However, in this particular circumstance, Walter is eligible for no-fault benefits. This means that several parties will also be involved in Walter's case, including insurance adjusters, rehabilitation insurance personnel, and defense and plaintiff counsel.

The case manager is in the process of juggling many balls to facilitate getting permission from the funder for additional services for Walter and his parents. The community team has made conducting its individual assessments a priority. The reporting lines will be complicated because of the pending litigation. The provision of supports for the family is of the utmost importance, as is the placement of an appropriate one-to-one rehabilitation worker. It is very important for the team to break down the conditions that are sensory overloading Walter. A neuropsychological assessment will reveal areas of deficit. The team will design a therapeutic regime that will facilitate improved function through the repetition of an assigned task. For other parts of the brain that have been shown to be severely damaged, modification of the environment and strategies to learn tasks in a new way will be included in the therapeutic regime. It is important to ensure that strategies and services be put in place before Walter returns to his parents' home.

Walter Dunbar: To-Do's

	Estimated amount of time
Set up a meeting with the insurance coordinator and the lawyer.	30 minutes
Set up team meeting with neuropsychologist and physiatrist.	15 minutes
Conduct team meeting with neuropsychologist and physiatrist.	1 hour
Request approval for a one-to-one worker.	15 minutes
Place the advertisement for the one-to-one worker.	30 minutes
Meet with the client and explain the need for a worker.	30 minutes
Go through the resumes and shortlist three.	1 hour
Call and interview three people shortlisted (1 hour per person).	3 hours
Set up meetings with two of the one-to-one workers and the client at separate times so that the client can choose the worker (three phone calls at 10 minutes per call).	30 minutes
Three client meetings (at 20 minutes per worker).	1 hour
Send summary to referral source and team members.	25 minutes
Meet with one-to-one rehabilitation worker.	1.5 hours
Write a brief first-month report and circulate to team members.	30 minutes

Client 2: Harry Thetics

Harry Thetics is a fun-loving 72-year-old widower. Harry was a police officer and he loves to reminisce about the old days, recounting tales of his colorful career to anyone who will listen.

Harry was married to Kathleen, the love of his life, for 37 years; he was devastated by her sudden death last year. Harry and Kathleen had met in high school and fell in love instantly. Despite his three loving adult sons, Harry has felt lost without Kathleen by his side. They were a team and Kathleen brought compassion and emotional security to any situation. Harry continued to live in the family home after Kathleen's passing.

It was fall and Harry was a little bored. He thought that on a nice sunny day he would get up on the roof and clean out the gutters; the big oak tree clogged the gutters every year.

For the past 10 years Harry had hired a company to provide this service—mostly at Kathleen's urging that he was just too old to get on the roof. "Too old," Harry thought. "Look at who went and died first," he said to himself as he raised his eyes to the heavens. Feeling slightly rebellious and with a skip in his step, Harry found his old wooden ladder. "This ought to do," Harry thought as he leaned the ladder against the house. He would tell the boys after he had finished this task, although they would be furious. The more Harry prepared to clean the gutters, the better he was feeling about himself, reclaiming his youth, so to speak. Harry gingerly ascended the ladder; when he was one rung away from the top, he heard a crack and his foot gave way as the rung fractured. Harry plunged to the ground.

A neighbor and his wife had just commented on that silly fool Harry "up on his roof at his age." As they peered out their window, they could not believe what they saw.

The ambulance arrived at City Hospital and Harry was immediately seen by a neurosurgeon, who determined that Harry had a Glasgow coma score of 13 and a compound fracture of his left nondominant humerus. The doctor was concerned about brachial plexus involvement. Harry was scheduled for surgery that evening.

Within 2 days Harry was able to converse with his sons, but he had no memory recall about how he was injured. Harry was very fatigued and the sons noticed that his personality had changed somewhat. Harry, usually so happy-go-lucky, appeared quite negative and agitated. He had also lost his sense of smell and could not taste his food well.

Harry stayed in an acute neurology ward for 2 weeks. He had surgery to his fractured arm and, thankfully, his brachial plexus was not affected. He did not receive a neuropsychological assessment in hospital but he did see an occupational therapist, who concluded that Harry was independent in all areas of self-care and independent living. Having been provided with aids and kitchen devices to assist with one-handed activity while his left arm is healing. The social worker was concerned about the family's remarks about Harry having a change in personality. Despite the plan to discharge Harry, the social worker pleaded the case for an outpatient neuropsychology assessment. In the meantime, she arranged for a community case manager, who is also a counselor, to follow up with Harry and his sons.

Prior to his fall, the family, along with Harry, had been in the process of exploring other living arrangements for him. Alvin, the eldest, owned and lived in a duplex; prior to Harry's fall, the family had discussed Harry's moving into the other side of the duplex. The case manager would continue to explore this idea with the family and advocate for appropriate supports. The case manager, along with the family doctor, would devise a plan.

Because the fall occurred in Harry's home, the social worker approached his homeowner insurance policy representative to explore any areas of potential funding. It would be important for the hospital to ensure that Harry was plugged into outpatient services prior to discharge as he might not have any formal funding and could easily slip through the cracks. Once the neuropsychological assessments were completed, a plan could be devised utilizing volunteers if necessary. It is also possible that, having been a member of the police force, Harry would be eligible for veterans affairs benefits. The social worker would also explore this option. At present there is high priority for making a decision about where Harry will live.

Harry Thetics: To-Do's

	Estimated amount of time
Set up client meeting.	10 minutes
Have a meeting with the client to discuss progress.	30 minutes
Schedule a neuropsychological assessment.	15 minutes
Call veterans affairs.	20 minutes
Call homeowner's policy representative.	30 minutes
Have a telephone call with the neurologist and physiatrist to discuss Harry's progress.	25 minutes
Have a discussion with the physiotherapist and ensure community follow-up.	15 minutes
Dictate report.	30 minutes
Proof the report.	10 minutes
Set up a call for a community case manager to recruit volunteers and take over the case.	45 minutes
Schedule a team meeting.	30 minutes
Meet with Alvin regarding housing.	1 hour

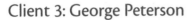

Client 3: George Peterson

George is 19 years old and he has been living on his own since leaving his fourth foster home at age 17. He has two biological siblings: Donna, age 14, and Emma, age 12. Donna and Emma had been assigned to another foster home when they were taken away from his biological mother and he does not know their whereabouts. George has had a troubled youth; he was bounced from foster home to foster home, resulting in a disposition that was not readily accepting and somewhat angry. It is thought that George suffered from fetal alcohol syndrome, but with little childhood documentation, this would, at best, be a guess.

George has an intrinsic dislike of anyone in authority. Despite his hard exterior George is a wounded, sensitive young man that feels that he does not belong anywhere. He was tired of being picked on and mocked at school for his tattered clothing, so he dropped out in grade 10 and took a job pumping gas at a local gas station.

George likes to spend time alone; he has one prized possession that he covets, having saved for almost a year to buy it. It is his white-water kayak. George lives in a community where the best rapids a young man could hope for are only 1 hour away. After another day of loneliness George decided to burn off some energy and, despite the spring runoff, tackle the rapids.

George had no use for rules—after all who would miss him if he was not around? The "rapids closed" sign only served to entice George toward the adventure.

George positioned himself in his kayak and secured his skirt. Filled with anticipation, he paddled out. "What a rush!" he called out to no one in particular. George had never seen the river this wild; too bad he could not share this with someone. He felt empowered as his strong arms guided his small but efficient watercraft.

George had been thinking about asking out a girl who had the night shift at the gas station; as he maneuvered his way through the water, dodging rocks and ducking as low lying branches brushed his head, his moment of daydreaming caught him unaware. The raging undercurrent in combination with the small upcoming waterfall was playing havoc with his small craft. Before George knew it he had capsized and little did he know that the branches of a tree were preventing him from doing the roll that he thought he had perfected. What seemed like an eternity passed before George lost consciousness.

Two paramedics out for an afternoon hike had enjoyed watching the skilled white-water kayaker; they were mortified as they witnessed the events transpire for George. The two paramedics sprang into action with little regard for their own safety. Within minutes they were able to rescue the body that had emerged from the kayak. George was clearly anoxic and unconscious but the paramedics bolted into action and within short order they were administering cardiopulmonary resuscitation. George regained consciousness by the time the ambulance arrived.

George was admitted to an acute neurology ward for observation; when they asked him about next of kin, the hospital staff were disturbed that this young man had no one. The two paramedics had stayed at his side because they were also concerned.

George was recovering well. It was difficult to say if he was experiencing any change in personality as it appeared that there was no one to verify what he was like before.

The two paramedics continued to visit George in hospital. Being risk takers themselves, they recognized a kindred spirit. In his gratitude, George warmed up for the first time in his life to these two heroes.

George informed the hospital staff that he was now having problems organizing his thoughts or planning a task. The hospital occupational therapist verified that these in fact were problems for George.

The hospital neuropsychologist was requested to conduct an assessment that identified areas of brain dysfunction.

The neuropsychological assessment did reveal two areas of concern: namely, global evidence of fetal alcohol symptomatology as well as areas of brain dysfunction related to anoxia. A case manager was assigned to organize a vocational plan for George. The good news was that the two paramedics were now providing a support system that George had never had. They were encouraging him to set his sights higher than being a gas station attendant. George was eager to attend vocational counseling and for the first time felt that circumstances were turning around for him. The case manager would need to move quickly, sourcing out funding from government sources such as human resources and development. George was recovering well but was still having some global problems with organization and sequencing. The hospital team was designing a plan to discharge George with the support of outpatient care until further funding could be secured. George had worked hard and it was felt by the hospital team that he could return to his basement suite, where he lived independently. The occupational therapist and neuropsychologist would follow up with George on an outpatient basis.

George Peterson: To-Do's

	Estimated amount of time
Set up a meeting with government agency for George.	10 minutes
Prepare for meeting and draw up agenda (dictation and proofing).	15 minutes
Have a meeting with brain injury association.	45 minutes
Once you have received approval from the government, review plan with the team.	1.5 Hours
Read the neuropsychology report.	30 minutes
Meet with the neuropsychologist to ensure that you understand his opinion and let him know that you are going to meet with human resources to confirm funding and will require his support.	30 minutes
Dictate outcome of that meeting.	10 minutes
Proof notes of meeting.	15 minutes
Schedule team meeting.	30 minutes

Client 4: Tom Miner

Tom is a 44-year-old gentleman who moved to British Columbia 30 years ago from Croatia. Tom's family fled the conflict in their home country; as a result Tom only has a grade 8 education. Tom loved the rural countryside that he grew up in. As a young, only child he enjoyed tending the sheep and hunting in the countryside with his father. Tom's father, Harmand, was a master taxidermist. Tom used to spend endless hours with his father after a hunt. Preparing the hides was heavy work, especially getting the large animal hides out of the big barrel where they soaked in salt brine.

When the family immigrated to Canada, they moved to Northern British Columbia. There was an exotic hunting lodge that was a favorite with big game hunters. Tom's father established his taxidermy business close by.

Tom joined his father in the family business; they worked side by side, enjoying each other's company as well as the work they were so passionate about.

Tom had met a young woman, Anne Marie, at a church social; they had been dating now for 3 years and Tom finally had the courage to ask for her hand in marriage.

Anne Marie was thrilled and a small family wedding took place 6 months later. She was now pregnant and planned on being a stay-at-home mom. The taxidermy business is doing very well and Tom's father has started to talk about retirement. They were discussing this as they drove home one evening in January. It was an especially cold evening; the wind was howling, whipping the snow in every direction and, as a result, visibility was poor—so poor in fact that Tom did not see the deer leap in front of his vehicle. The car skidded and plunged off an embankment. There were several calls to 911 as other vehicles stopped to see if they could provide some assistance. Within 8 minutes emergency crews had arrived. The car had rolled over several times and the jaws of life were required to allow the paramedics access to the passengers. It was clear that Tom's dad had not survived the crash. Tom was alive but unconscious. He was taken to the local hospital where the emergency team indicated that he had a Glasgow coma score of 9. Tom was stabilized enough to the point that he could be air lifted to a larger center.

Upon his arrival, the new team immediately prepared Tom for surgery to relieve the intracranial pressure.

Back home, Anne Marie and Tom's mother had been notified of Harmand's passing and Tom's injuries. The two women were in a state of shock as they planned to travel to Vancouver to be with Tom.

Tom remained in a coma for 6 days. When he emerged from his coma, he did not recognize the two women at his bedside. He was having problems with dysnomia. He was also struggling to find the right words to express himself. When the nurse asked if he would like some chicken broth, he responded by saying "car." Tom had not been apprised of his father's passing. Because of the hospital team's focus on executing life-saving measures to save Tom's life, it was not until Tom was conscious that the medical team realized that he had a great deal of shoulder pain. He had sustained an injury to his right shoulder girdle and was having difficulty maneuvering his right-dominant arm.

A team of professionals designed a program for Tom and the speech and language pathologist immediately set up a program for Tom, assisting, prompting, and cueing Tom in the identification of objects as well as the use for the object. Tom was having difficulty saying the word for toothbrush; for example, when asked what he would do with this object, he indicated that he would comb his hair with it. The speech pathologist educated Anne Marie and Tom's mother as well as other team members on Tom's difficulty with dysnomia, anomia, and anomic aphasia. She educated the women that, at least in the short term, Tom would have trouble using the right names for people, places, or things. Because of this he may experience halted speech as he tried to search for the correct word. She further explained that this difficulty might extend to writing as well as speech. She speculated that Tom may experience difficulty with reading as well. This could be further compounded by the fact that English was Tom's second language. The good news was that she felt that Tom's auditory comprehension was unaffected.

The speech pathologist was encouraging every person who interacted with Tom to do the following:

1. The use of semantic cues such as, for keys, *this is an object you use to open a door or, for a cup, this is used to hold coffee.*

2. The strategy of filling in the blank: *I am closing the ___.*

3. Phonemic cues: for instance, if Tom is having difficulty saying *brush*, the family and team can cue him with the sound *brrrrr.*

4. Antonyms naming the opposite: *it is not cold; it is ___*(hot).

5. Pictures to help Tom identify items, family members' names, and locations: It was through this process that Tom was informed of his father's death. He was devastated and blamed himself.

These communication hints were proving to be helpful not just to Tom but also to the family as it gave them a useful task to engage in while visiting and they could see the benefits. Other strategies they used were through general discussion, asking Tom questions that involved problem solving, such as "Thanksgiving is coming up, Tom. What holiday is next?" Through these exercises Tom's ability to communicate improved dramatically.

As Tom's speech was improving, the occupational therapist assessed Tom's ability to attend to functional activities of daily living. Cognitively, Tom was able to complete these tasks but his rotator cuff was causing a great deal of pain. The physical therapist was working on range of motion as well as strengthening. The physiatrist was guarded in his prognosis of Tom's rotator cuff injury and was suggesting to the team that an alternate form of employment would most likely need to be explored.

The neuropsychologist and the occupational therapist are in agreement with the physiatrist during a team meeting 6 weeks after Tom's accident. A candid discussion was had with Tom and the family about the realistic obstacles of Tom being able to return to work as a taxidermist, especially without the assistance of his father. Without the physical strength to lift the large animal hides out of the salt brine, there would be no business. The market for game foul was too small to support a family. The rotator cuff injury alone was enough reason for the team to feel that Tom should pursue another line of work; when this was coupled with the loss of his father as a partner and the cognitive challenges, it became a priority.

A vocational plan was set, taking into account Tom's age, that English was his second language, and that he had a grade 8 education.

The social worker was helping Tom with the grief over his father's death.

The hospital team was planning to discharge Tom; they were pleased with his cognitive improvement as well as his improvement with speech. His rotator cuff issue was not progressing as well. Prior to discharge, some final vocational preparations were being made before transference to the community team.

Because of the multifocus of the circumstances surrounding Tom's injury, many arrangements that were time sensitive required attention:

1. His father's death and the adjustment of Tom and family members
2. Anne Marie's pregnancy
3. The eventual career transition for Tom

Tom Miner: To-Do's

	Estimated amount of time
Set up a meeting with the no-fault adjuster.	15 minutes
Prepare for meeting and draw up agenda (dictation and proofing).	30 minutes
Have a meeting with WCB coordinator.	1 hour
Set up appointments with	
Vocational consultant	15 minutes
Employment counselor	15 minutes
Neuropsychologist	15 minutes
Read the neuropsychology consulting report.	45 minutes
Call the vocational consultant to ensure that you understand his opinion and let him know that you are going to meet with the insurance company to confirm funding and get his support.	15 minutes
Dictate outcome of that meeting.	15 minutes
Proof notes of meeting.	10 minutes
Write report and circulate to team.	30 minutes

Client 5: Richard Wain

Richard Wain is a 25-year-old young man who has a history of having sustained two traumatic brain injuries. The first was when he was a child of 13. At that time Richard had been riding his bike and was not wearing a helmet. He fell off his bike and was unconscious for about 3 hours. He was nauseous upon arrival to hospital, where he was said to have a Glasgow coma score of 14; however, nothing was clearly evident on the CAT scan. He stayed overnight for observation and was sent home to the care of his parents. Since that time Richard's parents have said that he was never the same. Richard states that he has no memory of the bicycle accident. Prior to this first diagnosed brain injury, Richard had been a joyful, outgoing boy who was very social and excelled in both school and sports.

When Richard returned home after the bicycle accident he appeared sullen and withdrawn to his parents. He preferred to isolate himself in his room at home. He said that he felt anxious around a lot of people and withdrew into his room, watching movies. His grades slipped and he grew more and more despondent.

Richard's friends did not understand the change in him and quickly lost interest and stopped coming by to visit. The teachers reported that Richard had become transient in his attendance at school. Richard's teachers observed that he was having difficulty focusing and attending to any given task. If there was any type of auditory stimulation, Richard withdrew into somewhat of a haze and appeared to shut down.

This first brain injury received little attention and eventually Richard was labeled as difficult, a slow learner, or a problem child.

As Richard struggled to assimilate cognitive information he became frustrated and withdrew into himself. As he grew older he developed into an introvert so very unlike who he was in his earlier days. His parents did not receive any information on brain injury and developed a belief system that Richard was a loner, perhaps with mental health issues.

Richard dropped out of school after limping through to grade 11. He was unable to maintain employment and at this present time was unemployed. When Richard was 24 he walked to the video store to pick up his week's supply of movies. As always, Richard was overwhelmed by the noise of the traffic. There was additional visual stimulation today: What would normally be considered a beautiful fall day was distracting Richard even more. As he meandered down the heavily treed street, a wind gust came up, stirring the fragile leaves into a flurry of abstract color as they fell to the ground.

Distracted by the visual stimulation, Richard failed to observe the red "do not walk" signal and continued walking to the store across the street. The driver of the vehicle forging through the green light was alarmed by the pedestrian who walked directly in front of her vehicle that was traveling at 80 miles per hour.

The driver did everything she could to avoid hitting Richard but to no avail. He lay motionless on the busy intersection. The paramedics arrived within minutes as their station was only around the corner. Richard was professionally attended to and arrived at the hospital within 10 minutes. The emergency team engaged in life-saving procedures and within 24 hours Richard had stabilized. However, he remained unconscious for 2 days. Richard's parents were panicked as they asked the doctors what to expect.

The neurologist informed the parents that Richard had sustained a blow to the front part of his brain and went on to further explain that Richard might demonstrate some personality traits that were not characteristic for him.

Days later, as the fog around Richards's cognition lifted, the parents understood what the neurologist had described. In the past Richard was not a person prone to swearing; however, now he would let out a prolific repertoire of profanities and, like a record that was skipping, he would perseverate on whatever term was the flavor of the hour. Richard was also having difficulty initiating tasks and had frequent angry outbursts.

At this point in the intervention process, Richard had been medically stabilized and would return home to the care of his parents.

Under a partial no-fault system Richard would receive some benefits for rehabilitation. The case manager had been invited to the hospital discharge meeting. A plan for intervention and family support was discussed at the meeting. The case manager recommended that additional clinical disciplines be added to the team. These recommendations were presented to the adjuster handling the funding of the no-fault insurance policy. It would be imperative as Richard returned home that supports were put in place and an intervention plan was well organized. In light of the fact that there was a previous brain injury, the sequelae of the first brain injury would be reviewed to avoid sensory overloading of Richard. The case manager was aware that the family was emotionally exhausted prior to this second brain injury and appropriate supports would be put in place to further allow them to support their son.

Richard Wain: To-Do's

	Estimated amount of time
Review medical records.	50 minutes
Educate the family.	1 hour
Set up team meeting.	30 minutes
Conduct a functional assessment.	2 hours
Conduct a full cognitive and sensory assessment.	2 hours
Contact the general practitioner and notify him of the team's recommendations.	10 minutes
Set out a therapeutic plan based on the team's assessment findings as well as the neuropsychological assessment.	1 hour
Set up interviews for one-to-one rehabilitation workers.	45 minutes
Set up meeting with rehabilitation worker and client.	15 minutes
Liaise with the brain injury support group.	20 minutes
Meet with a potential volunteer placement.	1 hour
Conduct meeting with rehabilitation worker and client.	1.5 hours
Design and set up an emotional therapy plan to develop self control.	2 hours
Conduct a team meeting.	1 hour
Meet with one-to-one rehabilitation worker.	1.5 hours

Client 6: Charles Locke

Charles Locke is a lighthearted 28-year-old who enjoys life to the fullest. Like many young men, he is a genius on the computer. From the time that Charles was a boy he had that entrepreneurial spirit. Charles's parents own and operate a television store. As a boy Charles learned very early on that you get paid if you work hard. His dad, Bob, was a self-made man and enjoyed educating Charles and his brother, Jack, on all aspects of running a business.

Jack was the athlete in the family and eventually went to Europe to join the world hockey league.

Charles, on the other hand, was the family academic; he had been a focused child and did well in school. He took on his first job as a newspaper boy when he was 11 years old. Charles saved his money and at the age of 16 purchased his first car. This discipline carried Charles through to university, where he earned a degree in business administration as well as a certificate in computer science with first-class honors.

Charles had been eager to join his father as a partner in the family business. He and his dad were extremely close and they enjoyed staying up late in the night to strategize a growth plan for the business. Both men dreamed of opening three stores and, at the height of their discussions, ramped up their enthusiasm by dreaming of becoming a franchise. Grace, Charles's mother, had taken such pleasure in watching Charles develop into the young man he had become today, and she could not have been more delighted about the business arrangement.

Second to business and computers, Charles's other passion was snowboarding. As children, Jack and Charles took to the slopes at the first sign of powder, often in the back country.

It had been a busy day in the store and Charles decided to take to the slopes that were close by for an evening of night boarding. It was a beautiful evening; the lights on the slopes gave the mountain a surreal quality. Charles loved night boarding because the crowds thinned out and left room on the slopes for speed. He had been boarding with his friend, Scott, but had lost sight of him. He mused that Scott must be in the trees as usual. Charles decided to board the lift line.

As Charles lay in hospital, he remembered nothing of that fateful day. Apparently Scott had come out of the trees and had not seen Charles; they collided at high speeds and Charles immediately lost consciousness. Scott was also injured in the collision. Upon arrival at Mountain General Hospital Charles began to experience a seizure. The emergency physician classified Charles as having a Glasgow coma score of 10. There were few adventitious sounds in both lungs, and a chest x-ray revealed consolidation in the right lower lobe, possibly due to pulmonary contusion. Charles's right forearm showed a fracture of the shaft of the ulna.

Charles is now 9 months post-injury and has returned home to live with his parents. His lung has healed nicely with no residual sequelae. His right arm is still sore and he takes anti-inflammatory medication for it during the winter and still attends physical therapy.

Charles has had a neuropsychological assessment that revealed some brain dysfunction impacting short-term memory, expressive language, and organization. He has not had another seizure and is on anti-convulsants at present. He complains of fatigue, dizziness, memory problems and difficulty carrying through with a task and organization.

Charles has been working with an occupational therapist, a neuropsychologist, and a social worker. The occupational therapist is concerned that Charles has returned to the family business too soon. There has been a large margin of error, in Charles performance at work particularly in the area of customer service. On several occasions Charles has answered the phone, left to check on the stock availability for the customer, and then never returned to the phone because he was distracted by other customers in the store. On another occasion, an individual wanted to exchange a television set; Charles replaced the television with one that was worth five times the original amount without charging the customer. He is feeling very discouraged.

The social worker has been meeting with Charles regularly. The occupational therapist has been working with Charles in regard to memory and organization. The OT has also conducted family education sessions for the family to assist in their understanding of Charles's difficulties.

The speech pathologist is helping Charles with expressive language.

The neuropsychologist, occupational therapist and vocational consultant are meeting with Charles to determine if this present career plan is within the realm of current possibility. This is a very active case and the case manager is facilitating the team's communication.

Charles Locke: To-Do's

	Estimated amount of time
Set team meeting.	1 hour
Ensure that all assessments and reports are circulated.	30 minutes
Educate family.	1.5 hours
Call neuropsychologist and vocational consultant.	20 minutes
Meet with father to discuss his observations and provide support.	1 hour
Meet with funder to discuss job retraining.	1.5 hours
Write report.	25 minutes
Set up meeting with neuropsychologist and vocational consultant.	30 minutes

Client 7: Gary McGeorge

Gary is a sweet 10-year-old boy. A history was obtained from Gary's mother (Sarah), grandmother (Lily), and sister (Emma). Gary's father was at work in the local sawmill and could not attend the meeting. Gary was born in Indiana to Sarah and Gary Sr. The family immigrated to Canada when Gary was 2 years old for his father's work. Gary's sister Emma was born 1 year later. The McGeorge family valued their time together and appreciated the simple things in life. Sundays were always a family day where they all enjoyed picnics by the lake or a game of lawn bowling in the backyard. Gary was very close to both his parents, but in particular to his father. Gary Sr. would always refer to Gary Jr. as his little namesake and that delighted the small boy.

Sarah was a stay-at-home mother by choice. The couple had decided early on that parenting was their biggest life responsibility and they wanted to devote as much time as possible to the children.

One sunny day in May while Emma was on a play date, Sarah was taking Gary Jr. to visit his grandmother, when a driver crossed over the median and hit them head on. Later, this driver was charged with drunk driving.

Sarah was saved by her airbag but Gary was thrown from his seat and lay unconscious as paramedics worked frantically to resuscitate him.

Upon arrival at emergency, Gary Jr. was determined to be semicomatose and flaccid in all four limbs, responding only to painful stimuli. The contusion on the right side of his head covered his ear and there was some blood in the external ear canal. The neurosurgeon suspected blood behind the eardrum and also noted bilateral orbital hematomas; however, pupil and eye movements were normal. The emergency room physician also noted a greenstick fracture of the right radius.

Gary Jr. is now 4 years into his recovery. He was 6 at the time of the motor vehicle accident and he is now 10. Gary has received the full gamut of service from his community clinical team. The clinical team includes a pediatric neuropsychologist, neurologist, physiatrist, social worker, speech pathologist, physical therapist, general practitioner, and occupational therapist; they have worked in collaboration with the insurance company and the plaintiff lawyer. Thankfully, little Gary was given an advance from the tort claim as well as benefits from the no-fault portion of the driver's insurance policy. Gary has had many struggles to overcome but he has worked hard and with the loving support of his family he is doing well.

At present, Gary Jr. is slightly hearing impaired; because this is coupled with difficulty in rote memory, auditory processing of language, spelling, reading, arithmetic, and gross motor co-ordination, Gary has been assigned a full-time learning assistant at school, where he is mainstreamed into a regular classroom. The community speech therapist will be discharging Gary to the care of the school speech and language pathologist.

The occupational therapist has been working with Gary through the use of remediated activity focusing on processing instruction and memory. The neuropsychologist has been instrumental in advocating to the school for additional services pursuant to his neuropsychological assessment. At present, this professional is working on a consultative basis offering guidance to the school staff.

The social worker has been actively assisting the family as well as Gary; this intervention has promoted acceptance and the family is doing well.

The physical therapist has designed an exercise regime to facilitate motor development and is assisting the school staff to integrate this program into the recess break.

The plaintiff lawyer is suggesting that it is time for the family to settle the legal claim. A team meeting has been requested so that the team can evaluate what transitions would take place and to strategize the anticipated monetary needs that Gary will require over his life. After the team meeting, final reports will be solicited and circulated to all of the community team and the findings will be incorporated into a cost-of-future-care analysis, which is being prepared by the case manager.

Gary McGeorge: To-Do's

	Estimated amount of time
Set up team meeting with the community team, school teacher and learning assistant, plaintiff lawyer, family, and Gary Jr.	1.5 hours
Prepare an agenda and circulate to the above mentioned requesting their input.	1 hour
Book boardroom for team meeting.	15 minutes
Conduct case review and re-assessment in preparation for the team meeting.	2 hours
Write report.	1.5 hours
Conduct team meeting.	1.5 hours
Write cost-of-future-care report.	11.5 hours
Meet with lawyer to prepare for court.	1.5 hours

Client 8: Portia Lavoire

Portia is a 23-year-old woman who had just returned from living abroad for 3 years. A straight-A student, Portia had been recruited by a modeling agency and decided to take the opportunity to move to Paris for 2 years.

After arriving home Portia enrolled in university to pursue a career in animal science. Upon her return she was living with her parents, Arthur and Agnes. The plan was to live at home with her parents until such time as her university education is completed.

Portia was driving home late one evening in December when her car hit a section of black ice and spun out of control and hit a tree.

Portia was not wearing a seat belt and for this reason she was thrown from her vehicle. Emergency crews arrived quickly and made every attempt to stabilize her condition. Upon arrival at Lakeview Jubilee Hospital, Portia was seen by a neurosurgeon and emergency physician, who diagnosed Portia as having:

1. A Glasgow coma score of 9
2. A grade 3 open Lisfranc fracture dislocation of her left foot
3. Fracture of her left tibia
4. Open tibial diaphyseal fracture

Portia's wounds were debrided, and she underwent an open reduction and internal fixation of the Lisfranc fracture dislocation and an intermeduliary nail was placed in her left tibia.

Portia was in hospital for 6 weeks, having sustained multiple injuries. Once Portia's surgical care was complete, she commenced an arduous rehabilitation regime. Her parents noted changes in her personality, clumsiness, accident proneness, and difficulty with organization. The hospital team agreed that Portia was ready for discharge from hospital but that she would require ongoing intervention from a community team including a neuropsychologist, physical therapist, occupational therapist, and, possibly, a one-to-one rehabilitation worker to carry out the team's therapeutic regime in the community setting.

The hospital discharge meeting concluded that a one-to-one worker could be funded by the insurance policy. The community team quickly assessed Portia and designed a community re-integration program focusing on:

1. Structuring activities of daily living and self-care
2. Ambulation and strength conditioning
3. Cognitive retraining with a focus on problem solving, sequencing, and organization

4. Proprioception, depth perception, and stereognosis
5. Emotional control
6. Grief counseling

The hospital discharge meeting effectively coordinated the hospital and community teams and a smooth transition was facilitated from hospital to the home. The community program has been designed and a one-to-one rehabilitation worker is in place. The case manager was assigned the task of supervising the overall program and meeting with the worker weekly. The physical therapist is seeing Portia in a clinic four times a week; the plan is to transition some of this program to a local gym with the one-to-one worker in attendance. A team conference needs to be scheduled in 3 weeks for input from all disciplines.

It is evident that the family will require more emotional support, and counseling has been suggested. Portia is grieving her physical loss and an appointment has been made for her to have 10 sessions with a clinical psychologist.

Portia Lavoire: To-Do's

	Estimated amount of time
Meet with the one-to-one rehabilitation worker.	1.5 hours
Schedule a team conference.	45 minutes
Set up appointment with the clinical psychologist.	15 minutes
Meet with the one-to-one worker.	1.5 hours
Meet with the one-to-one worker.	1.5 hours
Re-assess proprioception and stereognosis upgrade program.	1.5 hours
Meet with one-to-one rehabilitation worker.	1.5 hours
Write report.	30 minutes

Client 9: Karl Koster

Karl is a jovial butcher. Karl's ancestors hail from Germany. His aging mother resides with Karl, his wife Florence, and their two teenage daughters in a large metropolitan city. Karl is a traditional male and loves to work hard to provide for his family. In his spare time he enjoys hunting, fishing, and cross-country skiing, but his favorite activities are family gatherings where he relishes in cooking good German food.

Karl was coming home from the butcher shop in the early evening on a cold November night. He was walking to his car and, without notice, was attacked from behind with a sharp object.

Karl remembers nothing from the assault. The last thing he remembers was having lunch with his wife and mother. Karl had been brutally beaten in a robbery where not only his wallet was stolen but his butcher shop was also broken into.

Florence and the rest of the family were beside themselves with grief; not only were they terrified as to the reason for the assault but they were also concerned at the multiple injuries that Karl sustained. The hospital records showed:

1. Severe concussion
2. Fractured inferior pubis ramus left pelvis
3. Left rib fractures
4. Comminuted fracture right humerus
5. Displaced intercondylar fracture right elbow

Karl was treated in hospital for 5 weeks. At the point of discharge Karl was still experiencing pain in his pelvis and right arm. At this point he had undergone two surgeries and had sustained nerve damage to his right radial and ulnar nerves.

At the point of discharge from hospital Karl had undergone a neuropsychological evaluation. The primary concerns cited in this report were the following:

a. Concentration
b. Attention
c. Mobility
d. Bilateral dexterity

The physiatrist was encouraging a comprehensive home program and work hardening. All hospital team members—in particular, the neurologist—had reservations about Karl's ability to return to his previous occupation as a butcher.

A community case manager was invited to the hospital discharge meeting. Each hospital discipline discussed the objectives for the successful transition back home.

The following community re-integration plan was agreed upon:

1. The case manager would solicit funds from victims assistance.

2. Counseling would be put in place for Florence, Karl, and the two daughters.

3. The case manager would meet with workers' compensation to discuss options for job re-training.

4. A physical strength and tolerance program would be carried out by the community physical therapist.

5. The physiatrist and neurologist would follow up with the radial and ulnar nerve damage.

6. In due course, a work hardening program would be set up by the occupational therapist and neuropsychologist.

Karl Koster: To-Do's

	Estimated amount of time
Call victims assistance to set up meeting.	10 minutes
Have meeting with victims assistance.	1.5 hours
Call workers' compensation to set up meeting.	15 minutes
Set up team meeting.	45 minutes
Contact community mental health to set up counseling for Florence, Karl, and daughters.	15 minutes
Conduct team meeting.	1.5 hours
Design work hardening program; assess work environment.	2 hours
Meet with physical therapist to discuss progress.	20 minutes
Write report.	30 minutes
Attend meeting with workers' compensation.	1.5 hours
Call physiotherapist.	10 minutes
Meet with family.	1 hour

Client 10: Jim Breen

Jim Breen is a 17-year-old lad who resides outside Calgary on a ranch, with his mother, Bonnie, and father, Doyle. James is the oldest child of three; he has two younger brothers, Owen, and Brad. The family are true ranchers. They enjoy everything about life on a large working ranch. Doyle had been a chuck wagon champion in his younger years and all three boys had ambitions of participating in the Calgary Stampede. The two younger boys had aspirations to be chuck wagon drivers like their father, but Jim had already begun training as a bull rider. He loved the sheer adrenaline of getting on a powerful animal that flew out of the gate in a rage. Jim was already in the money and when he was not in school or working the animals, he was training with a professional.

One spring day after school, Jim saw a perfect opportunity to practice his new skill on his friend's bull. Without adequate supervision the ride did not go smoothly and within seconds he was bucked off, much to the delight of his observing school chums. Jim got up, brushed off his britches with as much dignity as he could muster, and walked away looking back to see where the bull was. The boys carried on down a dusty road to the Breen homestead. Jim had been quiet; when his friend Brad asked him if he was OK, he said "You bet. That bull didn't get the best of me." Within minutes Jim's balance was impaired and then he collapsed.

Upon admission to hospital it was determined that Jim had suffered an intracranial bleed and a skull fracture. The emergency team was hard at work to stabilize Jim. When he returned to his room, he was very foggy in his thinking and appeared irritated and agitated. The neurologist had indicated to Jim's parents that he expected that Jim could make a full recovery but that any contact or high-risk sports were out of the question. This news was very disturbing for Jim as well as his family.

Jim was discharged home and after 3 weeks he returned to school. The teachers noticed quite a dramatic decline in Jim's academic performance. Perhaps even more alarming was his mood. Jim was despondent and began to isolate himself.

The school staff were well aware of Jim's fall and they called a special parent–teacher conference. The teacher, principal, and school psychologist were present. After learning of the parents' concerns, they unanimously decided that the school counselor would solicit funding support from the Ministry of Education for an occupational therapist who would also serve as the case manager. The school would also contact the regional neuropsychologist to conduct a neuropsychology assessment.

Once funding was secure the occupational therapist commenced building a support system for Jim. Inclusive in this would be vocational counseling to explore other vocational and recreation pursuits that would not present any risk physically.

Jim Breen: To-Do's

	Estimated amount of time
Meet with school counselor.	1 hour
Contact the ministry of education and seek approval for an occupational therapy assessment.	30 minutes
Send referral to a community occupational therapist and provide a written report of expectations and goals.	30 minutes
Meet with Jim and conduct an extensive history.	2 hours
Set a follow-up meeting with the family, Jim, school personnel, psychologist, social worker, and neuropsychologist.	45 minutes
Conduct a team meeting.	1.5 hours
Write summary report.	1 hour
Meet with family.	1 hour

Client 11: Jane Dour

Jane Dour is a single 30-year-old who runs a successful catering business. Jane works long hours and has little time for socializing outside of work. Jane has always been organized and can plan an event that would be the social event of the season. She was becoming quite well known for her wedding planning skills. Always the peacemaker, Jane could calm the most anxious of brides. She was the type of person that made everyone feel welcome and she exudes confidence. Jane had a full roster for the next month. She was planning three major corporate Christmas parties for large oil and gas companies. She had also made the strategic error to plan a friend's Christmas wedding in Lake Tahoe.

Jane had great skill at multitasking, but this month she was beginning to look a little frayed. The oil companies expected perfection, and her friend's remote wedding was pushing her to the limit. Jane historically prepares the food with her catering staff for all of these events. Jane was working late 2 days before one of the Christmas parties, and she decided to do late night shopping for groceries to allow her to get an early start the next day. As Jane pulled out of the bulk food parking lot, she was having difficulty seeing over the stacks of boxes. She began to pull out seconds before she checked her rear view mirror; she collided with an oncoming delivery truck.

Jane was taken to emergency and diagnosed with a concussion and sent home. She attempted to engage in all of the necessary tasks required to carry out her commitments, but her staff were noticing a gross margin of error. In some recipes that required six ingredients, Jane would stop at two. She had taken the dark blue tablecloths home to launder and she could not understand what had happened to them: As she peered at the laundry water, the blue was bleeding out of the cloth. Jane called for help from her staff. Her staff member identified that Jane had indeed used bleach rather than laundry soap.

This loyal staffer told Jane not to worry—that she could handle all of these events. She then drove her to the hospital where she was admitted for observation. Jane recounted the events of the car accident as best she could, realizing that she remembered very little from that day. A case manager was assigned to backtrack and organize a full workup culminating in discharge to a community team that could assist Jane in cognitive retraining and work modification.

Jane Dour: To-Do's

	Estimated amount of time
Refer to neuropsychologist for assessment.	15 minutes
Contact occupational therapist for a full assessment including a work site evaluation.	10 minutes
Communicate with the family doctor.	10 minutes
Schedule a team meeting to discuss testing results.	45 minutes
Assist Jane in contacting the insurance company.	1 hour
Co-ordinate team meeting.	1 hour
Conduct team meeting.	1 hour
Write report and circulate to team.	30 minutes
Phone Jane to schedule an appointment.	10 minutes
Follow up with occupational therapist to discuss work site evaluation.	1 hour

Client 12: Mary Hopkins (Abeyance)

Mary Hopkins is a 55-year-old woman who had been referred to this case manager by her lawyer. The purpose of the referral was to set up a full community rehabilitation program. However, she is currently wait listed for surgery and anticipates getting called within the next 2 weeks. The lawyer has asked that she be placed on the master list for action to be taken 3 weeks from the referral date.

Mary Hopkins: To-Do's	
	Estimated amount of time
Follow up with lawyer as to the file status.	10 minutes

Client 13: Ethel Barnell (Pending)

Ethel sustained a brain injury 2 months ago and is now considering moving to be closer to her daughter. The hospital in her local community has made an inquiry as to this case manager's availability to take on Ethel's case. It is placed in pending status.

Ethel Barnell: To-Do's	
	Estimated amount of time
Follow up with referral source about the status of the case.	15 minutes

Client 14: Russell White

This file has settled and is now closed, no more billable time will be incurred however Russell White should still be included in the master list with a note that it has closed for 3 months thus the closed (1) closed (2) and closed (3). The purpose of this is strictly from an accounting perspective because disbursements may still be coming in such as phone bills or visa statements. At the end of three months the file will be removed from the system.

Russell White: To-Do's	
	Estimated amount of time
Follow up with referral source about the status of the case.	15 minutes

When a client is referred to the clinician, he or she enters the system by way of the master list. The clinical assessment then follows; this report will generate a list of to-do's that are immediately entered into the schedule based on the clinical timeline associated with the task and the urgency. As each new referral comes in, the process is repeated and the to-do's unfolding and recurring over the 4- to 6-year rehabilitation process continue to rotate through the 4-week prioritization system. To this end, nothing should take more than 4 weeks to the point of completion when using this system. This system provides:

1. Organization
2. Avoidance of procrastination
3. Cost effectiveness
4. Excellent and effective business and clinical practice
5. Allowance for unforeseen interruptions or crises
6. Prevention of clinician burnout

When coupled with the use of the quality statistics, this system provides a framework for the clinician to decide if there is space on the caseload to accept new referrals or, conversely, if there is not enough work to take measures to generate new referrals.

The process as referrals come in is as follows:

1. Give the referral source a quote for your service.
2. Assess the client.
3. Itemize all to-do's.
4. Assign the amount of time that you anticipate it will take to complete the task.
5. Color-code the priority of the task.
6. Project the overall time demands of your caseload on the first of each month, projecting the time that you will spend working with your clients.
7. On the last day of the month compare the time spent with the actual time billed.
8. Review quality statistics.

THE 4-WEEK SCHEDULE

The next step is to complete the 4-week schedule:

1. All items color coded red go into week 1 (Table 12.3, Weekly Schedule: Week 1, Red—27.58 hours).
2. All items color coded green go into week 2 (Table 12.4, Weekly Schedule: Week 2, Green—33.25 hours).
3. All items color coded blue go into week 3 (Table 12.5, Weekly Schedule: Week 3, Blue—25.8 hours).
4. All items color coded pink into week 4 (Table 12.6, Weekly Schedule: Week 4, Pink—16.25 hours).

Table 12.3 Weekly Schedule: Week 1 (Red)

Total hours = 27.58

Monday	Tuesday	Wednesday	Thursday	Friday	
Communication	Communication	Communication	Communication	Communication	8:00 a.m.
Set mtg: #1 Ins. co. and law. 30 min. #1 NP. and phys. 15 min. #2 With client 10 min.	#7 Set team mtg. 1.5 hr		# 8 Meet 1:1 wkr. 1.5 hrs.	#10 Meet Jim 2 hrs.	8:30 a.m.
					9:00 a.m.
#1 Req. approval for 1:1 worker 30 min.		#6 Set team mtg. 1 hr.			9:30 a.m.
#1 Place ad. 30 min.	#7 Prep mtg. 1 hr.		#6 Ed. fam. 1.5 hrs.		10:00 a.m.
#2 Sched. NP. and ax. 15 min. #4 Set mtg. voc. con. 15 min.		#9 Mtg. with VA 1.5 hrs.			10:30 a.m.
#2 Call HO pol. rep. 30 min.	#8 Sched. team conf. 45 min.			#10 Set team mtg. 45 min.	11:00 a.m.
Set mtg: #4 Adj. 15 min. #8 Clin. psych. 15 min.	#9 Set mtg. WCB 15 min.		#5 Ed. fam. 1 hr.		11:30 a.m.
Lunch	Lunch	Lunch	Lunch	Lunch	12:00 p.m.
#3 Set mtg. govt. 10 min. #3 Prepare for mtg. 15 min.	#1 Mtg. 1 hr. #1 Mtg. 1 hr.	#3 Design rev. plan 1.5 hrs.	#2 Mtg. with client	#11 Ref. to NP 15 min. #11 Call OT 10 min.	1:00 p.m.
#4 Prepare for mtg. 30 min.			#3 Mtg. TBI ass. 45 min.		1:30 p.m.
Set mtg: #4 Empl. couns. 15 min #4 NP. 15 min. #5 Team mtg. 30 min.	#9 Call VA 10 min. #9 Set team mtg. 45 min.				2:00 p.m.
		#5 Rev. meds. 50 min.	#4 Mtg. WCB co. 1 hr.		2:30 p.m.
	#10 Call MOH 30 min.				3:00 p.m.
#6 Set team mtg. 1 hr.	#2 Call VA 20 min.	#6 Circulate. rep. 30 min.	#10 Mtg. school couns. 1 hr.		3:30 p.m.
		#10 Ref. to OT 30 min.			4:00 p.m.
Communication	Communication	Communication	Communication	Communication	4:30 p.m.
					5:00 p.m.

Notes: Communication = check e-mails, text, return phone calls, check for messages.

Table 12.4 Weekly Schedule: Week 2 (Green)

Total hours = 33.25

Monday	Tuesday	Wednesday	Thursday	Friday	
Communication	Communication	Communication	Communication	Communication	8:00 a.m.
#1 Call ref. sources 1 hr.	#1 Int. 3 hrs.	#9 Design work prog. 2 hrs.	#1 Mtg. client 30 min.	#8 Meet 1:1–1.5 hrs.	8:30 a.m.
			#1 Mtg. client and wkr.: 1 hr.		9:00 a.m.
#1 Call wkrs. and client 30 min.					9:30 a.m.
#2 Phone neur. and phys. 25 min.		#10 Conduct team mtg. 1.5 hrs.	#3 Mtg. NP. 30 min.	#5 Conduct cog. ax. 2 hrs.	10:00 a.m.
#2 Phone phys o. 15 min. #4 Call voc. couns.15 min.			#11 Set team mtg. 1 hr.		10:30 a.m.
#4 Dictate outcome 15 min. #4 Proof 10 min. #5 Call GP 10 min.					11:00 a.m.
#7 Book boardroom 15 min.			#3 Dictate outcome 10 min. #3 Proof notes 10 min.		11:30 a.m.
Lunch	Lunch	Lunch	Lunch	Lunch	12:00 p.m.
#1 Shortlist resume 30 min.	#5 Meet vol. 1 hr.	#3 Read NP. rpt. 30 min.	#5 Conduct fct. ax. 2 hrs.	#6 Meet with funder 1.5 hrs.	1:00 p.m.
#5 Set up int. 1:1—45 min.	#5 Meet vol. 1 hr.	#4 Read NP. rpt. 45 min.			1:30 p.m.
	#7 Case rev. 2 hrs.				2:00 p.m.
#9 Call comm. hlth. 15 min. #10 Call fam. dr. 10 min.		#5 Design Th. plan 1 hr.	#5 Meet TBI sup. grp. 20 min.	#6 Write report. 25 min.	2:30 p.m.
#10 Sched. team mtg. 45 min.				#9 Team mtg. 1.5 hrs.	3:00 p.m.
	#1 Send out summary 25 min.	#10 Write summary rpt. 1 hr.	#11 Assist Jane re: ins. 1 hr.		3:30 p.m.
Communication	Communication	Communication	Communication	Communication	4:00 p.m.
					4:30 p.m.
					5:00 p.m.

Notes: Communication = check e-mails, text, return phone calls, check for messages.

Table 12.5 Weekly Schedule: Week 3 (Blue)

Total hours = 25.8

	Monday	Tuesday	Wednesday	Thursday	Friday	
Communication	Communication	Communication	Communication	Communication	Communication	8:00 a.m.
#2 Call comm. mgr. 45 min.	#7 Write COFC rpt. 2.5 hrs.	#7 Write COFC rpt. 1.5 hrs.	#5 Conduct mtg. 1:1 and client 1.5 hrs.	#7 Write COFC rpt. 2.5 hrs.		8:30 a.m.
						9:00 a.m.
#6 Call NP. and voc. couns. 20 min.						9:30 a.m.
#7 Write rpt. 1.5 hrs.						10:00 a.m.
			#6 Meet with father 60 min.			10:30 a.m.
						11:00 a.m.
Communication	Communication	Communication	Communication	Communication	Communication	11:30 a.m.
Lunch	Lunch	Lunch	Lunch	Lunch	Lunch	12:00 p.m.
#8 Reassess 1.5 hrs.	#7 Write COFC rpt. 2.5 hrs.	#1 Draft rpt. 30 min.	#7 Conduct team mtg. 1.5 hrs.	#7 Write COFC rpt. 2.5 hrs.		1:00 p.m.
		#2 Dictate rpt. 30 min.				1:30 p.m.
		#1 Proof rpt. 15 min. / #2 Proof rpt. 10 min.				2:00 p.m.
#10 Conduct team mtg. 1 hr.		#5 Conduct mtg. 1:1 and client 1.5 hrs.	#8 Meet 1:1 wkr. 1.5 hrs.			2:30 p.m.
						3:00 p.m.
#10 Write rpt. 30 min.			#9 Meet pt. 20 min.			3:30 p.m.
						4:00 p.m.
Communication	Communication	Communication	Communication	Communication	Communication	4:30 p.m.
						5:00 p.m.

Notes: Communication = check e-mails, text, return phone calls, check for messages.

251

Table 12.6 Weekly Schedule: Week 4 (Pink)   Total hours = 16.25

Time	Monday	Tuesday	Wednesday	Thursday	Friday
8:00 a.m.	Communication	Communication	Communication	Communication	Communication
8:30 a.m.	#2 Set team mtg. 30 min.	#11 Follow up OT. 1 hr.	#8 Meet with reh. wkr. 90 min.	#1 Meet 1:1 wkr. 90 min.	
9:00 a.m.	#3 Set team mtg. 30 min.				
9:30 a.m.	#6 Set mtg. NP. and voc. couns. 30 min.				#10 Meet with fam. 1 hr.
10:00 a.m.	#9 Call pt. 10 min. / #11 Call Jane; set mtg. 10 min.		#9 Meet WCCB 90 min.	#7 Meet law. court prep. 90 min.	
10:30 a.m.	#12 Call law. 10 min. / #13 Call ref. scurce 15 min.				#9 Meet with fam. 1 hr.
11:00 a.m.					
11:30 a.m.	Lunch	Lunch	Lunch	Lunch	Lunch
12:00 p.m.		#5 Conduct team mtg. 1 hr.	#1 Write rpt. 30 min.	#2 Meet with Alvin 1 hr.	
1:00 p.m.			#8 Write rpt. 30 min.	#5 Meet with wkr. 1.5 hrs.	
1:30 p.m.			#4 Write rpt. and circ. 30 min.		
2:00 p.m.					
2:30 p.m.					
3:00 p.m.					
3:30 p.m.					
4:00 p.m.					
4:30 p.m.	Communication	Communication	Communication	Communication	Communication
5:00 p.m.					

Notes: Communication = check e-mails, text, return phone calls, check for messages.

5. You will see that there is vacancy in each week; this allows for crises that may occur; if there are not any crisis items from the next week can be moved up. This type of scheduling is consistently avoiding procrastination. If the blue and green items are never moved up, they will eventually become a red out of urgency. This time management system avoids crisis living for the clinician, the client, and the family. It also allows time for ongoing public relations and it gives the clinician the necessary information to know whether the current caseload will allow enough time to take on new referrals.

6. It is important to build in time to allow for excellent communication. There should be two time allotments during the day that are designated for returning texts, e-mails, and phone calls. It is suggested that these be at the end of the morning and the end of the afternoon.

7. Modern communication and technology afford the health care provider instant communication; however, this can be very disruptive. Therefore, it is important to be disciplined in your use of instant communication. Texts, phone calls, and e-mails should be returned within the day they were received, but not necessarily in the instant that they were received.

Abbreviations for Time Management System

1:1	One to one	Couns.	Counselor
Ad.	Advertisement	Des.	Design
Adj.	Adjustor	Dr.	Doctor
Appt.	Appointment	Ed.	Educate
Ass.	Association	Empl.	Employment
Assist.	Assistant	Fam.	Family
Ax.	Assessment	Fct.	Functional
Circ.	Circulate	Govt.	Government
Clin.	Clinical	Hlth.	Health
Co.	Company	Hr.	Hour
COFC	Cost of future care	Int.	Interview
Cog.	Cognitive	Law.	Lawyer
Comm.	Community	Meds.	Medical record
Con.	Consultant	Mgr.	Case manager

Min.	Minutes	Reh.	Rehabilitation
MOH	Ministry of Health	Rep.	Representative
Mtg.	Meeting	Rev.	Review
Neur.	Neurologist	Rx.	Treatment
NP.	Neuropsychologist	Sched.	Schedule
OT	Occupational therapist	TBI	Traumatic brain injury
Ph.	Phone	Th.	Theory
Pol.	Policy	Tm.	Team
Prep.	Prepare	VA	Veterans affairs
Prog.	Program	Vic.	Victim
Psych.	Psychologist	Voc.	Vocational
Pt.	Physical therapist	Vol.	Volunteer
Ref.	Refer	WCB	Workers' Compensation Board
		Wkrs.	Workers

To take full advantage of the 4-week time management system, one must document the actual time spent to complete any given task, compare the time spent with industry standards and then compare one's own estimated time projections for future tasks (Tables 12.1 and 12.7). The actual time spent should match the time projections.

It is important that the funder not pay additional fees because of inexperience or disorganization on the part of the clinician. When a job task list is designed, it provides the quality control framework for time expenditure. The clinician then understands the expectation to stay on task. In the event that the task requires an inordinate amount of time, it is incumbent on the clinician to absorb the excess time spent unless previously authorized by the funder. Having clear parameters inspires the health care provider to become an excellent time manager.

QUALITY STATISTICS

In the author's experience, the following quality statistics are useful as a summary point on many levels (see Table 12.7):

1. This form is a great management tool to see if clinicians are effectively servicing their clients.
2. As sometimes happens in clinical practice, the professional may identify or enjoy working with one client over another. It is easy to see a month pass with a

Table 12.7 Quality Statistics

Name	File status	Projected hrs. including travel time over 4 weeks	Actual billed hrs. over 4 weeks	Discrepancy projected vs. actual billed	Explanation
Walter Dunbar	Active	12.67	14.5	1.83	Client required more time with 1:1 workers.
Harry Thetics	Active	5.34	7	1.66	Additional time required to recruit volunteers.
George Peterson	Active	4.59	6.5	1.91	Approval from government generated one additional meeting.
Tom Minor	Active	4.42	7.2	2.78	Additional meeting with vocational team.
Richard Wain	Active	15.84	5.3	−10.54	Because of urgency of McGeorge's COFC, these tasks did not get attended to.
Charles Locke	Active	6.75	7.2	0.45	Meeting with father took more time.
Gary McGeorge	Active	20.45	33.25	12.8	Discrepancy in medical opinions requiring clarification.
Portia Laviore	Active	9	8.9	−0.1	Meeting with worker took less time.
Karl Koster	Active	9.92	9.5	−042	Physical therapist was on vacation.
Jim Breen	Active	8.25	8.4	0.15	Meeting with school counselor took more time.
Jane Dour	Active	6	5.9	−0.1	Meeting with OT took less time.
Mary Hopkins	Abeyance	0.17	0.17		On target.
Ethel Barnell	Pending	0.25	0.25		On target.
Russell White	Closed				
Total estimated hours per day		103.65 ÷ 20 working days = 5.18 hrs/day	114.07 ÷ 20 working days = 5.7 hrs/day	10.42 ÷ 20 working days = 0.52 hrs/day	

wealth of time assigned to one client versus little time spent on another. There needs to be a means of ensuring that each client's needs have been identified and that the clinician has followed through in a timely, cost-effective manner. It is also important that every client receive the highest level of service at the most cost-effective rate. Some of the variations seen in clinical practice include:

a. An experienced clinician may take less time to complete any given task.

b. A less experienced clinician may take more time to complete a task.

c. Any therapist may avoid areas that he or she does not feel as confident in, and these tasks may be found in the procrastination bin.

d. Clients who are not in crisis may continually get bumped down the list and receive suboptimal care.

e. This screening tool can clearly provide indicators to the health care professional that he or she needs to take on no new cases or that he or she needs to engage in some public relations and marketing.

f. This screening tool allows health care providers to compare themselves against industry standards regarding the efficacy of the use of their time.

HOW TO PREPARE QUALITY STATISTICS

1. Each type of file should be separated by client name.

2. Use the job task list when estimating projected time requirements. This should be based on general industry standards based on the amount of time taken to complete the task by a clinician of good standing in the same discipline.

3. Calculate projected hours by the number of files, including travel time, and then add the hours.

4. If this is tracked over time, an organized clinician will find that he or she has projected accurately and that the projected time is in concert with the actual time.

5. If the time spent on the clinical files is over the projection and the actual time billed is under the projected time, chances are that this is a crisis-managed caseload.

6. If the time tracked is under the projection time as corroborated by the billing, these clients are not getting the care that they need.

7. This system creates a continual prompting for examination of quality and gives tools to the health care provider to stay on course.

The clinician who prepared the quality statistics in Table 12.7 was accurate in some projections and very inaccurate in others. The points of concern are as follows:

1. Regarding Walter, Harry, George, and Tom, there were less than 3 hours of differentiation from time spent to actual time billed. In these cases, the explanation is logical and, in cases such as these, the required time should have been anticipated in the original projection by the clinician.

2. In the case of Richard, the differentiation was over 10 hours, which is of concern because this is a very active file. With so many of the to-do's left unattended, this client is at risk for a crisis, which could also result in liability exposure for the clinician. Potentially, the reason that Richard did not get attended to would be because of the increased time expectation on the cost of future care for Gary.

3. The Gary M. file was also 12.8 hours over the projection and as a result was 12.8 hours over the quote. The clinician should have been well enough versed on this case to have anticipated the discrepancy in medical opinions. The suggestion to the clinician would be that, when scheduling a cost of future care, which can be anticipated well in advance, several days should be set aside to complete this project in one sitting during week 4 (pink) or week 3 (green). Ideally, a cost of future care should never end up in week 1 because the anticipated repercussion will be that other clients' needs will go unattended, leaving the clients at risk and the clinician exposed for liability.

4. Portia, Karl, Jim, and Jane were all slightly off the projected hours but had logical explanations. Overall, the clinician becomes better versed with his/her caseload, these differentials will reduce.

In general, the quality statistics on this caseload reflect that this is not a full caseload and that the clinician should be investing some time in public relations to generate more referrals. At least one of these cases is close to being closed freeing up more of the case manager's time. In almost half of these cases, the clinician was not anticipating tasks that would be required. It is important, when reviewing the files and preparing the to-do list, that any anticipated spinoff as a result of the listed to-do's has been allowed for and included. The time management in relationship to the McGeorge cost of future care resulted in poor clinical care for Mr. Wain and reduced billable hours.

SUMMARY

In summary, managing one's time when working with the traumatically brain injured is of the utmost importance. We can hinder our clients' progress and jeopardize our therapeutic relationship if our time is not managed properly. Clients may internalize any waiting period as lack of progress or of not being respected. We can reduce the stress on the client and on ourselves by utilizing this effective means of time management. The goal is to manage any client crisis without impacting other clients' needs. We do this by recognizing that there will be peaks and valleys in the recovery process. It is in anticipating the peaks and valleys and anticipating the time required to provide effective service at any given time that we can delegate a priority to the task. The color-coded system will ensure that anything with a top priority is dealt with in the current week. By the next week the second tier tasks become the top priority. In adhering to this color-coded system all tasks move up the priority list to be dealt with within a 4-week time frame. Clinically, we allow time to manage any crisis while avoiding being managed by the crisis.

From a business perspective, the effectiveness of the quality statistics is that the clinician can anticipate where he or she might run into trouble—whether in having too much work or, conversely, not enough work—thus apprising the clinician that it is time to engage in public relations and marketing.

Recording the status of the files and engaging in ongoing communication with the referral source will help clarify the future time requirements. The quality statistics are an indication of the estimated time required to provide quality clinical care against industry standards and against the estimated quote given to the funder at the time of the intake. In the event that the actual billed time exceeds the original quote, the clinician will either need to absorb the time if it was caused by poor time management, or renegotiate with the funder if additional clinical issues are the cause. It is imperative to follow the *rainbow effect* formula; a precursor to the effectiveness of the time management system is an intimate understanding of each case. When guided by the job task list, it keeps the health care professional on track and provides a structure in relationship to time and thus billing. The quality statistics predict the amount of time required by a client over the next 20 business days. This allows the clinician a window into future availability to take on new files. The quality statistics also compare actual time billed against the projection. If there are variables in the projected time and the actual time billed, this can indicate several things:

1. The clinician has either over- or underbilled.
2. The initial intake quote was not accurate and needs to be renegotiated.
3. The clinician requires assistance with time management.
4. The clinician has too many files.

The clinician's priority must be quality clinical care focused on the client's needs. We, the health care providers, must make every effort to facilitate a seamless therapeutic process, including unanticipated events.

CHAPTER 13

Diverse Funding

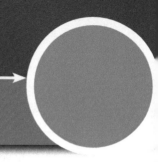

INTRODUCTION

The goal of this chapter is to streamline the arduous and oftentimes frustrating journey into where to look for funding. The previous chapters have focused predominantly on clients who have third-party liability. A brief review of motor vehicle scenarios will be included in this chapter.

The majority of this chapter will, however, focus on other pockets of monies that can be helpful to the under-insured brain-injured survivor. It is understood that, without financial support, the family will become the primary care provider, placing them at risk for burnout and increased risk of health problems. In the event that the family members become burnt out or become ill, the client is in the disadvantageous position of trying to cope on his or her own while dealing with the additional loss of the family support.

Without intervention and financial support, brain-injured clients may find that they no longer have the social or cognitive capabilities to make good choices.

Other cognitive impairments may make it virtually impossible for the individual to be a productive member of society. It is inherently understood that if the client is unable to care for his/her personal needs or to live independently, he or she is placed at risk.

The question is, what can be done in these cases?

The author's experience is primarily based in Canada; the funding search was conducted primarily for North America. However, the search words may be helpful for any nation; therefore, search words by category are included. In an effort to assist the process, the following areas of potential funding have been summarized and contact resources included in a suggested reading and website search at the end of the book.

The burden of brain injury is being felt in modern-day culture. Families and clients alike have a voice and that voice is being heard. It is interesting to note that there are pockets of money that can potentially be accessed if one just knows where to look.

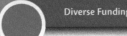

Many family members have taken on the role of advocacy and creative ideas are emerging as a result. In some instances, the very source of service delivery may have been spearheaded by families out of necessity.

I hope this chapter spawns an interest in searching for services outside the mainstream and will provide some fruit—especially to those clinicians and families advocating for those who do not have a third-party claim or who have exhausted their financial resources.

In the author's experience the most common expenses covering the gamut of potential needs for all levels of TBI fall into the categories, reviewed in Chapter 9, Table 9.1.

FUNDING SOURCES

It is recommended that early on in the process the health care providers introduce the client and family to the local and national brain injury associations; these organizations have become increasingly well versed in funding options.

One of the most common causes of traumatic brain injury is motor vehicle accidents. The following scenarios illustrate various policy structures used in motor vehicle insurance. It is important to recognize that while policies are written clearly, there are generally sections that are open to interpretation by the adjuster or major loss examiner issuing the funds. If a strong case can be made that the funds will mitigate the TBI survivor's situation, then flexibility in funding can oftentimes be achieved.

A multiple vehicle accident is when two or more cars are involved in a collision. Each driver should be carrying liability insurance and, hopefully, underinsured motorist protection insurance.

Scenario A

Bob carries $500,000 liability coverage and Sarah carries $3,000,000 liability coverage. Bob is speeding and runs through a red light illegally. Sarah is severely injured in the accident. Bob (defendant) is responsible for the accident and the resulting injuries and therefore is liable. Sarah (plaintiff) can make a claim against Bob's $500,000 policy. In some countries it would also be common for Sarah to file a lawsuit not just against Bob's insurance policy but also against Bob as an individual (assuming he has assets). To make a personal claim against an individual in Canada is not as common but is not unheard of either.

Scenario B

If Sarah were responsible for the accident (and therefore liable), and Bob were injured, Bob could make a claim against Sarah's $3,000,000 policy.

One can see from this example that there is a wide disparity on the limit that an injured party can sue for based on the insurance held by the other party. These examples shed light on how complicated insurance policies can be—even more so in the following scenario in which there is a multicar accident and the liability is shared.

Scenario C

In a multicar accident one driver (uninsured) was drinking, another driver ($1,000,000 limit) was speeding, and three drivers ($500,000, $1,000,000, and $5,000,000 limits) were obeying the law. The end result is a five-car pileup with three injured parties. In this case there is shared liability involving several insurance policies that vary in financial limits. It is to this end that plaintiff and defense lawyers are retained by the plaintiff and the defendant and tort actions commence.

TORT CLAIMS

A tort claim is the action taken by the plaintiff to claim damages against the defendant's insurance policy or personal assets. In the case of a TBI, the funds are needed very early on to cover medical expenses, wage loss, rehabilitation, and home and vehicle renovations and modifications.

In this case an advance from the tort claim can be requested by plaintiff counsel to assist the injured party's recovery process; the success of obtaining an advance from the tort is generally dependent on the strength of the claim, the cooperation of the defense lawyer, and the limits of the insurance policy.

The claim will generally focus on:

1. Non-pecuniary damages, such as pain and suffering
2. Wage loss
3. Future wage loss
4. Cost of future care

PARTIAL NO-FAULT SYSTEM

A partial no-fault system is where there is a tort claim. However, there is another section in the insurance policy allowing for the payment of medical and rehabilitation expenses incurred prior to the settlement of the claim with no liability considerations.

NO-FAULT SYSTEM

In a no-fault system the adversarial scenario of the plaintiff and defense generally does not take place, but rather the insurance policy agrees to pay within reasonable limits for the injured party's medical and rehabilitation expenses and agrees on a settlement. In these cases lawyers may or may not be involved depending generally on the severity of the injury. These types of insurance structures often have a ceiling; therefore, in some cases of catastrophic injury, a tort action may still commence.

GOVERNMENT FUNDING

The first point of searching for funds falls to the government websites. They are usually very user friendly, outlining criteria for eligibility and contact information. In a country where there is a socialized medical plan, many of the necessary interventions are available through government funding structures. There are, however, many divisions of health care; the suggested search words include the following:

• Home care	• Meal preparation	• Tax benefits program
• Long-term care	• Nursing home visits	• Supplemental security income
• Assisted living	• Home maintenance services	• Social security disability income
• Homemakers	• Financial aid programs	• Disability benefits
• Help at home	• Disability programs	• Social security
		• Registered disability savings plan

In some areas, if the options are explored, there may be a combination of government and co-pay opportunities. In many cases, it is as simple as asking the family doctor for a referral to the service; in other cases, assessment for eligibility may be based on needs and income level.

MEDICATION

There may be coverage for medications through an employer's policy, a spouse's policy, or through a government service. Ask a local pharmacist for the eligibility requirements and services. The search words include:

• Medication
• Pharmaceuticals
• Prescriptions
• Pharmacare
• Fair PharmaCare

VOCATIONAL RETRAINING

There are a variety of agencies focused on pre-vocational and work re-entry programs. It is a good idea to contact various government divisions focused on employment, such as human resources, employment and immigration, human resources and development, and welfare. These departments generally have employment counselors to talk to and may also have funds allocated for diagnostic vocational testing. The key search words include:

• Employment	• Work hardening programs
• Vocation	• Human resources
• Pre-vocation	• Skill development
• Employability	• Rehabilitation services
• Return to work	• Graduated return to work
	• Job retraining
	• Job re-entry

DISABILITY TAX CREDIT

There are many tax deductions for persons living with a disability. This, of course, will vary from country to country. Some categories found to be eligible for tax benefits may include the following search words:

• Education	• Permanent mobility impairment	• Personal care and supervision
• Textbooks	• Supplies	• Home-delivered meals
• Child disability benefits	• Specially equipped vehicles	• Recreational programs
• Children's art supplies	• Health care services	• Medical devices and supplies
• First-time home buyer	• Homemaker services	• Transportation
	• Attendant care	

WORKERS' COMPENSATION

Monies collected by employers go into a general fund known as the accident fund. These monies can be dispersed for a variety of services. Those insured under the Workers' Compensation Act can visit its website using these search words:

• Rehabilitation	• Temporary disability	• Job placement services
• Wage loss benefits	• Dependency benefits	• Case management
• Medical aid	• Physical restoration	• Help to find a new career
• Permanent disability	• Vocational evaluation	• Counseling
• Partial disability	• Rehabilitation	
	• Return to work	
	• Retraining	
	• Work-hardening program	

VETERANS AFFAIRS AND MILITARY BENEFITS

To receive a disability benefit, an individual must have a diagnosed medical condition or disability and be able to show that the condition or disability is related to his or her service. Search words include:

• Rehabilitation • Wage loss benefits • Medical aid • Permanent disability • Partial disability • Temporary disability • Dependency benefits • Physical restoration	• Vocational evaluation • Counseling • Job placement services • Mental health • Case management services • Monthly income • Retirement benefit • Health care benefit • Help to find a new career	• Vocational rehabilitation • Career transition programs • Return to work • Post-traumatic stress disorder • Adaptive lifestyle • TBI programs • Injured soldiers network • Disability compensation

ABORIGINAL AFFAIRS

It has been noted that there may be special benefits to first nations/aboriginal/native persons. The eligibility requirements appear to vary; to search applicability the following search words may be helpful:

• Employment • Vocation • Pre-vocation • Employability • Return to work • Work-hardening programs • Human resources • Skill development	• Rehabilitation services • Clinical psychology • Social work • Neuropsychology • Mental health therapist • Family support • Counseling

VICTIMS ASSISTANCE

Victims of violence may have very specific needs as well as the needs associated with traumatic brain injury. The following search criteria may be helpful:

• Mental health/counseling expenses • Pain and suffering	• Rehabilitation for disabled victims • Expenses to obtain documents

• Support for a child born as a result of a sexual assault • Lost wages for incapacitated or disabled victims • Lost support for dependents of victims • Funeral expenses	• Expenses to attend hearings • Services to replace work in the home previously performed by the victim • Property loss/damage

BLUE CROSS AND BLUE SHIELD

Services may be available through Blue Cross and Blue Shield; search words include:

• Vision care • Registered therapists • Health practitioners benefits • Naturopaths • Massage therapists • Physiotherapists • Chiropractors • Speech pathologists • Chiropodists/podiatrists • Osteopaths • Nursing benefits • Doctor's visits • Hospital expenses	• Psychologists • Audiologists • Acupuncturists • Registered dieticians • Hospital accommodation • Hospital daily cash benefit • Local ambulance benefits • Private-duty care • Prescriptions • Professional services

PRIVATE DISABILITY INSURANCE

Depending on the underwriter and the specific policy and coverage, some benefits may apply; search words include:

• Vision care • Registered therapists • Health practitioners benefits • Naturopaths • Massage therapists • Physiotherapists • Chiropractors • Speech pathologists • Chiropodists/podiatrists • Osteopaths • Nursing benefits • Doctor's visits	• Psychologists • Audiologists • Acupuncturists • Registered dieticians • Hospital accommodation • Hospital daily cash benefit • Local ambulance benefits • Private-duty care • Prescriptions • Hospital expenses • Professional services

HOMEOWNER INSURANCE

Depending on the policy and coverage, some benefits may apply. Many homeowners' policies provide coverage that will pay a certain amount of medical bills, regardless of how the injury occurred, so long as it happened on the premises of the homeowner. Accordingly, homeowner's insurance policies and any excess or umbrella policy should be carefully examined to determine whether or not there is medical coverage under the terms and provisions of that particular policy. This needs to be done promptly because many policies contain language requiring notice of injury or proof of claim being filed promptly.

TRAVEL INSURANCE

Depending on the policy and coverage, some benefits may apply.

ALTERNATE SOURCES OF FUNDING FOR SERVICE PROVISION

1. Government employment agencies such as the Office of Vocation and Rehabilitation may have a budget for diagnostic and vocational testing and may subcontract out to professionals with experience in traumatic brain injury. Check your government websites.

2. Government departments of education/special education may provide assessment, consultation, and additional classroom assistance for children with brain injuries. Check your Ministry of Education website.

3. Some government agencies in the departments of social service or welfare may provide additional services, including income assistance for individuals with brain injuries. Check your government website.

4. Nonprofit organizations, such as child care resources societies, child development centers, youth organizations, and organizations focused on the homeless, may have assistance for individuals with traumatic brain injury within their mandate and budget service provision. Check your community resource listings and nonprofit organization websites.

5. Private foundations may accept applications for funding.

6. Organizations such as brain trusts may have access to funding through application.

7. National, provincial, and state brain injury associations will have a wealth of information on how to apply and

access funding. They may also provide drop-in services and support groups as well as some professional service. (See additional resource material, Family Handouts Funding sources at **http://www.crcpress.com/product/ isbn/9781482228243.**)

PRIVATE FUNDING

Once the client is discharged to the community, it is quite common for the rehabilitation to be provided by private service providers. They would be funded either by an advance from the tort claim, through a settlement, or through the no-fault portion of the insurance policy. These companies may also provide some pro bono assistance if no other funding is available.

FUND-RAISING

The website of "HelpHOPElive" is unique in that it focuses on fund-raising, taking on the more difficult aspects of fund management and issuing tax receipts. It is based in the United States; the reason the author included it in this chapter is that it serves as a wonderful template for advocates in other countries— demonstrating what can be done in the arena of fund-raising. A visit to its user-friendly website is recommended.

HelpHOPELive is a nonprofit fund-raising solution for individuals and families with unmet medical bills related to a transplant, catastrophic injury such as traumatic brain injury, or illness. Drawing on decades of experience, they provide: personalized fund-raising guidance (one-on-one support); customized fund-raising materials (appeal letters, solicitation forms, event flyers); free web pages for online fundraising; traditional and social media support; ease of bill payment; tax deductibility and fiscal accountability; and more.

Celebrating 30 years of service, HelpHOPELive has provided more than $73 million in financial support, helping thousands of people nationwide in the United States to bridge the financial gap between what their health insurance will cover and what they actually need to heal, live and thrive. [58]

For more information, call 800.642.8399 or visit www.helphopelive.org. When searching this site be sure to visit their link to resource sites.

SUMMARY

The beginning of this chapter reviews various forms of third-party funding. There are also opportunities in a tort action to request an advance on the claim. In the author's experience, this may be possible with a larger, experienced law firm and when the limits of the policy are strong and the liability is clearly assigned to the defendant.

For those without a third-party claim, the situation becomes more complex but not impossible. The experience of sustaining a traumatic brain injury or advocating for a loved one who has had a TBI is troubling enough. When this is coupled with a lack of ability to pay for the much required medical and rehabilitation care, it can be devastating to the client and the family.

Given the rise in numbers of persons sustaining traumatic brain injuries, there are resources sprouting up from many arenas. The difficult aspect is understanding where to look for funds and determining if the survivor meets the eligibility requirements.

There are many resourceful and helpful organizations assisting the traumatically brain injured; they are listed in the suggested website section at the end of this book. The author also encourages attendance at brain injury conferences for families and survivors to keep in step with current resource developments.

The first recommended point of contact after the medical staff in hospital and the family doctor is the local and national brain injury associations. As the client's needs become more apparent, they can assist in directing the family to relevant organizations. If a case manager or social worker has been assigned to the case, this person will also be versed on current options for additional funding. It is important to identify that funding for these purposes does not refer to wage loss but rather intervention, medical/rehabilitation, and vocational costs.

These types of programs are ever changing and hopefully growing; this inventory was researched in August of 2013. The author suggests that the advocate continue to solicit information from various agencies to stay current. In the event that the TBI survivor does not fall within the eligibility requirements for the preceding list, we will move to one more option in Chapter 14, which is the use of volunteers.

CHAPTER 14

The Use of Volunteers

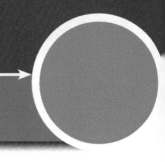

INTRODUCTION

There will be unfortunate situations where funding is not readily available and the needs of the client surpass what funding is available as described in Chapter 13.

There are still some creative options for accessing funding to finance service provision to the survivors of traumatic brain injury and their families. Volunteers are a wonderful way to augment the service roster. Through careful selection, education, and organization, this can be an effective means of recruiting manpower and facilitating service delivery. It is recommended if third-party funding is not available that this option commence early on in the process, to avoid the burden of care being placed entirely on family members for the reasons outlined in the previous chapters.

THE USE OF VOLUNTEERS

Recruiting Volunteers

When a tort claim is absent it can be a challenge to find the necessary resources to help your loved ones. The first step is to designate one person as the communications individual. This delegate will become the "go-to" person recruiting volunteers, communicating with the family, and, if agreed, meeting with the clinical team and setting up schedules for the volunteers as the professional team directs. This individual should be viewed as a trusted, competent person by the family and, ideally, not within the immediate family circle.

Steps to Recruiting Volunteers

1. Designate one person to the task of communication.
2. Based on the medical team's recommendations, develop a list of duties required of the volunteers such as:
   a. Meal preparation
   b. Transportation
   c. Assistance with child care

    d. Social interaction

    e. Exercise regime

    f. Tutorial assistance

    g. Assistance with activities of daily living

    h. Various rehabilitation tasks as assigned by the clinical team

    i. House cleaning

    j. Recreation

    k. Respite

3. Once the duties have been defined by the health care team, a system to develop a strategy to recruit volunteers should be implemented. The essential underpinning of using volunteers is to choose people that can make a reliable, consistent, regular, and long-term commitment. To this end it is often effective to solicit the volunteer pool from:

    a. Friends

    b. Relatives other than immediate family

    c. Neighbors

    d. Churches

    e. Rotary clubs

    f. Kinsmen

    g. Lions clubs

    h. Gyro clubs

    i. Brain injury association volunteers

    j. Other service groups

    k. University students

    l. College students

THE RECRUITMENT OF UNIVERSITY OR COLLEGE STUDENTS

University or college students who are in a program related to health care and psychology can be very helpful. It is possible, in concert with the faculty advisor, to design an independent study course. The person assigned to the task of communication can outline the expectation of the volunteer experience to approach the educational institute with. This course outline will offer a student or students the opportunity to gain course credit for time spent with the brain-injured client. Not only does the client gain the advantage of service very similar to a one-to-one rehabilitation worker, but the student also gains valuable clinical experience and course credit.

ORIENTATION AND EDUCATION OF VOLUNTEERS (See additional resource material, Family Handouts The Use of Volunteers at http://www.crcpress.com/product/isbn/9781482228243.)

Once the duties are defined and volunteers have been recruited, the same process of education as described in Chapter 5 should be provided to the volunteers with an assignment of duties and schedules.

It is suggested that a professional member of the clinical team in the hospital provide an educational session to all volunteers. This may be the assigned case manager, occupational therapist, neuropsychologist, or social worker. It is very important that the volunteers, like the one-to-one rehabilitation workers, do not do anything other than follow the instruction of the clinical team and report back to the team.

There should be regular access to the rehabilitation team for ongoing education and support.

SUMMARY

The use of volunteers can be a very effective way to provide service when funding is scarce. It assists in preventing the family from taking on this role, thus preserving the family unit and avoiding burnout for the loved ones of the survivor. There will be many people, especially in the early days, that will offer to help.

A list should be created of willing participants and, when they are ready the family should review the list and select those volunteers in whom they feel confident.

The most critical person is the volunteer who takes on the role of the "go-to" person. This person will function somewhat like a case manager. This individual should be competent, trustworthy, reliable, and, above all else, committed and organized.

This individual will need to have an excellent working knowledge of the goals set for the volunteers by the professional team. It is ideal if this person can have access to a member or members of the clinical team. In understanding the client's and family's needs, the go-to person can better solicit and recruit appropriate volunteers to work under the direction of the clinical team.

It can't be emphasized enough that commitment (just like in the case of the clinician) is critical for positive therapeutic outcomes. This go-to person will recruit volunteers, organize an educational session by a professional clinician, and co-ordinate scheduling of the volunteers.

When pairing the volunteers to each task, availability and commitment need to be clarified. If a commitment cannot be given to a time-consuming task, then another task less impactful on the client, such as providing one meal, should be assigned. To obtain commitment, having the volunteer benefit in some way such as gaining course credit, is helpful.

The health care provider and family will need to realize that there are increased liability risks when using volunteers and that appropriate measures will need to be taken from an insurance perspective to provide a comfort level to all involved.

The professional may need to inform his or her professional liability and malpractice provider that he or she will be supervising volunteers. The family should notify their homeowner insurance providers that volunteers will be working for them either in their home or away from the home. The same precaution needs to be taken for anyone providing transportation. One may choose to have the volunteers sign a waiver where applicable.

In short, the use of volunteers can be very effective in assisting the client and family with several tasks. With organization, commitment, and scheduling, the outcome can be remarkable. However, these scenarios are never clear-cut and all necessary precautions should be taken. The participation of the clinical team is imperative for support and guidance.

CHAPTER 15

Ethical Considerations

INTRODUCTION

The preceding chapters have reviewed how complex sustaining a traumatic brain injury can be—firstly for the survivor and secondly for the family. The section on the burden of proof (Table 0.1 in the Introduction) demonstrates the magnitude of the problem worldwide. The risks for the family are real and have been identified in Figure 7.2 and Table 7.3 in Chapter 7. Traumatic brain injury is not something that will go away; in fact, the World Health Organization's (WHO) estimate may be correct that "by 2020 TBI will surpass many diseases as the major cause of death and disability" [2, p. 164]. Collectively, we need to mobilize a worldwide strategy to deal with the increase in numbers of traumatic brain injuries. Considerations have been made toward traumatic brain injury as a "silent epidemic, as society is largely unaware of the magnitude of this problem" [8, p. 231]. Within industrialized countries "the number of productive years lost because of traumatic brain injury exceed[s] those of cancer, cerebrovascular disorders, and HIV/AIDS combined" [9, p. 1698]. This poses a challenge to society and health care systems around the world.

"The burden of TBI is manifest in all regions of the world, and is especially prominent in low and middle income countries. Even in high income countries, TBI management including intensive care differs across countries and best practices remain elusive. Access to tertiary neurosurgical and rehabilitation units is limited in rural environments and in the poorest regions of the world such as Sub-Saharan Africa. It is estimated that although over 80% of the world's people with disabilities live in LMIC [low middle income countries], only 2% have access to rehabilitation services. This lack of treatment and long term care service calls for comprehensive rehabilitative facilities based on trained manpower to enable and empower people affected by TBI to have an increased quality of life" [2, p. 350].

To manage the impact of TBI, action is required on the world stage at several levels. The research indicates that the incidence of TBI will increase and we are ill-equipped to deal with the ramifications. This increase in incidence will place a burden on health care, the social and criminal justice systems, the military, homeless programs, and the family unit.

PREVENTION IDENTIFICATION OF RISK FACTORS AND IMPROVEMENT OF PUBLIC POLICY

1. Prevent TBI through mandatory use of:
   a. Air bags
   b. Child seats
   c. Seat belts
   d. Bicycle, motorcycle, skateboard, hockey, and ski helmets

2. Impose strict regulations regarding the use of handheld devices while operating equipment and automobiles.

3. Impose and enforce strict regulations regarding speed controls.

4. Impose strict regulations regarding gun laws.

5. Provide education for anyone supervising an infant, baby, or toddler (prevention of shaken baby syndrome and falls).

6. Provide education on the risks of sustaining a traumatic brain injury as part of standard protocol in schools.

7. Impose and enforce regulations regarding the use of alcohol while driving, boating, or cycling.

8. Designate pedestrian crossings with clear signage including auditory crossing signals for the blind.

9. Provide safer road designs.

10. Resolution to civil unrest and war needs to be a priority for world leaders.

11. Provide education to those coaching athletes on the effect of cumulative concussive disorder. Clear guidelines need to be established regarding the time frame required to sit out of sporting activities post-concussion.

12. Provide education to those who have sustained one brain injury on the risk factors for sustaining subsequent TBIs.

INTERNATIONAL SHARING OF INFORMATION AND STANDARDS

Awareness and education should be shared by developed nations with governing bodies, brain injury associations, and citizens dealing with brain injury in under-developed nations.

"Developing countries face a double hazard with respect to TBI; they have a high preponderance of risk factors for TBI, while at the same time they are the least prepared to address TBI when they happen" [2, p. 350].

World statistics are just beginning to be compiled; this information should be shared globally. "Data on TBI is [*sic*] not specifically tracked at WHO although efforts are underway to improve this situation" [2, p. 351].

The following suggestions could be very helpful:

1. A means of communication for stakeholder networking among nations including national rosters of credible service providers

2. National criteria for service providers to outline educational expectations for anyone providing service to the traumatically brain injured across the medical, psychological, and rehabilitation disciplines

3. Provision and sharing of education to national brain injury associations and educational institutes for health care and education

4. Additional training for medical professionals, military personnel, homeless organizations, judges, lawyers, legal and justice institutes, and insurance providers, including prevention strategies and risks, clinical strategies to keep the family unit intact, and the prevention of health problems for primary loved ones

5. Standards of care and protocols to be developed nationally and shared through a worldwide network (possibly WHO), including protocols for prevention, reducing safety risks for the client to prevent second and third TBIs, rehabilitation, treatment, and family support

6. A system to provide a template of best practices to be created worldwide

7. A system of online learning, web-based education, and distance learning to be created and shared among nations for families, health care providers, clinicians, lawyers, judges, educators and funders

SPECIALIZED TRAINING

"Patients with moderate to severe TBI should be routinely followed up to assess their need for rehabilitation. There is strong evidence of benefit from formal interventions, particularly more intensive reprograms beginning when the patients are still in the acute ward" [1, p. 170].

Specialized education should be required for any clinician venturing into the arena of service provision for the traumatically brain injured, including:

1. Paramedics
2. Emergency/trauma personnel
3. Intensive care units, critical care, acute care, and hospital rehabilitation staff
4. Family doctors need to be well aware of TBI and be trained in the risks for the client and family. It is recommended that family doctors be educated to be able to provide the necessary support and be able to advocate for the client and family, acting as case managers once the community rehabilitation is completed.
5. Community rehabilitation clinicians (Table 2.2 in Chapter 2) require specialized training over and above their formal education and must have a working knowledge of traumatic brain injury rehabilitation prior to working with this population.
6. It is recommended that lawyers engaged in tort claims be specially trained and have an abundance of experience; the litigators should be in a financial position in their firm to retain the best medical experts. The case should also not be settled before the residual loss is established; this means that the lawyer needs to be in a financial position to work up the file without payment until the claim is settled (generally, 4–6 years post-trauma).
7. In light of the fact that over 80% percent of inmates in the criminal justice system have had at least one traumatic brain injury over their lifetime [59], judges need to be educated on TBI. Mandatory screening and intervention for TBI should be compulsory as the sentence is passed down for anyone who has demonstrated judgment, anger, impulse control problems, or behavioral issues.
8. Persons working in the criminal justice system should be well trained in TBI to discern what is, in fact, criminal psychopathology and what is a symptom of TBI. It is

recommended that programs of cognitive retraining be made available in the prison system and mandatory attendance be enforced for the TBI inmate.

9. It would be helpful for those persons working with the homeless to be well trained in TBI. With over 50% of the homeless having sustained a TBI prior to being homeless [4], those serving this struggling population need to be able to provide screening and intervention or have the ability to direct the TBI client to appropriate services. Life skills programs directed at cognitive remediation and teaching those skills necessary to live independently need to be introduced and made mandatory as part of the homeless shelter industry.

10. National military medical programs need standard protocols. Screening should ideally include a review of a soldier's previous health record, including loss of consciousness revealing any pre-existing TBIs prior to deployment. Secondly, any soldier who has been deployed and exposed to a blast, loss of consciousness, or a concussion should be screened for TBI and post-traumatic stress disorder (PTSD). Thirdly, specialized training programs need to be administered for returning veterans of war to treat TBI as well as PTSD. Lastly, veterans who have sustained a mild to moderate TBI should go through rigorous testing prior to returning to combat. "Of those reporting loss of consciousness, 43.9% met criteria for post-traumatic stress disorder (PTSD)" [60, p. 453].

"Because of improved protective equipment, a higher percentage of soldiers are surviving injuries that would have been fatal in previous wars. Head and neck injuries, including severe brain trauma, have been reported in one quarter of service members who have been evacuated from Iraq and Afghanistan. Concern has been emerging about the possible long-term effect of mild traumatic brain injury, or concussion, characterized by brief loss of consciousness or altered mental status, as a result of deployment related head injuries, particularly those resulting from proximity to blast explosions" [60, p. 454].

"All admitted patients who have been exposed to a blast are routinely evaluated for brain injury; 59 percent of them have been given a diagnosis of TBI…Of these injuries, 56 percent are considered moderate or severe, and 44 percent are mild" [61, p. 2045].

11. Insurance agents, adjusters, and major loss examiners may very well be the frontline personnel who have authority over the allocation of funds available for community rehabilitation for the TBI survivor. It is critical to provide valuable education to these parties—namely, in the arena of assistance for the family, secondary losses, and assistance to reduce financial pressure so that the client can focus all energy on getting well.

12. Insurance corporations could serve their subscribers well in learning that high-end provision of service by well educated health care providers improves outcomes over the long term for the client and reduces family health problems, burnout, and family breakdown, thus reducing the overall loss.

Protocols and policies to remove barriers reducing financial stress need to be in place. Ideally, medical/rehabilitation trained personnel should be hired within insurance corporations to foster a corporate climate of assisting the client and family to mitigate their circumstances.

BARRIERS

There are many barriers to establishing consistent standards of care for TBI survivors and their families.

One barrier worth noting is that of the financial burden. As indicated in the preceding chapters, families who have experienced the crisis of a loved one having sustained a TBI are more often than not faced with negative financial implications, creating more stress and hardship. If the primary bread winner is injured, there is a loss of salary compounding the expense of medical care.

Mild to moderate TBI often goes undiagnosed and unattended. These families are not offered treatment, often resulting in financial crisis, family breakdown, and poor outcomes for the TBI survivor. If the injury occurred in a country where the client and family need to finance the medical care themselves, the repercussions can be devastating. If the client is insured, it is common that delays may occur in financial assistance, making it difficult for the client to meet the family's monthly financial obligations.

Many times the insurance provider has caveats in the policy that may disqualify an injured party to receive the benefits needed, thus creating more stress and strain for the client and family.

In the event of a tort claim, the lawyer retained will need the skill to negotiate an advance from the tort action to assist the client financially during the 4-to 6-year rehabilitation process.

The reality is that our universal health care systems are exhausted in many nations. The expectation that existing government health policies can support the rising long-term community rehabilitation needs of the traumatically brain injured client are most likely unrealistic.

In the author's experience, most of the financial support for the long-term rehabilitation needs of the client in developed nations are supported through those third-party funding sources listed in Figure 4.1 (Chapter 4).

It therefore becomes incumbent on the third-party funder to bear the responsibility of selecting highly trained and specialized, committed health care professionals who have the skill to achieve positive clinical outcomes.

Mandatory specialized training for all health care clinicians working with TBI clients should be required prior to entry into the realm of service delivery to the traumatically brain injured.

It is recommended that additional courses, including efficacy in business practice and time management, be offered at a university level to any clinician interested in pursuing a career in the service delivery to the traumatically brain injured. Ideally, this would be augmented with in-house training in rehabilitation corporations.

For those clients that do not have any third-party funding, assistance will still be required. Programs on fundraising and education on the use of alternate forms of service such as volunteers and students should be made available, possibly through the brain injury associations.

It is the author's opinion that socially conscious, private, professional and rehabilitation companies develop a social policy to provide some pro bono assistance to clients that do not have third-party funding, thus allowing for professional input for the families and volunteers.

SELECTION OF COMMUNITY SERVICE PROVIDERS

In North America most service provision falls within the private sector for the community extended portion of traumatic brain injury intervention. There may be a tendency for some professionals such as neuropsychologists, clinical psychologists, occupational therapists, speech therapists, social workers, etc. to maintain a full-time, part-time or three-quarter time job at a government agency, while also taking on a client or clients who have sustained a traumatic brain injury in the private sector.

I hope this book has served to educate the professional sector on the risk factors associated with taking on one or two TBI clients while being committed to employment elsewhere. Our clients deserve our best. The motivation should never be the financial reimbursement we may make by serving them. Our motivation should be service delivery, in that we will reap our reward. We must be available to all parties involved in any particular client case. Our absence if we have another commitment to another job will result in not being available for the client, the family, the team meetings, phone calls, and the other clinicians involved in the client's community care, compromising the client's clinical care and outcome not to mention the family unit.

If we have a legal obligation to another job, it is difficult if not impossible to fulfill this ethical responsibility.

Finally, is the duration of our commitment. As clinicians, ideally, we will develop a specialty in the area of traumatic brain injury and continue working in it as a career. Our clients will require in the community, a 4-to 6-year intervention plan, and the research is clear that continuity is important for successful clinical outcomes. If we are not available to give expert witness testimony, our clients can be negatively impacted. If we move from job to job, the client will suffer more loss and less continuity and familiarity and will regress if we leave before the therapy is complete. One should not embark on this journey with a client if one cannot fulfill the obligation to completion.

Of course, there are exceptions to this cardinal rule. A care provider may unexpectedly move or become ill, or there is the rare case that the client and therapist cannot connect. But these should be exceptions and not rule. In the event of these cases, great attention should be made to the transference of the file to an appropriate replacement.

"There are a number of organizations and institutions involved in care, research and prevention of neurotrauma such as the European Brain Injury Society, the International Brain Injury Association, the Neurotrauma Society, the International Association for the Study of Traumatic Brain Injury and Rehabilitation International. Clearly collaboration between such bodies with clear leadership from an international organization such as the WHO is required. Joint programs between developed and developing countries should also be encouraged at both regional and national levels.

It is crucial to plan comprehensive TBI prevention, management and rehabilitation programs around the world, especially in developing countries, that are evidence based. Such programs may involve many different operational layers—research, policy formulation, public and political education, publicity campaigns, legislation, changes in manufacturing practice, as well as environmental and system modification" [2, p. 351].

SUMMARY

In final summary, a traumatic brain injury is a devastating life event that could impact any of us at any given time. We all have loved ones that provide stability to our environment as we do for them; if someone we love sustains a traumatic brain injury or if we ourselves sustain a TBI, our life will be impacted. The question is, will this be a life circumstance that makes the very life experience richer or will it unravel our relationships and cause despair? In your reading this book I trust that the risks have become clear. However the prevailing hope also should be clear. We as humans are resilient; if we, the health care providers, create an environment of healing, then healing can take place. We need to return our clients to a place of hope—the place of the human spirit, that place where love and hope reside.

Not one of us is exempt from life experiences, and TBI could happen to any of us. It is to this end that we should understand that if we were in our client's shoes, we would want the best for ourselves and our families; we would appreciate the education and intervention that would help us to cope and remain connected. We would want our health care providers to be committed through the duration of the recovery process. If we adopt the stance of treating others the way that we would want to be treated ourselves, then we position our clients, their families, and ourselves on a rewarding journey where the resilience of the human spirit will inspire and move us. To all of those clients with whom I have had the privilege to walk with through the journey of recovery, you are the inspiration for this book.

GLOSSARY OF TERMS

Abstract reasoning: A concept or idea not related to any specific instance or object that potentially can be applied to many different situations or objects. Persons with cognitive deficits often have difficulty understanding abstract concepts [28].

Acquired brain injury: Damage to the brain that occurs after birth and is not related to a congenital or a degenerative disease. These impairments may be temporary or permanent and cause partial or functional disability or psychosocial maladjustment [28].

Agnosia: Impairment of the ability to recognize, or comprehend the meaning of various sensory stimuli not attributable to disorders of the primary receptors or general intellect; agnosias are receptive defects caused by lesions in various portions of the cerebrum [28].

Ambulatory: Walking about or able to walk about; denoting a patient who is not confined to bed or hospital as a result of disease or surgery [28].

Amnesia: A disturbance in the memory of stored information of very variable durations, minutes to months, in contrast to short-term memory, manifest by total or partial inability to recall past experiences [28].

Aneurysm: Circumscribed dilation of an artery or a cardiac chamber, in direct communication with the lumen, usually resulting from an acquired or congenital weakness of the wall of the artery or chamber [28].

Anoxia: A condition in which there is an absence of oxygen supply to an organ's tissues, although there is adequate blood flow to the tissue [28].

Anterograde amnesia: Amnesia in reference to events occurring after the trauma or disease that caused the condition [28].

Apathy: Indifference; absence of interest in the environment. Often one of the earliest signs of cerebral disease [28].

Aphasia: Impaired or absent comprehension or production of or communication by speech, reading, writing, or signs, caused by an acquired lesion of the dominant cerebral hemisphere [28].

> **Auditory:** An impairment in comprehension of the auditory forms of language and communication, including the ability to write from dictation in the presence of normal hearing. Spontaneous speech, reading, and writing are not affected.

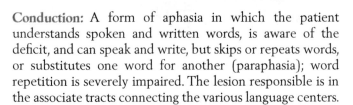

Conduction: A form of aphasia in which the patient understands spoken and written words, is aware of the deficit, and can speak and write, but skips or repeats words, or substitutes one word for another (paraphasia); word repetition is severely impaired. The lesion responsible is in the associate tracts connecting the various language centers.

Crossed: Aphasia in a right-handed person due to a solely right cerebral lesion.

Global: All aspects of speech and communication are severely impaired. At best, patients can understand or speak only a few words or phrases; they can neither read nor write.

Motor: A type of aphasia in which there is a deficit in speech production or language output, often accompanied by a deficit in communicating by writing, signs, or other manifestations. The patient is aware of the impairment.

Nominal: An aphasia in which the principal deficit is difficulty in naming people and objects seen, heard, or felt due to lesions in various portions of the language area.

Pure: Rare aphasias affecting only one type of communication (e.g., reading), whereas related communication forms (such as writing and auditory comprehension) remain intact.

Semantic: Aphasia in which objects are correctly named; little disturbance is found in the articulation of words; individual words are understood, but the broader meaning of what is heard cannot be grasped.

Sensory: Aphasia with impairment in the comprehension of spoken and written words, associated with effortless, articulated, but paraphrastic speech and writing; malformed words, substitute words, and neologisms are characteristic. When the condition is severe and speech is incomprehensible, it is called jargonaphasia. The patient often appears unaware of the deficit.

Syntactic: Aphasia in which the words are fairly well pronounced but are spoken in short phrases or poorly constructed sentences without articles, prepositions, or conjunctions.

Transcortical: An aphasia in which the unaffected motor and sensory language areas are isolated from the rest of the hemispheric cortex. Subdivided into transcortical sensory and transcortical motor aphasias.

Apraxia: A disorder of voluntary movement consisting of impairment of the performance of skilled or purposeful movements, notwithstanding the preservation of comprehension, muscular power, sensibility, and coordination in general that results from acquired cerebral disease. Or, a psychomotor defect in which the proper use of an object cannot be carried out although the object can be named and its uses described [28].

> **Constructional:** Apraxia manifested as an impairment in activities such as building, assembling, and drawing; caused by parietal lobe lesions.

> **Ideokinetic:** A form of apraxia in which simple acts cannot be performed, presumably because the connections between the cortical centers that control volition and the motor cortex are interrupted.

Ataxic dysarthria: Dysarthria caused by cerebellar lesions [28].

Atrophy: A wasting of tissues, organs, or the entire body, as from death and reabsorption of cells, diminished cellular proliferation, decreased cellular volume, pressure, ischemia, malnutrition, lessened function, or hormonal changes [28].

Attention: The act or state of attending; the application of the mind to any object of sense or thought [62].

Awareness: A condition of being alert and cognizant of one's surroundings and external phenomena, as well as one's personal state [28].

Balance: The system that depends on vestibular function, vision, and proprioception to maintain posture, navigate in one's surroundings, coordinate motion of body parts, modulate fine motor control, and initiate the vestibulooculomotor reflexes [28].

Benign positional vertigo: Brief attacks of paroxysmal vertigo and nystagmus that occur solely with certain head movements or positions (e.g., with neck extension); due to labyrinthine dysfunction [28].

Berry aneurysm: A small saccular aneurysm of a cerebral artery that resembles the fruit; can rupture causing a subarachnoid hemorrhage [28].

Bilateral: Relating to or having two sides [28].

Blood clot: The coagulated phase of blood; the soft, coherent, jelly-like red mass resulting from the conversion of fibrinogen to fibrin, thereby entrapping the red blood cells (and other formed elements) within the coagulated plasma [28].

Brain concussion: A clinical syndrome, usually due to head trauma, characterized by immediate but transient impairment

---

Note: [62]. By permission. From *Merriam-Webster's Medical Dictionary*, @ 2006 by Merriam-Webster, Inc. (www.merriam-webster.com).

of cerebral function, principally alteration of consciousness, but also disturbance of vision and equilibrium, without any detectable structural brain damage [28].

Brain contusion: A bruising, usually of the surface of the brain, with infarction of brain parenchyma and extravasation of blood but without rupture of the pia-arachnoid; healing results in a superficial depressed sclerotic area, possibly with incorporated meninges [28].

Brain stem: The part of the brain composed of the midbrain, pons, and medulla oblongata and connecting the spinal cord with the forebrain and cerebrum [62].

CAT scan: A sectional view of the body constructed by computed tomography—called also CT scan [62].

Cerebellum: A large dorsally projecting part of the brain concerned especially with the coordination of muscle and the maintenance of bodily equilibrium, situated between the brain stem and the back of the cerebrum and formed in humans of two lateral lobes and a median lobe [62].

Cerebral hypoxia: Cerebral hypoxia occurs where there is not enough oxygen getting to the brain [62].

Cerebral spinal fluid: A fluid largely secreted by the choroid plexuses of the ventricles of the brain, filling the ventricles and the subarachnoid cavities of the brain and spinal cord [28].

Closed head injury: A head injury in which continuity of the scalp and mucous membranes is maintained [28].

Cognition: Generic term embracing the mental activities associated with thinking, learning, and memory [28].

Cognitive impairment: Cognitive impairment describes the decline in cognitive functions like memory, selective attention, executive control, or conscious perception [64].

Coma: A state of profound unconsciousness from which one cannot be roused; may be due to the action of an ingested toxic substance or of one formed in the body, due to trauma, or to disease [28].

Computed tomography (CT): An x-ray examination technique in which only structures in a particular plane produce clearly focused images [63].

Concussion: A violent shaking or jarring or an injury of a soft structure, such as the brain, resulting from a blow or violent shaking [28].

Congenital aneurysm: Localized dilation of a cerebral vessel; usually a berry aneurysm [28].

Conjugate movement: Rotation of the two eyes in the same direction [28].

Consciousness: The state of being aware, or perceiving physical facts or mental concepts; a state of general wakefulness and responsiveness to environment; a functioning sensorium [28].

Consecutive aneurysm: Two or more aneurysms along the path of blood flow [28].

Contracture: Static muscle shortening due to tonic spasm or fibrosis, to loss of muscular balance, to the antagonist being paralyzed, or to a loss of motion of the adjacent joint [28].

Contusion: Any mechanical injury (usually caused by a blow) resulting in hemorrhage beneath unbroken skin [28].

Countercoup injury of the brain: An injury occurring beneath the skull opposite to the area of impact [28].

Coup injury of the brain: An injury occurring directly beneath the skull at the area of impact [28].

Decerebrate posturing: Posturing manifested by the obtunded patient extending arms laterally away from the center of the body in response to noxious stimuli, with flexed wrists outward [28].

Decerebrate rigidity: A postural change that occurs in some comatose patients, consisting of episodes of opisthotonos, rigid extension of the limbs, internal rotation of the upper extremities, and marked plantar flexion of the feet; produced by a variety of metabolic and structural brain disorders [28].

Decorticate posturing: Posturing manifested by the obtunded patient pulling arms and hands medially toward the center (core) of the body in response to noxious stimuli [28].

Decorticate rigidity: A unilateral or bilateral postural change, consisting of the upper extremities flexed and adducted and the lower extremities in rigid extension; due to structural lesions of the thalamus, internal capsule, or cerebral white matter [28].

Diffuse aneurysm: An aneurysm that has enlarged and spread to the surrounding tissues as a consequence of a contained rupture of its walls [28].

Diffuse axonal injury: An injury caused by shaking or strong rotation of the head by physical forces, such as with a car crash. Injury occurs because the unmoving brain lags behind the movement of the skull, causing nerve structures to tear. The tearing of the nerve tissue disrupts the brain's regular communication and chemical processes [65].

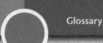

Diplegia: Paralysis of corresponding parts on both sides of the body [28].

Diplopia: The condition in which a single object is perceived as two objects [28].

Disinhibition: Removal of an inhibition, such as by a toxic or organic process or removal of an inhibitory effect by a stimulus, as when a conditioned reflex has undergone extinction but is restored by some extraneous stimulus [28].

Disorientation: Loss of the sense of familiarity with one's surroundings (time, place, and person); loss of one's bearings [28].

Distractibility: A disorder of attention in which the mind is easily diverted by inconsequential occurrences; seen in mania and attention deficit disorder [28].

Dorsi flexion: Upward movement (extension) of the foot or toes or of the hand or fingers [28].

Dysarthria: A disturbance of speech due to emotional stress, to brain injury, or to paralysis, incoordination, or spasticity of the muscles used for speaking [28].

Dysmetria: An aspect of ataxia in which the ability to control the distance, power, and speed of an act is impaired. Usually used to describe abnormalities of movement caused by cerebellar disorders [28].

Ectatic aneurysm: An aneurysm in which all the coats of the artery, although stretched, are unruptured [28].

Emotional amnesia: Psychological etiology of forgetting or repressing of emotion [28].

Emotional labiality: Emotional labiality is a disorder characterized by involuntary emotional displays of mood that are overly frequent and excessive, often the result of various neuropathologies [66].

Equilibrium: The condition of being evenly balanced; a state of repose between two or more antagonistic forces that exactly counteract each other [28].

Evoked potential: Registration of the electrical responses of active brain cells as detected by electrodes placed on the surface of the head at various places. The evoked potential, unlike the waves on an EEG, is elicited by a specific stimulus applied to the visual, auditory, or other sensory receptors of the body. Evoked potentials are used to diagnose a wide variety of central nervous system disorders [28].

Expressive language: Expressive language refers to the way a person expresses himself or herself for everyday wants, needs, and feelings. Spoken, written, and body language, including facial expressions and sign language, are all abilities considered to be expressive language skills [67].

Flaccidity: The condition or state of being flaccid [28].

Flexion–extension injury: Forceful sequential application of a forward and backward movement of the unsupported head that may produce an injury to the cervical spine or the brain [28].

Frontal lobe: The anterior division of each cerebral hemisphere having its lower part in the anterior fossa of the skull and bordered behind by the central sulcus [62].

Frontal lobe syndrome: Frontal lobe syndrome (FLS) is a cluster of behavioral, affective, and cognitive symptoms resulting from pathological processes that destroy or interfere with the function of the gray matter of the prefrontal areas of the frontal lobes. Although the quantity, severity, and variety of observable features can vary considerably across cases, it is the ensemble of deficits that is known as FLS. Behavioral and affective characteristics of FLS may include abulia, apathy, lack of concern, confabulation, perseverative responding, loss of spontaneity, inability to maintain goal-directed behavior, motor impersistence, utilization behavior, environmental dependency, stimulus-bound behavior, disorganization, inability to modify behavior to accommodate new information, risk-taking behavior, disinhibition, restlessness, distractibility, hypomania, social inappropriateness, witzelsucht, tactlessness, lack of behavioral restraint, inappropriate sexual behavior/conversation, poor self-awareness, diminished empathy, boastfulness, capriciousness, delusions, puerility, mood incongruent affect, emotional incontinence, constricted range or poor modulation of emotional expression, euphoria, aggression, and irritability. Cognitive deficits may include impairments in attention, working memory, short-term memory, set-shifting, abstract reasoning, judgment, ability to suppress inappropriate responses, verbal and design fluency, strategizing and planning capacity, and capacity for temporal arrangement. FLS is not generally associated with loss of basic sensory or motor capacities or with obvious impairment of speech. FLS may be present with lesions of varying size and location within the prefrontal cortices due to brain injury, tumors, infarcts, seizures, and degenerative or developmental conditions. Furthermore, although FLS can occur from both unilateral and bilateral damage, bilateral lesions often produce more clinically obvious and behaviorally complex deficits [68].

Glasgow Coma Scale: A scale that is used to assess the severity of a brain injury that consists of values from 3 to 15 obtained by summing the ratings assigned to three variables depending

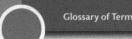
on whether and how the patient responds to certain stimuli by opening the eyes, giving a verbal response, and giving a motor response. A low score (3 to 5) indicates a poor chance of recovery and a high score (8 to 15) indicates a good chance of recovery [62].

Head injury: Any injury to the head, whether associated with a skull fracture or not. Patients with head injuries should be assessed for signs of neurological damage, which may not develop at once. Patients who, after a head injury, are or have been unconscious, who are drowsy, vomiting, confused, or who have any focal neurological signs—for example, blurred vision or a motor or sensory malfunction—should be seen by a doctor. Particular care should be taken with individuals who have consumed alcohol and sustained a head injury in a fight, fall, or vehicle accident. Symptoms indicative of a severe head injury may be attributed (wrongly) to the effects of alcohol and crucial time may be lost in treating the injury [63].

Hemianopia: Loss of vision for one-half of the visual field of one or both eyes [28].

Hemiparesis: Weakness affecting one side of the body [28].

Hemiplegia: Paralysis of one side of the body [28].

Hemiplegic: Relating to hemiplegia [28].

Hemorrhage: An escape of blood from the intravascular space, or, to bleed [28].

Hypertonic: Having a greater degree of tension or having a greater osmotic pressure than a reference solution, which is ordinarily assumed to be blood plasma or interstitial fluid; refers more specifically to a fluid in which cells shrink [28].

Hypoxia: Decrease below normal levels of oxygen in inspired gases, arterial blood, or tissue, without reaching anoxia [28].

Inattention: Lack of attention; negligence [28].

> **Selective:** An aspect of attentiveness in which a person attempts to ignore or avoid perceiving that which generates anxiety.

> **Sensory:** The inability to feel a tactile stimulus when a similar stimulus, presented simultaneously in a homologous area of the body, is perceived.

Infraclinoid aneurysm: An intracranial aneurysm occurring below the level of the anterior clinoid process of the sphenoid bone [28].

Insight: Self-understanding as to the motives and reasons behind one's own actions or those of another [28].

Interdisciplinary: Denoting the overlapping interests of different fields of medicine and science [28].

Intracerebral hemorrhage: Occurs into the substance of the cerebrum, usually in the region of the internal capsule by the rupture of the lenticulostriate artery [28].

Intracranial: Within the cranium, usually meaning within the cranial cavity [28].

Intracranial aneurysm: Any aneurysm located within the cranium [28].

Intracranial pressure: Pressure within the cranial cavity [28].

Ipsilateral: On the same side, with reference to a given point (e.g., a dilated pupil on the same side as an extradural hematoma with contralateral limbs being paretic) [28].

Ischemia: Local loss of blood supply due to mechanical obstruction (mainly arterial narrowing or disruption) of the blood vessel [28].

Lacunar amnesia: Amnesia in reference to isolated events [28].

Learning: Generic term for the relatively permanent change in behavior that occurs as a result of practice [28].

Lethargic: Relatively mild impairment of consciousness resulting in reduced alertness and awareness; this condition has many causes but is ultimately due to generalized brain dysfunction [28].

Lower motor neuron dysarthria: Dysarthria caused by dysfunction of the motor nuclei and the lower pons or medulla, or other neural connections, central and peripheral to the muscles of articulation [28].

Magnetic resonance imaging (MRI): A diagnostic radiologic modality, using nuclear magnetic resonance technology, in which the magnetic nuclei (especially protons) of a patient are aligned in a strong, uniform magnetic field, absorb energy from tuned radiofrequency pulses, and emit radiofrequency signals as their excitation decays. These signals, which vary in intensity according to nuclear abundance and molecular chemical environment, are converted into sets of tomographic images by using field gradients in the magnetic field, which permits three-dimensional localization of the point sources of the signals [28].

Memory: General term for the recollection of that which was earlier experienced or learned, or, the mental information processing system that receives (registers), modifies, stores, and retrieves informational stimuli; composed of three stages: encoding, storage, and retrieval [28].

> **Long term (LTM):** The phase of the memory process considered the permanent storehouse of information that has been registered, encoded, passed into the short-term memory, coded, rehearsed, and finally transferred and stored

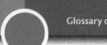

for future retrieval; material and information retained in LTM underlie cognitive abilities.

Remote: Memory for events of long ago as opposed to recent events.

Short term (STM): That phase of the memory process in which stimuli that have been recognized and registered are stored briefly; decay occurs rapidly, sometimes within seconds, but may be held indefinitely by using rehearsal as a holding process by which to recycle material over and over through STM.

Miliary aneurysm: Dilation in the diameter of small arteries and arterioles secondary to lipohyalinosis from long-standing hypertension; associated with intracerebral hematomas [28].

Monoplegia: Paralysis of one limb [28].

Motor control: The operations of the nervous system that regulate the timing and the amount of contraction of muscles necessary to produce smooth and coordinated movement of the body [29].

Fine: Refers to precise and subtle movements such as in threading a needle or rolling or stacking coins [29].

Gross: Involves large, strong movements such as walking, reaching, grabbing, etc. [29].

Motor planning: Motor planning can be broadly defined as the capacity to plan the necessary steps to achieve purposeful movements [69].

Neglect: To disregard or ignore; to fail to perform a duty or to give due attention or care [28].

Nystagmus: Involuntary rhythmic oscillation of the eyeballs, either pendular or with a slow and fast component [28].

Horizontal nystagmus: Left and right motion.

Rotary nystagmus: Clockwise and counterclockwise motion.

Vertical nystagmus: Up and down motion.

Occipital lobe: The occipital lobe is the most posterior lobe of the cerebral hemispheres and is primarily related to visual processing [71].

Open head injury: A head injury in which there is a loss of continuity of scalp or mucous membranes; the term is sometimes used to indicate a communication between the exterior and the intracranial cavity [28].

Organizing: To provide with or to assume a structure [28].

Orientation: The recognition of one's temporal, spatial, and personal relationships and environment [28].

Paranoid: Relating to or characterized by paranoia or having delusions of persecution [28].

Paraplegia: Paralysis of both lower extremities and, generally, the lower trunk [28].

Parietal lobe: The middle division of each cerebral hemisphere that is situated behind the central sulcus, above the sylvian fissure, and in front of the parieto-occipital sulcus that contains an area concerned with bodily sensations [62].

Perception: The mental process of becoming aware of or recognizing an object or idea; primarily cognitive rather than affective or conative, although all three aspects are manifested [28].

Perseveration: The constant repetition of a meaningless word or phrase or the duration of a mental impression, measured by the rapidity with which one impression follows another as determined by the revolving of a two-colored disc. Or, in clinical psychology, the uncontrollable repetition of a previously appropriate or correct response, even though the repeated response has since become inappropriate or incorrect [28].

Plantar flexion: Bending the foot or toes toward the plantar surface [28].

Positive emission tomography (PET) scan: Creation of tomographic images revealing certain biochemical properties of tissue by computer analysis of positrons emitted when radioactively tagged substances are incorporated into the tissue. Radiotracers used in PET are analogues of physiologic or pharmaceutical agents into which positron-emitting isotopes with short half-lives (2–110 minutes) have been incorporated. Radioisotopes are produced artificially by bombarding stable isotopes with a proton beam generated by a cyclotron. The uptake and metabolism of these positron emitters mimic, at least in part, those of the radio stable natural substances to which they are analogous. Concentrated in particular organs or tissues and incorporated into metabolic processes, they can reflect biochemical function or dysfunction. The glucose analogue 2-(fluorine-18)fluoro-2-deoxy-d-glucose (FDG) is widely used to locate zones of heightened energy metabolism. When a positron emitted by a radiotracer collides with an electron, the particles annihilate each other and two gamma rays are discharged in opposite directions (at 180°). After intravenous administration of the radiotracer, the subject is positioned within a scanner consisting of a ring of scintillation crystals that convert gamma rays into flashes of visible light. These flashes are detected and recorded electronically, and a computer program assembles the data into a three-dimensional image, color-coded to reflect concentration density [28].

Post-traumatic amnesia: Discrimination and memory loss that occur with injury and may persist for weeks or months—usually regarded as an indicator of eventual recovery. It affects the organization and retrieval of information about events occurring after the point at which injury occurred [29].

Problem solving: Problem solving is the process of constructing and applying mental representations of problems to finding solutions to those problems that are encountered in nearly every context [70].

Proprioception: A sense or perception, usually at a subconscious level, of the movements and position of the body, and especially its limbs, independently of vision; this sense is gained primarily from input from sensory nerve terminals in muscles and tendons (muscle spindles) and the fibrous capsule of joints combined with input from the vestibular apparatus [28].

Quadriplegia: Paralysis of all four limbs [28].

Ranchos los Amigos scale: A tool that is used to determine various levels of functional recovery from traumatic brain injury (see Chapter 3, Appendix 3F) [29].

Range of motion: Refers to movement of a joint (important to prevent contractures) [28].

> **Active:** Amount of motion at a given joint when the subject moves the part voluntarily.

> **Passive:** Amount of motion at a given joint when the joint is moved by an external force or therapist.

Retrograde amnesia: Amnesia with reference to events that occurred before the trauma or disease that caused the condition [28].

Ruptured aneurysm: An aneurysm that is hemorrhaging into its wall or surrounding tissue, representing a true surgical emergency [28].

Scanning: The act of imaging by traversing with an active or passive sensing device, often identified by the technology or device employed [28].

Secondary gain: Interpersonal or social advantages (e.g., assistance, attention, sympathy) gained indirectly from organic illness [28].

Sensorimotor: Functioning in both sensory and motor aspects of bodily activity [62].

Sequencing: The determination of the sequence of subunits in a macromolecule [28].

Shunt: To bypass or divert or a bypass or diversion of fluid to another fluid-containing system by fistulation or a prosthetic device. The nomenclature commonly includes origin and terminus (e.g., atriovenous, splenorenal, ventriculocisternal) [28].

Single-photon emission computerized tomography (SPECT) scan: A SPECT scan lets a doctor analyze the function of some internal organs. A SPECT scan is a type of nuclear imaging test, which uses a radioactive substance and a special camera to create three-dimensional pictures [28].

Skull fracture: A break of the cranium resulting from trauma [28].

Somatosensory: Sensation relating to the body's superficial and deep parts as contrasted to specialized senses such as sight [28].

Spasticity: One type of increase in muscle tone at rest; characterized by increased resistance to passive stretch, velocity dependence, and asymmetry about joints (greater in the flexor muscles at the elbow and the extensor muscles at the knee). Exaggerated deep tendon reflexes and clonus are additional manifestations [28].

Spontaneous recovery: The return of the conditioned response, after apparent extinction, in the presence of the conditioned stimulus without the unconditioned stimulus also being present [28].

Stereognosis: Ability to perceive or the perception of material qualities (as shape) of an object by handling or lifting it: tactile recognition [62].

Strabismus: A manifest lack of parallelism of the visual axes of the eyes [28].

Tactile: Relating to touch or to the sense of touch [28].

Temporal lobe: A large lobe of each cerebral hemisphere that is situated in front of the occipital lobe and contains a sensory area associated with the organ of hearing [62].

Tinnitus: Perception of a sound in the absence of an environmental acoustic stimulus. The sound can be a pure tone or noise, including ringing, whistling, hissing, roaring, or booming, in the ears. Tinnitus is usually associated with a loss of hearing. The site of origin of the sound percept may be in the central auditory pathways even if the initial lesion is in the end organ of the auditory system [28].

Traumatic brain injury: The loss or disturbance of memory after an insult or injury to the brain of the type that accompanies a traumatic head injury or excessive use of alcohol, after the cessation of ingestion of alcohol or other psychoactive drugs, or loss or disturbance of memory of the type seen in hysteria and other forms of dissociative disorder [28].

Tremor: Repetitive, often regular oscillatory movements caused by alternate or synchronous, but irregular contraction of opposing muscle groups; usually involuntary. Or, minute ocular movement occurring during fixation on an object [28].

Unilateral: Confined to one side only [28].

Verbal apraxia: A speech disorder in which phonemic substitutions are constantly used for the desired syllable or word [28].

Vestibular: Relating to a vestibule, especially the vestibule of the ear [28].

Visual field deficit: Occurs when a person is not visually perceiving information in a particular area of the visual field. It commonly involves either the left or right portion of the visual field. [29].

REFERENCES

1. World Health Organization. 2006. Neurological disorders: Public health challenges. Geneva: World Health Organization Press.

2. Hyder, A. A., Wunderlich, C. A., Puvanachandra, P., Gururaj, G., and Kobusingye, O. C. 2007. The impact of traumatic brain injuries: A global perspective. *Neurorehabilitation* 22 (5): 341–353.

3. Gargollo, P. C., and Lipson, A. C. 2007. Brain trauma, concussion and coma: The Dana guide. Available at http://www.dana.org/news/brainhealth/detail.aspx?id=9790 (accessed September 10, 2013).

4. Hwang, S. W., Colantonio, A., Chiu, S., Tolomiczenki, G., Kiss, A., Cowan, L., et al. 2008. The effect of traumatic brain injury on the health of homeless people. *Canadian Medical Association Journal* 179 (8): 779–784.

5. Langlois, J. A., Rutland Brown, W., and Wald, M. M. The epidemiology and impact of traumatic brain injury: A brief overview. *Journal of Head Trauma Rehabilitation*. Highlights from the 2nd Federal TBI Interagency Conference 21 (5): 375–378, September/October 2006.

6. Vanderploeg, R. D., Belanger, H. G., and Curtiss, G. 2009. Mild traumatic brain injury and posttraumatic stress disorder and their associations with health symptoms. *Archives of Physical Medicine & Rehabilitation* 90 (7): 1084–1093.

7. Thompson, J. 2008. Persistent symptoms following mild traumatic brain injury (mTBI)—A resource for clinicians and staff. Available at http://www.veterans.gc.ca/pdf/pro_research/mtbi-report-sep08.pdf (accessed September 8, 2013).

8. Roozenbeek, B., Maas, A. I., and Menon, D. K. 2013. Changing patterns in the epidemiology of traumatic brain injury. *Nature Reviews Neurology* 9 (4): 231–236.

9. Tuominen, R., Joelsson, P., and Tenovuo, O. 2012. Treatment costs and productivity losses caused by traumatic brain injuries. *Brain Injury* 26 (13–14): 1697–1701.

10. BrainTrust Canada Association. 2012. The facts about brain injury. Available at http://www.vistacentre.ca/_files/statistics.pdf (accessed September 1, 2013).

11. Feigin, V. L., Theadom, A., Barker-Collo, S., Starkey, N. J., McPherson, K., Kahan, M., et al. 2013. Incidence of traumatic brain injury in New Zealand: A population-based study. *Lancet Neurology* 12 (1): 53–64.

12. Mavis, I., and Akyildiz, D. 2013. Misconceptions about brain injury in Turkey. *Brain Injury* 27 (5): 587–595.

13. Tiret, L., Hausherr, E., Thicoipe, M., Garros, B., Maurette, P., Castel, J. P., et al. 1990. The epidemiology of head trauma in Aquitaine (France), 1986: A community-based study of hospital admissions and deaths. *International Journal of Epidemiology* 19 (1): 133–140.

14. Andelic, N. 2013. The epidemiology of traumatic brain injury. *Lancet Neurology* 12 (1): 28–29.

15. Das, A., Botticello, A. L., Wylie, G. R., and Radhakrishnan, K. 2012. Neurologic disability: A hidden epidemic for India. *Neurology* 79 (21): 2146–2147.

16. Andersson, E. H., Bjorklund, R., Emanuelson, I., and Stalhammar, D. 2003. Epidemiology of traumatic brain injury: A population based study in western Sweden. *Acta Neurologica Scandinavica* 107 (4): 256–259.

17. Kübler-Ross, E. 1997. *Living with death and dying.* New York: Touchstone.

18. Kübler-Ross, E. 1997. *On children and death.* New York: Touchstone.

19. Kübler-Ross, E., and Kessler, D. 2005. *On grief and grieving: Finding the meaning of grief through the five stages of loss.* New York: Scribner.

20. David B. Wright Memorial Foundation. 2011. Five stages of grief by Elisabeth Kübler-Ross, http://www.davidbwrightmemorial-foundation.org/Pages/FiveStagesofGrief.aspx (accessed August 13, 2013).

21. Verhaeghe, S., Defloor, T., and Grypdonck, M. 2005. Stress and coping among families of patients with traumatic brain injury: A review of the literature. *Journal of Clinical Nursing* 14 (8): 1004–1012.

22. Levy, D. 2011. Grey matter: A neurosurgeon discovers the power of prayer...One patient at a time. Carol Stream, IL: Tyndale House Books.

23. Cloud, H., and Townsend, J. 1992. Boundaries: When to say yes, when to say no to take control of your life. Grand Rapids, MI: Zondervan Publishing House.

24. Peck, S. 1993. Further along the road less traveled: The unending journey toward spiritual growth. New York: Simon & Schuster.

25. Kübler-Ross, E. 1972. The family physician and the dying patient. *Canadian Family Physician* 18 (10): 79–83.

26. Government of Saskatchewan. 2012. Alcohol, drugs and your health. Available at http://www.health.gov.sk.ca/alcohol-and-drugs-after-brain-injury (accessed August 12, 2013).

27. Statistics Canada. 2011. National Occupational Classification (NOC). Available at http://www.statcan.gc.ca/concepts/occupation-profession-eng.htm (accessed August 12, 2013).

28. Stedman, T. L. 2011. Stedman's online medical dictionary, 28th ed. Philadelphia: PA: Lippincott, Williams & Wilkins.

29. BrainTrust Canada Association. n.d. Family guide to the rehabilitation phase of brain injury. Available at http://www.braintrust-canada.com/files/3713/4100/6242/familyguiderehab.pdf (accessed August 12, 2013).

30. Van Der Kwaak, A., Ferris, K., and Dekker, L. 2010. Sexuality and counseling: Building evidence of good practice. Available at http://www.kit.nl/net/KIT_Publicaties_output/ShowFile2.aspx?e=1635 (accessed August 12, 2013).

31. Matsuka, K. M., and Christiansen, C. I I. 2011. A proposed model of lifestyle balance. *Journal of Occupational Science* 15:9–19.

32. Headway. 2013. Rehabilitation and continuing care after brain injury. Available at https://www.headway.org.uk/rehabilitation.aspx (accessed August 13, 2013).

33. Thompson, J. N., Majumdar, J., Sheldrick, R., and Morcos, F. 2013. Acute neurorehabilitation versus treatment as usual. *British Journal of Neurosurgery* 27 (1): 24–29.

34. Murphy, L. D., McMillan, T. M., Greenwood, R. J., Brooks, D. N., Morris, J. R., and Dunn, G. 1990. Services for severely head-injured patients in north London and environs. *Brain Injury* 4 (1): 95–100.

35. Prang, K. H., Ruseckaite, R., and Collie, A. 2012. Healthcare and disability service utilization in the 5-year period following transport-related traumatic brain injury. *Brain Injury* 26 (13–14): 1611–1620.

36. Eisen, M. L., Goodman, G. S., Qin, J., Davis, S., and Crayton, J. 2007. Maltreated children's memory: Accuracy, suggestibility, and psychopathology. *Developmental Psychology* 43 (6): 1275–1294.

37. Jacobs, B., van Ekert, J., Vernooy, L. P., Dieperink, P., Andriessen, T. M., Hendriks, M. P., et al. 2012. Development and external validation of a new PTA assessment scale. *BMC Neurology* 12:69.

38. Zafonte, R. D., Mann, N. R., Millis, S. R., Black, K. L., Wood, D. L., and Hammond, F. 1997. Posttraumatic amnesia: Its relation to functional outcome. *Archives of Physical Medicine & Rehabilitation* 78 (10): 1103–1106.

39. Jennett, B., and Bond, M. 1975. Assessment of outcome after severe brain damage. *Lancet* 1 (7905): 480–484.

40. Jennett, B., Teasdale, G., Galbraith, S., Braakman, R., Avezaat, C., Minderhoud, J., et al. 1979. Prognosis in patients with severe head injury. *Acta Neurochirurgica*—Supplementum 28 (1): 149–152.

41. Teasdale, G., and Jennett, B. 1974. Assessment of coma and impaired consciousness. A practical scale. *Lancet* 2 (7872): 81–84.

42. Zafonte, R. D., Hammond, F. M., Mann, N. R., Wood, D. L., Black, K. L., and Millis, S. R. 1996. Relationship between Glasgow coma scale and functional outcome. *American Journal of Physical Medicine & Rehabilitation* 75 (5): 364–369.

43. Schmidt, A. Rancho Los Amigos scale synopsis. Unpublished, used with permission, 2013.

44. Dennis, K. C. 2009. Current perspectives on traumatic brain injury. *ASHA Access Audiology* 8 (4).

45. Wilson, B. A., Evans, J. J., Emslie, H., Balleny, H., Watson, P. C., and Baddeley, A. D. 1999. Measuring recovery from post traumatic amnesia. *Brain Injury* 13 (7): 505–520.

46. Hagen, C., Malkmus, D., and Durham, P. 1979. Levels of cognitive functioning. *Rehabilitation of the Head Injured Adult: Comprehensive physical management*, Downey, CA, Professional Staff Association of Rancho Los Amigos National Rehabilitation Center.

47. Holmes, T. H., and Rahe, R. H. 1967. The social readjustment rating scale. *Journal of Psychosomatic Research* 11:213–218.

48. Bohnen, N., Twijnstra, A., and Jolles, J. 1992. Post-traumatic and emotional symptoms in different subgroups of patients with mild head injury. *Brain Injury* 6 (6): 481–487.

49. Mayo Clinic. 2013. Traumatic brain injury. Available at http://www.mayoclinic.com/health/traumatic-brain-injury/DS00552/DSECTION=symptoms (accessed September 5, 2013).

50. Kolakowsky-Hayner, S. A., Miner, K. D., and Kreutzer, J. S. 2001. Long-term life quality and family needs after traumatic brain injury. *Journal of Head Trauma Rehabilitation* 16 (4): 374–385.

51. Davis, L. C., Sander, A. M., Struchen, M. A., Sherer, M., Nakase-Richardson, R., and Malec, J. F. 2009. Medical and psychosocial predictors of caregiver distress and perceived burden following traumatic brain injury. *Journal of Head Trauma Rehabilitation* 24 (3): 145–154.

52. Lander, L., Howsare, J., and Byrne, M. 2013. The impact of substance use disorders on families and children: From theory to practice. *Social Work in Public Health* 28 (3–4): 194–205.

53. Vernig, P. M. 2011. Family roles in homes with alcohol-dependent parents: An evidence-based review. *Substance Use and Misuse* 46 (4): 535–542.

54. Kiresuk, T. J., and Sherman, R. E. 1968. Goal attainment scaling: A general method for evaluating comprehensive community mental health programs. *Community Mental Health Journal* 4 (6): 443–453.

55. Lefaivre, C. Amended goal attainment scale. Unpublished; used with permission, 2013.

56. Blue, I. A. 1986. Cross-examining the expert. *Advocates' Quarterly* 7:13.

57. Clark, J. 2011. Techniques in crossing the scientific witness. CBA spring advocacy program. Advocacy for the courts in intellectual property matters: The art of cross-examination http://www.cba.org/cba/cle/PDF/ADVO11_Clark_Paper.pdf 1–13.

58. Shensky, S. Overview of HelpHopeLive. Unpublished, used with permission, 2013.

59. Wald, M. M., Helgeson, S. R., and Langois, J. A. 2007. Traumatic brain injury among prisoners. *Brain Injury Professional* (5): 22–25.

60. Hoge, C. W., McGurk, D., Thomas, J. L., Cox, A. L., Engel, C. C., and Castro, C. A. 2008. Mild traumatic brain injury in U.S. soldiers returning from Iraq. *New England Journal of Medicine* 358 (5): 453–463.

61. Okie, S. 2005. Traumatic brain injury in the war zone. *New England Journal of Medicine* 352 (20): 2043–2047.

62. Medline Plus: A U.S. service of the National Library of Medicine National Institutes of Health. Medical Dictionary. 2012. Available at http://www.nlm.nih.gov/medlineplus/mplusdictionary.html (accessed October 17, 2013).

63. Macpherson, G. 2004. *Black's medical dictionary*, 40th ed. London. A&C Black, imprint of Bloomsbury Publishing Plc.

64. Godde, B. 2013. Springer reference: Encyclopedia of Neuroscience. Available at http://www.springerreference.com/docs/html/chapterdbid/114664.html (accessed October 23, 2013).

65. Brain Injury Association of America. 2013. An overview of diffuse axonal injury. Available at http://www.biausa.org/tbims-abstracts/an-overview-of-diffuse-axonal-injury?A=SearchResult&SearchID=7257364&ObjectID=2758774&ObjectType=35 (accessed October 17, 2013).

66. Bolt, N. 2013. Springer reference: Encyclopedia of child behavior and development. Available at http://www.springerreference.com/docs/html/chapterdbid/180016.html (accessed October 23, 2013).

67. Frazier, M. S. 2013. Springer reference: Encyclopedia of child behavior and development. Available at http://www.springerreference.com/docs/html/chapterdbid/180040.html (accessed October 24, 2013).

68. Krch, D. Springer Reference: Encyclopedia of Clinical Neuropsychology. 2013; Available at http://www.springerreference.com/docs/html/chapterdbid/184544.html (accessed October 24, 2013).

69. Zampella, C., and Bennetto, L. 2013. Springer reference: Encyclopedia of autism spectrum disorders. Available at http://www.springerreference.com/docs/html/chapterdbid/334299.html (accessed October 24, 2013).

70. Jonassen, D. H., and Hung, W. 2013. Springer Reference: Encyclopedia of the science of learning. Available at http://www.springerreference.com/docs/html/chapterdbid/319628.html (accessed October 24, 2013).

71. Noggle, C. A. 2013. Springer Reference: Encyclopedia of child behavior and development. Available at http://www.springerreference.com/docs/html/chapterdbid/180016.html (accessed October 24, 2013).

FURTHER READING

Abrahams, P. 2007. *How the body works: A comprehensive illustrated encyclopedia of anatomy.* London, UK: Amber Books Ltd.

Attendant Care and Physical Disability Unit, Ageing Disability and Home. 2011. Care and support pathways for people with an ABI: Referral and service options.

Bergman, P., and Moore, A. 2010. *Nolo's deposition handbook,* 5th ed. Berkeley, CA: Nolo Press.

Black, C. 1999. *Changing course: Healing from loss, abandonment and fear.* Bainbridge, WA: Mac Publishing.

Bryant, R. A., Marosszeky, J. E., Crooks, J., and Gurka, J. A. 2000. Posttraumatic stress disorder after severe traumatic brain injury. *American Journal of Psychiatry* 157 (4): 629–631.

Canada Revenue Agency. 2012. Medical and disability-related information. Available at: http://www.cra-arc.gc.ca.ezproxy.library.ubc.ca/E/pub/tg/rc4064/rc4064-12e.pdf (accessed September 26, 2013).

Cloud, H., and Townsend, J. 1992. *Boundaries: When to say yes, when to say no to take control of your life.* Grand Rapids, MI: Zondervan Publishing House.

Giffords, G., and Kelly, M. 2011. *Gabby.* New York: Scribner.

Kiresuk, T. J., and Sherman, R. E. 1968. Goal attainment scaling: A general method for evaluating comprehensive community mental health programs. *Community Mental Health Journal* 4(6).

Levy, D. 2011. *Gray matter: A neurosurgeon discovers the power of prayer… One patient at a time.* Carol Stream, IL: Tyndale House Books.

Matuska, K. 2012. Validity evidence of a model and measure of life balance. *OTJR: Occupation, Participation and Health* 32 (1): 229–237.

McCracken, T. O. 2011. *Anatographica: A fantastic three dimensional journey into the body.* Powder Springs, GA: Creation Book Publishers.

McMillan, B. 2008. *The illustrated atlas of the human body.* London, UK: Weldon Owen.

National Institute for Health and Clinical Excellence. 2007. Head injury: Triage, assessment, investigation and early management of head injury in infants, children and adults, 1–19.

Osborne, C. 1998. *Over my head: A doctor's own story of head injury from the inside looking out.* Kansas City, MO: Andrew McMeel Publishing.

Peck, S. 1993. *Further along the road less traveled: The unending journey toward spiritual growth.* New York: Simon & Schuster.

Sullivan, C. 2008. *Brain injury survival kit: 365 tools and tricks to deal with cognitive functional loss.* New York: Demos Health.

Wagman, P., Hakansson, C., Jacobsson, C., Falkmer, T., and Bjorklund, A. 2012. What is considered important for life balance? Similarities and differences among some working adults. *Scandinavian Journal of Occupational Therapy* 19 (4): 377–384.

Wong, P. P., Dornan, J., Schentag, C. T., Ip, R., and Keating, M. 1993. Statistical profile of traumatic brain injury: A Canadian rehabilitation population. *Brain Injury* 7 (4): 283–294.

Woodruff, L., and Woodruff, B. 2008. *In an instant: A family's journey of love and healing.* New York: Random House.

Wu, X., Hu, J., Zhuo, L., Fu, C., Hui, G., Wang, Y., Yang, W., Teng, L., Lu, S., and Xu, G. 2008. Epidemiology of traumatic brain injury in eastern China, 2004: A prospective large case study. *Journal of Trauma-Injury Infection & Critical Care* 64 (5):1313–1319.

Yuan, Q., Liu, H., Wu, X., Sun, Y., Yao, H., Zhou, L., and Hu, J. 2012. Characteristics of acute treatment costs of traumatic brain injury in Eastern China—A multi-centre prospective observational study. *Injury* 43 (12): 2094–2099.

Zur, B. M., Laliberte, Rudman D., Roy, R. A., and Wells, J. L. 2013. Components of cognitive competence predictive of occupational competence in persons with dementia: A Delphi study. *Canadian Journal of Occupational Therapy* 80 (2): 71–81.

SUGGESTED WEBSITES

The Able Trust. 2013. Available at http://www.abletrust.org/ (accessed October 24, 2013).

Acoustic Neuroma Association. What is an acoustic neuroma? 2013. Available at http://www.anausa.org/index.php/overview (accessed November 15, 2013).

Adaptive Sports Centre. 2013. Available at http://www.adaptivesports.org/ (accessed October 24, 2013).

AHEDD. 2013. What would you like to accomplish? Available at http://www.ahedd.org/index.html (accessed October 24, 2013).

American Association of People with Disabilities. 2013. Redefine disability. Available at http://www.aapd.com/ (accessed October 24, 2013).

American Association of State Compensation Insurance Funds. Available at http://www.aascif.org/index.php (accessed September 19, 2013).

American Occupational Therapy Association (AOTA) Inc. Home. Available at http://www.aota.org/ (accessed October 19, 2013).

American Spinal Injury Association. 2013. Recovery through discovery. Available at http://www.asia-spinalinjury.org/ (accessed October 24, 2013).

Association of Workers Compensation Boards of Canada. Canadian Workers Compensation 101. 2007. Available at http://www.awcbc.org/en/canadianworkerscompensation101.asp (accessed September 19, 2013).

Beach, J., and Friendly, M. Child care fee subsidies in Canada. Childcare Resource and Research Unit http://www.childcarequality.ca/wdocs/QbD_FeeSubsidies_Canada.pdf (pp. 1–20).

Brain Injury Resource Center. 2012. Available at http://www.headinjury.com/ (accessed October 24, 2013).

Brain and Spinal Injury Trust Fund Commission. 2013. How to apply. Available at http://www.ciclt.net/sn/adm/editpage.aspx?ClientCode=bsitf&FileName=LPhowtoapply.txt (accessed October 24, 2013).

Brain Trauma Foundation. Improving the outcome of traumatic brain injury patients. Available at http://www.braintrauma.org (accessed November 15, 2013).

Brainline.org. 2013. Preventing, treating and living with traumatic brain injury. Available at http://www.brainline.org/ (accessed October 24, 2013).

Canadian Resource Centre for Victims of Crime. 2012. Financial Assistance. Available at http://crcvc.ca/for-victims/financial-assistance/ (accessed September 19, 2013).

Canada Revenue Agency. 2012. Medical and disability-related information. Available at http://www.cra-arc.gc.ca/E/pub/tg/rc4064/rc4064-12e.pdf (accessed September 26, 2013).

Caregiver Resource Network. n.d. Available at http://www.caregiverresource.net/ (accessed October 19, 2013).

Caring Voice Coalition. 2013. Available at http://www.caringvoice.org/ (accessed October 19, 2013).

Centre for Neuroskills. 2013. Brain injury. Available at http://neuroskills.com/brain-injury/ (accessed September 11, 2013).

Christopher & Dana Reeve Foundation. 2013. Today's care. Tomorrow's cure. Available at http://www.christopherreeve.org/site/c.ddJFKRNoFiG/b.4048063/k.C5D5/Christopher_Reeve_Spinal_Cord_Injury_and_Paralysis_Foundation.htm (accessed October 24, 2013).

Darrell Gwynn Foundation. 2013. Available at http://darrellgwynnfoundation.org/ (accessed October 24, 2013).

Defence and Veterans Brain Injury Centre. 2013. Available at http://www.dvbic.org/ (accessed October 19, 2013).

Family Caregiver Alliance. Family caregiver navigator. Available at http://www.caregiver.org/caregiver/jsp/fcn_content_node.jsp?nodeid=2083 (accessed October 19, 2013).

Federal Evidence Review. 2013. Federal rules of evidence. Available at http://federalevidence.com/rules-of-evidence#Rule703 (accessed October 19, 2013).

Fighting Back Scholarship Program. 2013. Welcome to the Fighting Back Scholarship Program. Available at http://www.fightingbacksp.org/ (accessed October 24, 2013).

Find a caregiver. Home. 2013. Available at http://findacaregiver.com/ (accessed October 19, 2013).

Foundation for Rehabilitation Equipment & Endowment. n.d. Helping adults achieve independence through mobility. Available at http://www.free-foundation.org/ (accessed October 24, 2013).

GiveTech.org. 2003. Access for all. Available at http://www.givetech.org/ (accessed October 24, 2013).

Government of Canada. 2013. National Defense and the Canadian Armed Forces: The guide to benefits, programs and services for CAF members and their families. Available at http://www.forces.gc.ca/en/caf-community-benefits-ill-injured-deceased/guide.page (accessed October 10, 2013).

Health Advocate. 2013. Health advocate: Helping America to better navigate healthcare...personally. Available at http://www.healthadvocate.com/ (accessed October 19, 2013).

Health Canada. 2012. Your health benefits: A guide for First Nations to access non-insured health benefits. Available at http://www.hc-sc.gc.ca/fniah-spnia/alt_formats/pdf/pubs/nihb-ssna/yhb-vss/nihb-ssna-yhb-vss-eng.pdf (accessed September 26, 2013).

———. 2013. First Nations and Inuit health. Available at http://www.hc-sc.gc.ca/fniah-spnia/nihb-ssna/index-eng.php (accessed September 26, 2013).

Healthcare Hospitality Network. Healthcare hospitality network. n.d. Available at http://www.nahhh.org/ (accessed November 14, 2013).

HelpHOPELive. Catastrophic injury patients. Available at http://www.helphopelive.org/services/catastrophic-injury-patients/ (accessed September 26, 2013).

Human Resources and Skill Development Canada. 2005. If you have an accident: What to do and how to do it. Available at http://www.labour.gc.ca/eng/health_safety/compensation/pubs_wc/pdf/accident.pdf (accessed September 24, 2013).

Hunt, G. 2013. The national alliance for caregiving. Available at http://www.caregiving.org/ (accessed October 19, 2013).

Internal Revenue Agency of the United States of America. 2013. More information for people with disabilities. Available at http://www.irs.gov/Individuals/More-Information-for-People-with-Disabilities (accessed September 26, 2013).

Joni and friends. 2013. Christian fund for the disabled (CFD). Available at http://www.joniandfriends.org/help-and-resources/organizations/christian-fund-disabled/ (accessed October 24, 2013).

Lewin, E. 2012. Welcome to Nancy's house. Available at http://www.nancys-house.org/ (accessed October 19, 2013).

National Council on Independent Living. 2013. Welcome to the independent living movement. Available at http://www.ncil.org/ (accessed October 24, 2013).

National Mobility Equipment Dealers Association. 2013. The best source for wheelchair accessible vehicles. Available at http://www.nmeda.com/ (accessed October 24, 2013).

National Neurotrauma Society. 2013. Available at http://www. neurotraumasociety.org/ (accessed November 12, 2013).

National Rehabilitation Information Center. Welcome to the National Rehabilitation Information Center! Available at http://www.naric. com/ (accessed November 15, 2013).

Office of Justice Programs. Office for victims of crime: Victim compensation. Available at http://ovc.ncjrs.gov/topic.aspx?topicid=76 (accessed September 19, 2013).

Official US Government Site for Medicare. What is Medicare? Available at http://www.medicare.gov/sign-up-change-plans/decide-how-to-get-medicare/whats-medicare/what-is-medicare.html (accessed September 26, 2013).

Patient Advocate Foundation. 2012. National financial resource directory. Available at http://www.patientadvocate.org/NURD/index2. php?application=financial (accessed October 10, 2013).

Patient Services Inc. 2013. Available at https://www.patientservicesinc. org/ (accessed October 19, 2013).

Perspectives Network. 2013. Survive with pride. Available at http://www. tbi.org/ (accessed November 14, 2013).

Rosen, J. A. 2013. The Schwartz center for compassionate healthcare. Available at http://www.theschwartzcenter.org/ (accessed October 19, 2013).

Schorr, A. 2013. Patient power. Available at http://www.patientpower. info/ (accessed October 19, 2013).

Service Canada. 2013. People serving people. Available at http:// www.servicecanada.gc.ca/eng/lifeevents/disability.shtml (accessed September 25, 2013).

University of Washington. n.d. Models systems knowledge translation center. Available at http://uwmsktc.washington.edu/ (accessed October 24, 2013).

US Department of Education. 2010. Centers for independent living. Available at http://www2.ed.gov/programs/cil/index.html (accessed November 14, 2013).

US Department of Health and Human Services. 2013. Fact sheet: The affordable care act and American Indian and Alaska Native people. Available at http://www.hhs.gov/healthcare/facts/factsheets/2011/03/americani ndianhealth03212011a.html (accessed September 25, 2013).

US Department of Health and Human Services. n.d. Agency for healthcare research and quality: Advancing excellence in healthcare. Available at http://www.ahrq.gov/ (accessed November 15, 2013).

US Department of Veteran Affairs. 2013. Compensation. Available at http:// www.benefits.va.gov/COMPENSATION/types-compensation.asp (accessed September 26, 2013).

Veterans Affairs Canada. 2012. Disability benefits. Available at http://www. veterans.gc.ca/eng/services/disability-benefits (accessed September 19, 2013).

Well Spouse Association. 2013. Well spouses speak. Available at http:// www.wellspouse.org/ (accessed October 19, 2013).

Wishart, S., and McKimm, M. 2010. Expert medical witnesses: Scientists or advocates? Available at http://medicalmisdiagnosisresearch. wordpress.com/2010/11/05/expert-medical-witnesses-scientists-or-advocates/ (accessed October 19, 2013).

APPENDIX: BRAIN INJURY ASSOCIATIONS

Brain Injury Associations in Canada

Brain Injury Association of Canada

Head office located in Ottawa, Ontario, 440 Laurier Ave, Suite 200, K1R 7X6

Phone: 613-762-1222

E-mail: info@biac-aclc.ca

Website: http://biac-aclc.ca

British Columbia Brain Injury Association

Box 143, 11948 207th Street, Maple Ridge, BC V2X 1X7

Phone: 604-465-1783

Phone: 877-858-1788

Fax: 888-429-0656

Website: www.bcbraininjuryassociation.com

Northern Brain Injury Association

1237 4th Avenue, Prince George, BC, V2L 3J5

Phone: 250-562-4673

E-mail: info@nbia.ca

Website: http://nbia.ca/?page_id=39

The Brain Injury Association of Alberta (BIAA)

4916 50th Street, Red Deer, Alberta, T4N 1X7

Phone: 403-309-0866

E-mail: admin@biaa.ca

Website: http://www.biaa.ca/contact.html

Brain Care Centre ARR

#229, 10106 111th Ave, Edmonton, Alberta, T5G 0B4

Phone: 780-477-7575

E-mail: shamim@braincarecentre.com

Website: http://www.braincarecentre.com/

Saskatchewan Brain Injury Association ARR

P. O. Box 3843, Regina, Saskatchewan, S4P 3Y3

Phone: 306-373-1555

E-mail: none provided

Website: http://www.sbia.ca/contact.aspx

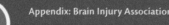

Brain Injury Association of Prince Edward Island
  81 Prince St., Suite 5, Charlottetown Prince Edward Island, C1A 4R3
  Phone: 902-314-4228
  E-mail: info@biapei.com
  Website: http://www.biapei.com/

Ontario Brain Injury Association Main Office ARR
  PO Box 2338, St. Catharines, Ontario, L2R 7R9
  Phone: 905-641-8877
  E-mail: obia@obia.on.ca
  Website: http://www.obia.ca

Manitoba Brain Injury Association
  204-825 Sherbrook Street, Winnipeg, Manitoba, R3A 1M5
  Phone: 204-975-3280
  E-mail: mbia@mymts.net
  Website: http://www.mbia.ca/wp/contact-us/

The Brain Injury Association of New Brunswick
  19 King, Sackville, New Brunswick, B4L 3G5
  Phone: 506-939-3101
  E-mail: none provided
  Website: http://biac-aclc.ca/new-brunswick

Newfoundland and Labrador Brain Injury Association
  PO Box 21063, St. Johns, Newfoundland and Labrador, A1A 5B8
  Phone: 709-579-3070
  E-mail: nlbia2011@gmail.com
  Website: http://www.nlbia.ca/contact/

Brain Injury Association of Nova Scotia
  PO Box 8804, Halifax, Nova Scotia, B3K 5M4
  Phone: 902-473-7301
  E-mail: info@braininjuryns.com
  Website: http://braininjuryns.com/contact-us/

BRAIN INJURY ASSOCIATIONS IN THE UNITED STATES

Brain Injury Association of America (United States)
  Head office: 1608 Spring Hill Road, Suite 110, Vienna, VA 22182

Phone: 703-761-0750

E-mail: braininjuryinfo@biausa.org

Website: http://www.biausa.org

Alabama (no affiliate office; see BIA head office information)

Head office: 1608 Spring Hill Road, Suite 110, Vienna, VA 22182

Phone: 800-444-6443

E-mail: braininjuryinfo@biausa.org

Website: http://www.biausa.org

Alaska (no affiliate office; see BIA head office information)

Head office: 1608 Spring Hill Road, Suite 110, Vienna, VA 22182

Phone: 800-444-6443

E-mail: braininjuryinfo@biausa.org

Website: http://www.biausa.org

Arizona (no affiliate office; see BIA head office information)

Head office: 1608 Spring Hill Road, Suite 110, Vienna, VA 22182

Phone: 800-444-6443

E-mail: braininjuryinfo@biausa.org

Website: http://www.biausa.org

Arkansas (no affiliate office; see BIA head office information)

Head office: 1608 Spring Hill Road, Suite 110, Vienna, VA 22182

Phone: 800-444-6443

E-mail: braininjuryinfo@biausa.org

Website: http://www.biausa.org

BIA of California

3501 Mall View Rd Suite 115, Box 397, Bakersfield, CA 93306

Phone: 661-872-4903

E-mail: pdaoutis@biacal.org

Website: http://www.biacal.org

Colorado (no affiliate office; see BIA head office information)

Head office: 1608 Spring Hill Road, Suite 110, Vienna, VA 22182

Phone: 800-444-6443

E-mail: braininjuryinfo@biausa.org

Website: http://www.biausa.org

Connecticut (no affiliate office; see BIA head office information)
Head office: 1608 Spring Hill Road, Suite 110, Vienna, VA 22182

Phone: 800-444-6443

E-mail: braininjuryinfo@biausa.org

Website: http://www.biausa.org

BIA of Delaware
840 Walker Road, Suite A, Dover, DE 19904

Phone: 302-346-2083

E-mail: director@biade.org

Website: http://www.biade.org

BIA of Florida
1637 Metropolitan Boulevard, Suite B, Tallahassee, FL 32308

Phone: 850-410-0103

E-mail: biaftalla@biaf.org

Website: http://www.biaf.org

BIA of Georgia
1441 Clifton Road NE, Atlanta, GA 30322

Phone: 404-712-5504

E-mail: info@braininjurygeorgia.org

Website: http://www.braininjurygeorgia.org

BIA of Hawaii
420 Kuwili Street, Suite 103, Honolulu, HI 96817

Phone: 808-436-8977

E-mail: biahi@hawaiiantel.net

Website: http://www.biausa.org/Hawaii/

Idaho (no affiliate office; see BIA head office information)
Head office: 1608 Spring Hill Road, Suite 110, Vienna, VA 22182

Phone: 703-761-0750

E-mail: braininjuryinfo@biausa.org

Website: http://www.biausa.org

BIA of Illinois
PO Box 64420 Chicago, IL 60664-0420

Phone: 800-699-6443

E-mail: info@biail.org

Website: http://www.biail.org

BIA of Indiana
 9020 Crawfordsville Road
 Indianapolis, IN 46234
 Phone: 317-356-7722
 E-mail: lmiller@biai.org
 Website: http://www.biai.org

Iowa (no affiliate office; see BIA head office information)
 Head office: 1608 Spring Hill Road, Suite 110, Vienna, VA 22182
 Phone: 800-444-6443
 E-mail: braininjuryinfo@biausa.org
 Website: http://www.biausa.org

BIA of Kansas and Greater Kansas City
 6701 W 64th Street, Suite 120, Overland Park, KS 66202
 Phone: 913-754-8883
 E-mail: rabramowitz@biaks.org
 Website: http://www.biaks.org

Kentucky (no affiliate office; see BIA head office information)
 Head office: 1608 Spring Hill Road, Suite 110, Vienna, VA 22182
 Phone: 800-444-6443
 E-mail: braininjuryinfo@biausa.org
 Website: http://www.biausa.org

BIA of Louisiana
 8325 Oak Street, New Orleans, LA 70118
 Phone: 504-982-0685
 E-mail: info@biala.org
 Website: http://www.biala.org

Maine (no affiliate office; see BIA head office information)
 Head office: 1608 Spring Hill Road, Suite 110, Vienna, VA 22182
 Phone: 800-444-6443
 E-mail: braininjuryinfo@biausa.org
 Website: http://www.biausa.org

BIA of Maryland
 2200 Kernan Drive, Baltimore, MD 21207
 Phone: 410-448-2924
 E-mail: info@biamd.org
 Website: http://www.biamd.org

BIA of Massachusetts

30 Lyman Street, Westborough, MA 01581

Phone: 508-475-0032

E-mail: biama@biama.org

Website: http://www.biama.org

BIA of Michigan

7305 Grand River, Suite 100, Brighton, MI 48114-7379

Phone: 810-229-5880

E-mail: info@biami.org

Website: http://www.biami.org

Minnesota (no affiliate office; see BIA head office information)

Head office: 1608 Spring Hill Road, Suite 110, Vienna, VA 22182

Phone: 703-761-0750

E-mail: braininjuryinfo@biausa.org

Website: http://www.biausa.org

BIA of Mississippi

PO Box 55912, Jackson, MS 39296-5912

Phone: 601-981-1021

E-mail: ljenkins@msbia.org or dpierce@msbia.org

Website: http://www.msbia.org

BIA of Missouri

2265 Schuetz Road, St. Louis, MO 63146

Phone: 314-426-4024

E-mail: info@biamo.org

Website: http://www.biamo.org

Montana (no affiliate office; see BIA head office information)

Head office: 1608 Spring Hill Road, Suite 110, Vienna, VA 22182

Phone: 703-761-0750

E-mail: braininjuryinfo@biausa.org

Website: http://www.biausa.org

BIA of Nebraska

2424 Ridge Point Circle

Lincoln, NE 68512

Phone: 402-423-2463

E-mail: peggy@biane.org

Website: http://www.biane.org

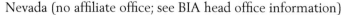

Nevada (no affiliate office; see BIA head office information)

Head office: 1608 Spring Hill Road, Suite 110, Vienna, VA 22182

Phone: 800-444-6443

E-mail: braininjuryinfo@biausa.org

Website: http://www.biausa.org

BIA of New Hampshire

109 North State Street, Suite 2, Concord, NH 03301

Phone: 603-225-8400

E-mail: mail@bianh.org

Website: http://www.bianh.org

New Jersey (no affiliate office; see BIA head office information)

Head office: 1608 Spring Hill Road, Suite 110, Vienna, VA 22182

Phone: 800-444-6443

E-mail: braininjuryinfo@biausa.org

Website: http://www.biausa.org

New Mexico (no affiliate office; see BIA head office information)

Head office: 1608 Spring Hill Road, Suite 110, Vienna, VA 22182

Phone: 800-444-6443

E-mail: braininjuryinfo@biausa.org

Website: http://www.biausa.org

BIA of New York State

10 Colvin Avenue, Albany, NY 12206-1242

Phone: 518-459-7911

E-mail: info@bianys.org

Website: http://www.bianys.org

BIA of North Carolina

PO Box 10912, Raleigh, NC 27605

Phone: 919-833-9634

E-mail: sandra.farmer@bianc.net

Website: http://www.bianc.net

North Dakota (no affiliate office; see BIA head office information)

Head office: 1608 Spring Hill Road, Suite 110, Vienna, VA 22182

Phone: 703-761-0750

E-mail: braininjuryinfo@biausa.org

Website: http://www.biausa.org

BIA of Ohio

PO Box 21325, Columbus, OH 43221

Phone: 614-481-7100

E-mail: Help@biaoh.org

Website: http://www.biaoh.org

BIA of Oklahoma

3015 E. Skelly Drive, #135, Tulsa, OK 74105

Phone: 800-444-6443

E-mail: brainhelp@braininjuryoklahoma.org

Website: http://www.braininjuryoklahoma.org

Oregon (no affiliate office; see BIA head office information)

Head office: 1608 Spring Hill Road, Suite 110, Vienna, VA 22182

Phone: 800-444-6443

E-mail: braininjuryinfo@biausa.org

Website: http://www.biausa.org

BIA of Pennsylvania, Inc.

950 Walnut Bottom Road, Suite 15-229 Carlisle, PA 17015

Phone: 866-635-7097

E-mail: admin@biapa.org

Website: http://www.biapa.org

BIA of Rhode Island

935 Park Avenue, Suite 8, Cranston, RI 02910-2743

Phone: 401-461-6599

E-mail: braininjuryctr@biaofri.org

Website: http://www.biaofri.org

BIA of South Carolina

800 Dutch Square Boulevard, Suite B-225, Columbia, SC 29210

Phone: 803-731-9823

E-mail: scbraininjury@bellsouth.net

Website: http://www.biausa.org/SC/

South Dakota (no affiliate office; see BIA head office information)

Head office: 1608 Spring Hill Road, Suite 110, Vienna, VA 22182

Phone: 800-444-6443

E-mail: braininjuryinfo@biausa.org

Website: http://www.biausa.org

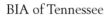

BIA of Tennessee

955 Woodland Street, Nashville, TN 37206

Phone: 615-248-2541

E-mail: director@BraininjuryTN.org

Website: http://www.BrainInjuryTN.org

Brain Injury Association of America—Texas Division

603 Louis Henna Blvd, Suite 197, Round Rock, TX 78664

Phone: 800-444-6443

E-mail: braininjuryinfo@biausa.org

Website: http://www.biausa.org/Texas/index.htm

Utah (no affiliate office; see BIA head office information)

Head office: 1608 Spring Hill Road, Suite 110, Vienna, VA 22182

Phone: 800-444-6443

E-mail: braininjuryinfo@biausa.org

Website: http://www.biausa.org

BIA of Vermont

PO Box 482, Waterbury, VT 05676

Phone: 802-244-6850

E-mail: support1@biavt.org

Website: http://www.biavt.org

BIA of Virginia

1506 Willow Lawn Drive, Suite 212, Richmond, VA 23230

Phone: 804-355-5748

E-mail: info@biav.net

Website: http://www.biav.net

BIA of Washington, DC (District of Columbia)

1232 Seventeenth Street NW, Washington, DC 20036

Phone: 202-659-0122

E-mail: info@biadc.org

Website: http://www.biadc.org

Washington (no affiliate office; see BIA head office information)

Head office: 1608 Spring Hill Road, Suite 110, Vienna, VA 22182

Phone: 703-761-0750

E-mail: braininjuryinfo@biausa.org

Website: http://www.biausa.org

West Virginia (no affiliate office; see BIA head office information)

Head office: 1608 Spring Hill Road, Suite 110, Vienna, VA 22182

Phone: 800-444-6443

E-mail: braininjuryinfo@biausa.org

Website: http://www.biausa.org

Wisconsin (no affiliate office; see BIA head office information)

Head office: 1608 Spring Hill Road, Suite 110, Vienna, VA 22182

Phone: 800-444-6443

E-mail: braininjuryinfo@biausa.org

Website: http://www.biausa.org

Wyoming (no affiliate office; see BIA head office information)

Head office: 1608 Spring Hill Road, Suite 110, Vienna, VA 22182

Phone: 800-444-6443

E-mail: braininjuryinfo@biausa.org

Website: http://www.biausa.org

BRAIN INJURY ASSOCIATIONS IN EUROPE

Austria: Austrian Federation of Traumatic Brain Injured People and Friends

Association: Selbst Hilfe Gruppe Schadel Hirn Trauma

Lascygasse 20/18 A-1170 Vienna, Austria

Phone: +43 664 323 3632

E-mail: shg-sht@gmx.at

Website: www.shg-sht.at

Belgium: Le NOYAU (not listed)

Czech Republic: Cerebrum

Krizikova 56/75a 186 00 Prague 8, Czech Republic

Phone: +420 226 807 048

E-mail: info@cerebrum2007.cz

Website: www.cerebrum2007.cz

Denmark: Danish Brain Injury Association

Hjerneskadeforeningen

Broendby Moellevej 8 2605 Broendby, Denmark

Phone: +45 4343 2433

E-mail: info@hjerneskadeforeningen.dk

Website: www.hjerneskadeforeningen.dk

Finland: Aivovammaliitto Ry

Nordenskioldinkatu 18 A 00250 Helsinki, Finland

Phone: +358 09 8366 580

E-mail: aivovammaliitto@aivovammaliitto.fi

Website: http://www.aivovammaliitto.fi/

France: UNAFTC

91-93 rue Damremont, 75018 Paris, France

Phone: +33 153 806 603

E-mail: unaftc@wanadoo.fr

Website: www.traumacranien.org

Germany: SelbstHilfeVerband— Forum Gehirn e. V.

Schnorringer Weg 1 51597 Morsbach- Erblingen Germany

Phone: not listed

E-mail: info@shv-forum-gehirn.de

Website: http://www.shv-forum-gehirn.de/

Iceland: Hugarfar

Address: Melabraut 23 170 Seltjarnarnes, Iceland

Phone: +354 661 5522

E-mail: hugarfar@hugarfar.is

Website: www.hugarfar.is

Ireland: Headway

Unit 1-3 Manor Street Business Park off Shea's Lane Manor Street Dublin 7, Ireland

Phone: +353 181 020 66

E-mail: info@headway.ie

Website: www.headway.ie

Italy: Federazione Nazionale Associazioni Trauma Cranico (FNATC)

Via Roma 9 21040 Carnago (varese), Italy

Phone: +393282133412 (Leorin)

Phone: +393343178202 (Fogar)

E-mail: info@associazionitraumi.it

Website: www.associazionitraumi.it

Netherlands: Cerebraal
Palestinastraat 1b 3533EH Utrecht, Netherlands
Phone: +31 030 296 65 75
E-mail: secr@cerebraal.nl
Website: http://www.cerebraal.nl/

Poland: Cerebrum
Portugual: Novamente
Estrada da Malveira da Serra Edificio Cadin, sala 10 2750-782 Cascais, Portugal
Phone: +351 919 437 335
E-mail: geral@novamente.pt
Website: www.novamente.pt

Slovenia: Drustvo Vita
Dunajska 106 1000 Ljubljana, Slovenia
Phone: +386 404 551 49
E-mail: drustvo.vita92@gmail.com
Website: www.vita-poskodbe-glave.si

Spain: Federacion Espanola de Dano Cerebral (FEDACE)
C/Pedro Teixeira 8, planta 10 28020 Madrid, Spain
Phone: +34 914 178 905
E-mail: info@fedace.org
Website: www.fedace.org

Sweden: Hjarnskadeforbundet Hjarnkraft
Nybohovsgrand 12, 1 tr., SE 117 63 Stockholm, Sweden
Phone: +46 844 745 30
E-mail: info@hjarnkraft.nu
Website: www.hjarnkraft.nu

Switzerland: Fragile Suisse
Beckenhofstrasse 70 8006 Zurich, Switzerland
Phone: +41 44 360 30 60
E-mail: mail@fragile.ch
Website: www.fragile.ch

United Kingdom: Headway
190 Bagnall Road, Old Basford, Nottingham NG6 8SF United Kingdom
Phone: +44 020 854 596 40
E-mail: chiefexec@headway.org.uk
Website: www.headway.org.uk

BRAIN INJURY ASSOCIATIONS IN AUSTRALIA

Australian Capital Territory: The National Brain Injury Foundation

> Phone: 02 6282 2880

New South Wales: Brain Injury Association of NSW

> Suite 102, Level 1, 3 Carlington Road, Epping, NSW 2121 Australia
>
> Phone: 02 9868 5261 or 1800 802 840
>
> E-mail: mail@biansw.org.au
>
> Website: http://www.biansw.org.au/

Northern Territory (1): Somerville Community Services

> Website: http://www.somerville.org.au/ (see website for listing by city)

Northern Territory (2): Integrated Disability Action

> Unit 4, Nightcliff Community Centre, 18 Bauhinia Street, Nightcliff, NT 0810
>
> Phone: 08 8948 5400
>
> E-mail: office@idainc.org.au
>
> Website: http://www.idainc.org.au/

Queensland: Synapse (Brain Injury Association of Queensland)

> Level 1 262 Montague Road, West End, Qld 4101
>
> Phone: 07 3137 7400 or 1800 673 074
>
> E-mail: online submission form
>
> Website: http://synapse.org.au/

South Australia: Brain Injury Network of SA

> 70 Light Square, Adelaide, SA 5000
>
> Phone: 08 8217 7600 or 1300 733 049
>
> E-mail: info@binsa.org
>
> Website: http://www.binsa.org/

Tasmania: Brain Injury Association of Tasmania

> Selfs Point Road, Cornelian Bay, TAS 7008
>
> Phone: 03 6278 7299
>
> E-mail: eo@biat.org.au
>
> Website: http://www.biat.org.au/

Victoria: Brainlink

> 54 Railway Road, Blackburn, Victoria 3130
>
> Phone: 03 9845 2950 or 1800 677 579

E-mail: online submission form
Website: http://www.brainlink.org.au/

Western Australia: Headwest
645 Canning Highway, Alfred Cove, WA 6154
Phone: 08 9330 6370 or 1800 626 370
E-mail: admin@headwest.asn.au
Website: http://www.headwest.asn.au/

BRAIN INJURY ASSOCIATIONS IN NEW ZEALAND

Auckland: Auckland Brain Injury Association
PO Box 99-765 Newmarket, Auckland 1149
Phone: 09 520 4807
E-mail: information@brain-injury.org.nz
Website: http://www.brain-injury.org.nz

Bay of Plenty: Bay of Plenty Brain Injury Association
C/O Hillier Centre, PO Box 10050, Mt. Maunganui
Phone: 07 572 4547
E-mail: liaison.headwaybop@brain-injury.org.nz

Bay of Plenty: Eastern Bay of Plenty Brain Injury Association
PO Box 528, Whakatane
Phone: 07 307 1447
E-mail: braininjury@drct.co.nz
Website: http://www.drct.co.nz

Canterbury: Brain Injury Association (Canterbury/West Coast) Inc.
PO Box 342, Christchurch 8140
Phone: 03 365 3262
E-mail: canterbury@brain-injury.org.nz
Website: http://www.brain-injury.org.nz

Gisborne: Gisborne Brain Injury Association
448 Palmerston Road, Gisborne
Phone: 06 868 8708
E-mail: liaison.gisborne@brain-injury.org.nz

Hawkes Bay: Hawkes Bay Brain Injury Association
605 Willowpark Road, South Akina, Hastings
Phone: 06 878 6875
E-mail: liaison@braininjuryhb.co.nz

Lakes: Rotorua Brain Injury Association
C/O Community House 1, 115 Haupapa Street, Rotorua
Phone: 07 350 1251
E-mail: liaison.rotorua@brain-injury.org.nz
Website: http://www.brain-injury.org.nz

Manawatu-Whanganui: Central Districts Brain Injury Association
PO Box 1054, Palmerston North 4440
Phone: 06 354 3540
E-mail: liaison.cd@brain-injury.org.nz

Nelson: Nelson Brain Injury Association
PO Box 1419, Nelson
Phone: 03 546 6656
E-mail: nelson@brain-injury.org.nz

Northland Brain Injury Association
PO Box 4001, Kamo, Whangarei
Phone: 09 459 5013
E-mail: northland@brain-injury.org.nz

Otago: Otago Brain Injury Association
PO Box 5222, Dunedin
Phone: 03 471 6156
E-mail: liaison.dunedin@brain-injury.org.nz

Wanganui Brain Injury Association
PO Box 102, Wanganui
Phone: 06 347 9721
E-mail: liaison.whanganui@brain-injury.org.nz

Wellington: Wellington Brain Injury Association
PO Box 12-180 Thorndon, Wellington
Phone: 04 473 5004
E-mail: liaison.wellington@brain-injury.org.nz

BRAIN INJURY ASSOCIATION IN INDIA

India Head Injury Foundation
138, Sunder Nagar, New Delhi 110 003, India
Phone: 91 11 2987 1955
E-mail: ihif@indianheadinjuryfoundation.org
Website: http://indianheadinjuryfoundation.org/

INDEX